Birth Asphyxia

Editors

BEENA D. KAMATH-RAYNE
ALAN H. JOBE

CLINICS IN PERINATOLOGY

www.perinatology.theclinics.com

Consulting Editor
LUCKY JAIN

September 2016 • Volume 43 • Number 3

ELSEVIER

1600 John F. Kennedy Boulevard • Suite 1800 • Philadelphia, Pennsylvania, 19103-2899

http://www.theclinics.com

CLINICS IN PERINATOLOGY Volume 43, Number 3
September 2016 ISSN 0095-5108, ISBN-13: 978-0-323-46263-1

Editor: Kerry Holland
Developmental Editor: Casey Jackson

Clinics in Perinatology (ISSN 0095-5108) is published quarterly by Elsevier Inc., 360 Park Avenue South, New York, NY 10010-1710. Months of issue are March, June, September, and December. Business and Editorial Offices: 1600 John F. Kennedy Blvd., Ste. 1800, Philadelphia, PA 19103-2899. Customer Service Office: 3251 Riverport Lane, Maryland Heights, MO 63043. Periodicals postage paid at New York, NY and additional mailing offices. Subscription prices are $290.00 per year (US individuals), $502.00 per year (US institutions), $340.00 per year (Canadian individuals), $614.00 per year (Canadian institutions), $420.00 per year (international individuals), $614.00 per year (international institutions), $100.00 per year (US students), and $195.00 per year (Canadian and international students). International air speed delivery is included in all Clinics subscription prices. All prices are subject to change without notice. **POSTMASTER:** Send address changes to *Clinics in Perinatology*, Elsevier Health Sciences Division, Subscription Customer Service, 3251 Riverport Lane, Maryland Heights, MO 63043. **Customer Service: Telephone: 1-800-654-2452** (U.S. and Canada); **1-314-447-8871** (outside U.S. and Canada). **Fax: 1-314-447-8029. E-mail: journalscustomerservice-usa@elsevier.com** (for print support); **journalsonlinesupport-usa@elsevier.com** (for online support).

Reprints. For copies of 100 or more, of articles in this publication, please contact the Commercial Reprints Department, Elsevier Inc., 360 Park Avenue South, New York, NY 10010-1710. Tel. 212-633-3874; Fax: 212-633-3820; E-mail: reprints@elsevier.com.

Clinics in Perinatology is also published in Spanish by McGraw-Hill Interamericana Editores S.A., P.O. Box 5-237, 06500 Mexico D.F., Mexico.

Clinics in Perinatology is covered in *MEDLINE/PubMed (Index Medicus) Current Contents, Excepta Medica, BIOSIS and ISI/BIOMED.*

Contributors

CONSULTING EDITOR

LUCKY JAIN, MD, MBA
Richard W. Blumberg Professor and Interim Chair, Emory University School of Medicine, Department of Pediatrics, Executive Medical Director and Interim Chief Academic Officer, Children's Healthcare of Atlanta, Atlanta, Georgia

EDITORS

BEENA D. KAMATH-RAYNE, MD, MPH
Associate Professor of Pediatrics, Perinatal Institute and Global Child Health Center, Cincinnati Children's Hospital Medical Center, Cincinnati, Ohio

ALAN H. JOBE, MD, PhD
Professor of Pediatrics, Perinatal Institute, Cincinnati Children's Hospital Medical Center, Cincinnati, Ohio

AUTHORS

SHABINA ARIFF, MBBS, FCPS
Department of Paediatrics and Child Health, The Aga Khan University, Karachi, Pakistan

SARA K. BERKELHAMER, MD
Clinical Associate Professor of Pediatrics, University at Buffalo, Buffalo, New York

ZULFIQAR A. BHUTTA, FRCPCH, PhD
Professor, Center of Excellence in Women and Child Health, Department of Paediatrics and Child Health, The Aga Khan University, Karachi, Pakistan; Director, Research Centre for Global Child Health, Toronto, Ontario, Canada

DARA BRODSKY, MD
Associate Director of the NICU, Beth Israel Deaconess Medical Center; Assistant Professor of Pediatrics, Harvard Medical School, Boston, Massachusetts

LINA F. CHALAK, MD, MSCS
Associate Professor, Department of Pediatrics, University of Texas Southwestern Medical Center, Dallas, Texas

VANN CHAU, MD
Division of Neurology (Pediatrics), The Hospital for Sick Children, University of Toronto and Neuroscience and Mental Health Research Institute, Toronto, Ontario, Canada

HANNAH C. GLASS, MDCM, MAS
Associate Professor, Departments of Neurology and Pediatrics, Benioff Children's Hospital; Department of Epidemiology and Biostatistics, University of California San Francisco, San Francisco, California

ROBERT L. GOLDENBERG, MD
Department of Obstetrics and Gynecology, Columbia University, New York, New York

MARGO S. HARRISON, MD
Instructor, Department of Obstetrics and Gynecology, Columbia University, New York, New York

CHRISTINA A. HERRERA, MD
Fellow, Department of Obstetrics and Gynecology, University of Utah, Salt Lake City, Utah; Department of Maternal Fetal Medicine, Intermountain Healthcare, Murray, Utah

NOAH H. HILLMAN, MD
Associate Professor, Department of Pediatrics, Saint Louis University, St Louis, Missouri

STUART B. HOOPER, PhD
The Ritchie Centre, MIMR-PHI Institute of Medical Research, Monash Institute of Medical Research, Monash University, Melbourne, Victoria, Australia

SANDRA E. JUUL, MD, PhD
Professor, Division of Neonatology, Department of Pediatrics, University of Washington, Seattle, Washington

BEENA D. KAMATH-RAYNE, MD, MPH
Associate Professor of Pediatrics, Perinatal Institute and Global Child Health Center, Cincinnati Children's Hospital Medical Center, Cincinnati, Ohio

STEVEN J. KORZENIEWSKI, PhD
Assistant Professor, Department of Obstetrics and Gynecology, Wayne State University School of Medicine, Detroit, Michigan

ABBOT R. LAPTOOK, MD
Women and Infants Hospital of Rhode Island; Professor of Pediatrics, Warren Alpert Medical School, Brown University, Providence, Rhode Island

JOY LAWN, FRCPCH, MPH, PhD
Professor, Director of MARCH Center, London School of Hygiene and Tropical Medicine, London, United Kingdom

ANNE CC LEE, MD, MPH
Associate, Department of Pediatric Newborn Medicine, Brigham and Women's Hospital, Boston, Massachusetts

RYAN M. McADAMS, MD
Associate Professor, Division of Neonatology, Department of Pediatrics, University of Washington, Seattle, Washington

ELIZABETH M. McCLURE, PhD
Senior Research Epidemiologist, Research Triangle Institute, Social, Statistical and Environmental Health Sciences, Research Triangle Park, North Carolina

STEPHANIE L. MERHAR, MD, MS
Division of Neonatology, Cincinnati Children's Hospital Medical Center, Perinatal Institute, Cincinnati, Ohio

SARAH U. MORTON, MD, PhD
Fellow, Harvard Neonatal-Perinatal Medicine Training Program, Department of Neonatology, Children's Hospital, Boston, Massachusetts

SUSAN NIERMEYER, MD, MPH
Professor of Pediatrics, University of Colorado, Aurora, Colorado

TRACEY ONG, PhD
The Ritchie Centre, Hudson Institute of Medical Research, Clayton, Victoria, Australia

ATHINA PAPPAS, MD
Professor, Department of Pediatrics, St. John Hospital and Medical Center, Wayne State University School of Medicine, Detroit, Michigan

JEFFREY M. PERLMAN, MB ChB
Division Chief, Division of Newborn Medicine, Komansky Center for Children's Health, New York Presbyterian Hospital; Professor of Pediatrics, Weill Cornell Medicine, New York, New York

GRAEME R. POLGLASE, PhD
Associate Professor, The Ritchie Centre, Hudson Institute of Medical Research, Clayton, Victoria, Australia

MATTHEW A. RAINALDI, MD
Division of Newborn Medicine, Komansky Center for Children's Health, New York Presbyterian Hospital; Assistant Professor of Pediatrics, Weill Cornell Medicine, New York, New York

DAVID H. ROWITCH, MD, PhD
Department of Paediatrics, University of Cambridge, Cambridge, United Kingdom; Department of Pediatrics and Neurological Surgery, University of California San Francisco, San Francisco, California

ROBERT M. SILVER, MD
Professor, Department of Obstetrics and Gynecology, University of Utah, Salt Lake City, Utah; Department of Maternal Fetal Medicine, Intermountain Healthcare, Murray, Utah

KRISTINA SOBOTKA, PhD
Institute of Neuroscience and Physiology, The Sahlgrenska Academy, University of Gothenburg, Göteborg, Sweden

ARJAN B. TE PAS, MD, PhD
Division of Neonatology, Department of Pediatrics, Leiden University Medical Centre, Leiden, The Netherlands

Contents

The physiology of the fetus is fundamentally different from the neonate, with both structural and functional distinctions. The fetus is well-adapted to the relatively hypoxemic intrauterine environment. The transition from intrauterine to extrauterine life requires rapid, complex, and well-orchestrated steps to ensure neonatal survival. This article explains the intrauterine physiology that allows the fetus to survive and then reviews the physiologic changes that occur during the transition to extrauterine life. Asphyxia fundamentally alters the physiology of transition and necessitates a thoughtful approach in the management of affected neonates.

The pathophysiology of asphyxia generally results from interruption of placental blood flow with resultant fetal hypoxia, hypercarbia, and acidosis. Circulatory and noncirculatory adaptive mechanisms exist that allow the fetus to cope with asphyxia and preserve vital organ function. With severe and/or prolonged insults, these compensatory mechanisms fail, resulting in hypoxic ischemic injury, leading to cell death via necrosis and apoptosis. Permanent brain injury is the most severe long-term consequence of perinatal asphyxia. The severity and location of injury is influenced by the mechanisms of injury, including degree and duration, as well as the developmental maturity of the brain.

Perinatal asphyxia is a general term referring to neonatal encephalopathy related to events during birth. Asphyxia refers to a deprivation of oxygen for a duration sufficient to cause neurologic injury. Most cases of perinatal asphyxia are not necessarily caused by intrapartum events but rather associated with underlying chronic maternal or fetal conditions. Of intrapartum causes, obstetric emergencies are the most common and are not always preventable. Screening high-risk pregnancies with ultrasound, Doppler velocimetry, and antenatal testing can aid in identifying fetuses at risk. Interventions such as intrauterine resuscitation or operative delivery may decrease the risk of severe hypoxia from intrauterine insults and improve long-term neurologic outcomes.

Stillbirths are among the most common pregnancy-related adverse outcomes but are more common in low-income and middle-income countries than in high-income countries. In high-income countries, most stillbirths occur early in the preterm period, whereas in low-income and middle-income countries, most occur in term or in late preterm births. In low-income and middle-income countries, conditions, such as prolonged or obstructed labor, placental abruption, preeclampsia/eclampsia, fetal growth restriction, fetal distress, breech and other abnormal presentations, and multiple births, are associated with stillbirth. In high-income countries, placental abnormalities are the most common associations. Globally, fetal asphyxia is likely the most common final pathway to stillbirth.

Historically, recommendations for neonatal resuscitation were largely based on dogma, but there is renewed interest in performing resuscitation studies at birth. The emphasis for resuscitation following birth asphyxia is administering effective ventilation, as adequate lung aeration leads not only to an increase in oxygenation but also increased pulmonary blood flow and heart rate. To aerate the lung, an initial sustained inflation can increase heart rate, oxygenation, and blood pressure recovery much faster when compared with standard ventilation. Hyperoxia should be avoided, and extra oxygen given to restore cardiac function and spontaneous breathing should be titrated based on oxygen saturations.

The cardiovascular response to asphyxia involves redistribution of cardiac output to maintain oxygen delivery to critical organs such as the adrenal gland, heart, and brain, at the expense of other organs such as the gut, kidneys and skin. This redistribution results in reduced perfusion and localized hypoxia/ischemia in these organs, which, if severe, can result in multiorgan failure. Liver injury, coagulopathy, bleeding, thrombocytopenia, renal dysfunction, and pulmonary and gastrointestinal injury all result from hypoxia, underperfusion, or both. Current clinical therapies need to be considered together with therapeutic hypothermia and cardiovascular recovery.

Neonatal encephalopathy (NE) is a major cause of neonatal mortality and morbidity. Therapeutic hypothermia (TH) is standard treatment for newborns at 36 weeks of gestation or greater with intrapartum hypoxia-related NE. Term and late preterm infants with moderate to severe encephalopathy show improved survival and neurodevelopmental outcomes at 18 months of age after TH. TH can increase survival without increasing major disability, rates of an IQ less than 70, or cerebral palsy. Neonates with severe NE remain at risk of death or severe neurodevelopmental impairment. This review discusses the evidence supporting TH for term or near term neonates with NE.

Although therapies in addition to whole-body cooling are being developed to treat the neonate at risk for hypoxic-ischemic encephalopathy, we have no quickly measured serum inflammatory or neuronal biomarkers to acutely and accurately identify brain injury or to follow the efficacy of therapy. This review covers inflammatory serum biomarkers in the setting of birth asphyxia that can help assess the degree or severity of encephalopathy at birth and neurodevelopmental outcomes. These biomarkers still need to be independently validated in large cohorts before they are ready for clinical implementation in practice.

Hypoxic-ischemic encephalopathy is associated with a high risk of morbidity and mortality in the neonatal period. Long-term neurodevelopmental disability is also frequent in survivors. Conventional Magnetic Resonance Imaging (MRI) defines typical patterns of injury that reflect specific pathophysiologic mechanisms. Advanced magnetic resonance techniques now provide unique perspectives on neonatal brain metabolism, microstructure, and connectivity. The application of these imaging techniques has revealed that brain injury commonly occurs at or near the time of birth and evolves over the first weeks of life. Amplitude-integrated electroencephalogram and near-infrared spectroscopy are increasingly used as bedside tools in neonatal intensive care units to monitor brain function.

Birth asphyxia, also termed perinatal hypoxia-ischemia, is a modifiable condition as evidenced by improved outcomes of infants $\geq$36 weeks' gestation provided hypothermia treatment in randomized trials. Preterm animal models of asphyxia in utero demonstrate that hypothermia can provide short-term neuroprotection for the developing brain, supporting the interest in extending therapeutic hypothermia to preterm infants. This review focuses on the challenge of identifying preterm infants with perinatal asphyxia, the neuropathology of hypoxic-ischemic brain injury across extreme, moderate, and late preterm infants, and patterns of brain injury, use of therapeutic hypothermia, and approach to patient selection for neuroprotective treatments among preterm infants.

Neonatal encephalopathy due to intrapartum events is estimated at 1 to 2 per 1000 live births in high-income countries. Outcomes have improved over the past decade due to implementation of therapeutic hypothermia, the only clinically available neuroprotective strategy for hypoxic-ischemic encephalopathy. Neonatal encephalopathy is the most common condition treated within a neonatal neurocritical care unit. Neonates with encephalopathy benefit from a neurocritical care approach due to prevention of secondary brain injury through attention to basic physiology, earlier recognition and treatment of neurologic complications, consistent management using guidelines and protocols, and use of optimized teams at dedicated referral centers.

Neonatal encephalopathy among survivors of presumed perinatal asphyxia is recognized as an important cause of cerebral palsy (CP) and neuromotor impairment. Recent studies suggest that moderate to severe neonatal encephalopathy contributes to a wide range of neurodevelopmental and cognitive impairments among survivors with and without CP. Nearly 1 of every 4 to 5 neonates treated with hypothermia has or develops CP. Neonatal encephalopathy is diagnosed in only approximately 10% of all cases. This article reviews the long-term cognitive outcomes of children with presumed birth asphyxia and describes what is known about its contribution to CP.

Almost one quarter of newborn deaths are attributed to birth asphyxia. Systematic implementation of newborn resuscitation programs has the potential to avert many of these deaths as basic resuscitative measures alone can reduce neonatal mortality. Simplified resuscitation training provided through *Helping Babies Breathe* decreases early neonatal mortality and stillbirth. However, challenges remain in providing every newborn the needed care at birth. Barriers include ineffective educational systems and programming, inadequate equipment, personnel and data monitoring, and limited political and social support to improve care. Further progress calls for renewed commitments to closing gaps in the quality of newborn resuscitative care.

Intrapartum-related neonatal deaths include live-born infants who die in the first 28 days of life from neonatal encephalopathy or die before onset of neonatal encephalopathy and have evidence of intrapartum injury.

A smaller portion of the population in poorer countries has access to basic obstetric and postnatal care causing neonatal mortality rates to be higher. Presence of a skilled birth attendant and provision of basic emergency obstetric care can reduce intrapartum birth asphyxia by 40%. With the announcement of Sustainable Development Goals and global Every Newborn Action Plan, there is hope that interventions around continuum of care will save lives.

PROGRAM OBJECTIVE
The goal of *Clinics in Perinatology* is to keep practicing perinatologists, neonatologists, obstetricians, practicing physicians and residents up to date with current clinical practice in perinatology by providing timely articles reviewing the state of the art in patient care.

TARGET AUDIENCE
Perinatologists, neonatologists, obstetricians, practicing physicians, residents and healthcare professionals who provide patient care utilizing findings from *Clinics in Perinatology*.

LEARNING OBJECTIVES
Upon completion of this activity, participants will be able to:
1. Review the pathophysiology and diagnosis of birth asphyxia.
2. Discuss the obstetric, cardiovascular, and neurological aspects of birth asphyxia and neonatal encephalopathy.
3. Review the short and long term cognitive outcomes of birth asphyxia.

ACCREDITATION
The Elsevier Office of Continuing Medical Education (EOCME) is accredited by the Accreditation Council for Continuing Medical Education (ACCME) to provide continuing medical education for physicians.

The EOCME designates this enduring material for a maximum of 15 *AMA PRA Category 1 Credit*(s)™. Physicians should claim only the credit commensurate with the extent of their participation in the activity.

All other health care professionals requesting continuing education credit for this enduring material will be issued a certificate of participation.

DISCLOSURE OF CONFLICTS OF INTEREST
The EOCME assesses conflict of interest with its instructors, faculty, planners, and other individuals who are in a position to control the content of CME activities. All relevant conflicts of interest that are identified are thoroughly vetted by EOCME for fair balance, scientific objectivity, and patient care recommendations. EOCME is committed to providing its learners with CME activities that promote improvements or quality in healthcare and not a specific proprietary business or a commercial interest.

The planning committee, staff, authors and editors listed below have identified no financial relationships or relationships to products or devices they or their spouse/life partner have with commercial interest related to the content of this CME activity:
Shabina Ariff, MBBS, FCPS; Sara K. Berkelhamer, MD; Zulfiqar A. Bhutta, FRCPCH, PhD; Dara Brodsky, MD; Lina F. Chalak, MD, MSCS; Vann Chau, MD; Anjali Fortna; Robert L. Goldenberg, MD; Margo S. Harrison, MD; Christina A. Herrera, MD; Noah H. Hillman, MD; Kerry Holland; Stuart B. Hooper, PhD; Lucky Jain, MD, MBA; Sandra E. Juul, MD, PhD; Beena D. Kamath-Rayne, MD, MPH; Steven J. Korzeniewski, PhD; Abbot R. Laptook, MD; Joy Lawn, FRCPCH, MPH, PhD; Anne CC Lee, MD, MPH; Ryan M. McAdams, MD; Elizabeth M. McClure, PhD; Stephanie L. Merhar, MD, MS; Sarah U. Morton, MD, PhD; Palani Murugesan; Susan Niermeyer, MD, MPH; Tracey Ong, PhD; Athina Pappas, MD; Jeffrey M. Perlman, MB ChB; Graeme R. Polglase, PhD; Matthew A. Rainaldi, MD; David H. Rowitch, MD, PhD; Robert M. Silver, MD; Kristina Sobotka, PhD; Megan Suermann; Arjan B. te Pas, MD, PhD.

The planning committee, staff, authors and editors listed below have identified financial relationships or relationships to products or devices they or their spouse/life partner have with commercial interest related to the content of this CME activity:
Hannah C. Glass, MDCM, MAS has research support from the National Institutes of Health; Pediatric Epilepsy Research Foundation; and Cerebral Palsy Alliance.
Alan H. Jobe, MD, PhD is a consultant/advisor for CHIESI Farmaceutici S.p.A., and has research support from CHIESI Farmaceutici S.p.A.; Fisher & Paykel Healthcare Limited; Merck & Co., Inc.; and GSK group of companies.

UNAPPROVED/OFF-LABEL USE DISCLOSURE
The EOCME requires CME faculty to disclose to the participants:
1. When products or procedures being discussed are off-label, unlabelled, experimental, and/or investigational (not US Food and Drug Administration [FDA] approved); and
2. Any limitations on the information presented, such as data that are preliminary or that represent ongoing research, interim analyses, and/or unsupported opinions. Faculty may discuss information about

pharmaceutical agents that is outside of FDA-approved labelling. This information is intended solely for CME and is not intended to promote off-label use of these medications. If you have any questions, contact the medical affairs department of the manufacturer for the most recent prescribing information.

TO ENROLL

To enroll in the *Clinics in Perinatology* Continuing Medical Education program, call customer service at 1-800-654-2452 or sign up online at http://www.theclinics.com/home/cme. The CME program is available to subscribers for an additional annual fee of $235 USD.

METHOD OF PARTICIPATION

In order to claim credit, participants must complete the following:
1. Complete enrolment as indicated above.
2. Read the activity.
3. Complete the CME Test and Evaluation. Participants must achieve a score of 70% on the test. All CME Tests and Evaluations must be completed online.

CME INQUIRIES/SPECIAL NEEDS

For all CME inquiries or special needs, please contact elsevierCME@elsevier.com.

CLINICS IN PERINATOLOGY

THE CLINICS ARE AVAILABLE ONLINE!
Access your subscription at:
www.theclinics.com

Foreword

Birth Asphyxia and the Inextricable Intersection of Fetal and Neonatal Physiology

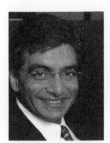

Lucky Jain, MD, MBA
Consulting Editor

Nearly fifty years ago, Patrick and colleagues[1] reported on a series of experiments in which they first asphyxiated and then resuscitated mature fetal lambs and rhesus monkeys. Their results led to a remarkable appreciation of the time sequence of physiologic changes in the minutes following birth asphyxia. In the words of Dr Dawes,[2] "the object we had in mind in working on acute anoxia after birth has been to discover what factors limit survival ... and to find out whether it is possible so to modify them, that survival may ensue after a period of anoxia which would otherwise be fatal, or which would have caused permanent cerebral damage." They described in extensive detail the occurrence of a prolonged period of apnea succeeded by continuous abnormal breathing, as a "warning of what may be encountered in the human fetus."[1] While our understanding of these events has evolved over time, fundamental observations made during that time remain largely unchanged and have shaped our interventions to prevent this catastrophic occurrence.

Yet an estimated 4 million newborns, equal to nearly all of the births in the United States each year, die worldwide of birth asphyxia.[3] This is despite the significantly better appreciation of higher fetal and neonatal vulnerability in the perinatal period, increased availability of trained personnel, and widespread acceptance of the Neonatal Resuscitation Program offered by the American Academy of Pediatrics. Many of these deaths are preventable, reminding us of the work that remains to be accomplished. In a previous writing on this subject, I have referred to the lessons we can and should learn from the remarkable success achieved in how serious trauma is managed in the battlefields today.[4] Interventions of unproven value or ones that actually do harm have no place in what we offer to these vulnerable neonates in the golden minutes after birth (**Fig. 1**).[5] Decades after the studies of Dawes and others,

Clin Perinatol 43 (2016) xv–xvii
http://dx.doi.org/10.1016/j.clp.2016.06.003
0095-5108/16/$ – see front matter © 2016 Published by Elsevier Inc.

perinatology.theclinics.com

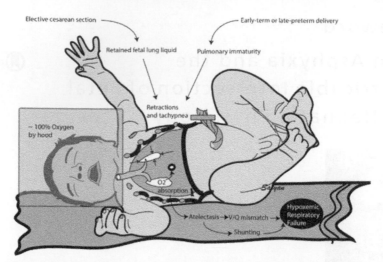

Fig. 1. Absorption atelectasis—administration of a high concentration of inspired oxygen without positive pressure in an infant with respiratory distress can lead to nitrogen washout and alveolar collapse. Atelectasis can result in V/Q mismatch, shunting, and hypoxemic respiratory failure with persistent pulmonary hypertension. (*Adapted from* Lakshminrusimha S, Saugstad OD. The fetal circulation, pathophysiology of hypoxemic respiratory failure and pulmonary hypertension in neonates, and the role of oxygen therapy. J Perinatol 2016;36:S6; with permission.)

lack of response after 10 minutes of complete asphyxia (or stillbirth) bodes poorly for chances of meaningful survival.[6]

In this issue of *Clinics in Perinatology*, Drs Kamath-Rayne and Jobe have put a together a state-of-the-art compilation of articles related to birth asphyxia. The articles offer a comprehensive review of physiologic changes that precede and follow birth asphyxia, and interventions that can help ameliorate them. I want to thank the editors, authors, and the publishing team at Elsevier (Kerry Holland and Casey Jackson) for addressing this topic of great importance in this issue of the *Clinics in Perinatology*.

Lucky Jain, MD, MBA
Emory University School of Medicine
Department of Pediatrics
Children's Healthcare of Atlanta
2015 Uppergate Drive
Atlanta, GA 30322, USA

E-mail address:
ljain@emory.edu

REFERENCES

1. Patrick JE, Dalton KJ, Dawes GS. Breathing patterns before death in fetal lambs. Am J Obstet Gynecol 1976;125:73–8.

2. Dawes GS. Anoxia and survival after birth. Proc R Soc Med 1960;53:1039–41.

3. Black RE, Cousens S, Johnson HL, et al. Child Health Epidemiology Reference Group of WHO UNICEF: global, regional, and national causes of child mortality in 2008: a systematic analysis. Lancet 2010;375:1969–87.

4. Jain L. The neonatal golden hour. Clin Perinatol 2012;39:xiii–xiv.
5. Lakshminrusimha S, Saugstad OD. The fetal circulation, pathophysiology of hypoxemic respiratory failure and pulmonary hypertension in neonates, and the role
   of oxygen therapy. J Perinatol 2016;36:S3–11.
6. Jain L, Ferre C, Vidyasagar D, et al. Cardiopulmonary resuscitation of apparently
   stillborn infants: survival and long-term outcome. J Pediatr 1991;118:778–82.

Preface

Birth Asphyxia—Providing Care for Mothers, Fetuses, and Newborns Across the Perinatal Continuum

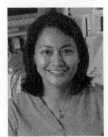
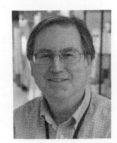

Beena D. Kamath-Rayne, MD, MPH   Alan H. Jobe, MD, PhD
Editors

Birth asphyxia accounts for approximately 23% of the 3.6 million neonatal deaths per year and may occur in the antenatal, intrapartum, or postpartum period. Therefore, we envisioned that a *Clinics in Perinatology* issue devoted to this important topic should contain articles relevant to the obstetrician, neonatologist, and pediatrician who may care for the pregnant woman, fetus, and newborn across this time period.

For this issue, we included topics that would broadly approach birth asphyxia and appeal to the target audience. The logical progression of this issue takes the reader through a review of the pathophysiology of asphyxia, and possible cardiovascular alterations during asphyxia that may contribute to ongoing multiorgan dysfunction. Our obstetrical colleagues then reviewed possible interventions in the obstetrical period for detection and prevention of asphyxia and a discussion of stillbirth (the hidden birth asphyxia). For the neonatologist and pediatrician, we included articles that discuss neonatal encephalopathy, a summary of results of trials on therapeutic hypothermia, what unanswered questions remain about therapeutic hypothermia, and a description of other novel therapeutics that may add to our standard of care. Coverage of possible future directions in the management of birth asphyxia included a review of biomarkers in neonatal encephalopathy, imaging, and other diagnostics (such as amplitude integrated EEG) for determining long-term outcome. In thinking about how to specifically improve long-term outcomes of asphyxiated infants, we also included a discussion of the role of the neuro-NICU, and what is known about the longer-term outcomes of these infants, including the contribution of birth asphyxia to cerebral palsy. Finally, given that most asphyxia-related mortality occurs in low-resource settings, we felt it appropriate to close with articles that discussed the prevention and treatment of these

Clin Perinatol 43 (2016) xix–xx
http://dx.doi.org/10.1016/j.clp.2016.06.002   **perinatology.theclinics.com**

deaths in such settings, and the challenges in neonatal resuscitation in low-resource settings.

We thank the distinguished authors that stepped up to provide their state-of-the-art expertise to cover these topics. We hope that you will find the issue to be engaging, informative, and stimulating for moving forward to fill the ongoing research gaps that remain regarding this important topic.

Beena D. Kamath-Rayne, MD, MPH
Cincinnati Children's Hospital Medical Center
MLC 7009, 3333 Burnet Avenue
Cincinnati, OH 45229, USA

Alan H. Jobe, MD, PhD
Cincinnati Children's Hospital Medical Center
MLC 7009, 3333 Burnet Avenue
Cincinnati, OH 45229, USA

E-mail addresses:
Beena.Kamath-Rayne@cchmc.org (B.D. Kamath-Rayne)
Alan.Jobe@cchmc.org (A.H. Jobe)

Fetal Physiology and the Transition to Extrauterine Life

Sarah U. Morton, MD, PhD[a],*, Dara Brodsky, MD[b]

KEYWORDS

- Fetal physiology • Intrauterine circulation
- Transition from intrauterine to extrauterine life • Transition physiology

KEY POINTS

- The intrauterine circulation diverts blood away from the fetal lungs via 2 right-to-left shunts.
- Ductus venosus blood is diverted through the foramen oval into the left atrium and most right ventricular output is shunted via the ductus into the descending aorta.
- The accumulation of fetal lung fluid within the fetal airways is critical for fetal lung development.
- The transition to extrauterine life is characterized by changes in circulatory pathways, initiation of ventilation and oxygenation via the lungs, and many changes in metabolism.

INTRODUCTION

The physiology of the fetus is fundamentally different from the neonate with both structural and functional distinctions. The transition from intrauterine to extrauterine life requires rapid, complex, and well-orchestrated steps to ensure neonatal survival. It is critical that neonatal care providers have a clear understanding of fetal and normal transitional physiology so that they can recognize deviations from typical physiology and manage these scenarios appropriately.[1] Asphyxia fundamentally alters the physiology of transition and necessitates a thoughtful approach in the management of affected neonates.

Disclosure Statement: Neither of the authors or any member of their families have a financial relationship or interest with any proprietary entity producing health care goods or services related to the content of this activity. The authors do not include any discussion or reference of commercial products or services.
[a] Harvard Neonatal-Perinatal Medicine Training Program, Department of Neonatology, Children's Hospital, Enders 9, 300 Longwood Avenue, Boston, MA 02216, USA; [b] Beth Israel Deaconess Medical Center, Harvard Medical School, Boston, MA 02115, USA
* Corresponding author.
E-mail address: sarah.morton@childrens.harvard.edu

Clin Perinatol 43 (2016) 395–407
http://dx.doi.org/10.1016/j.clp.2016.04.001
0095-5108/16/$ – see front matter © 2016 Elsevier Inc. All rights reserved.
perinatology.theclinics.com

FETAL PHYSIOLOGY
Cardiac Development

The human fetal circulation begins when the heart first beats at approximately 22 days of gestation. Gas exchange is initially provided by both the yolk sac and the placenta until the placenta becomes dominant at 10 weeks' gestation. Because oxygenated maternal blood mixes with poorly oxygenated blood within the free-flowing placental space, the oxygen content of blood provided to the fetus is lower than the maternal uterine arterial blood, causing the fetus to live in a relatively hypoxemic environment. Because the fetal lungs do not contribute to intrauterine oxygenation, there are several intrauterine shunts designed to direct blood away from the fetal lungs. Unique aspects of the fetal circulation (and other organ systems) are summarized in **Box 1**.

Our initial knowledge about the human fetal circulation was obtained from data in fetal sheep.[2] Recently, ultrasonography and MRI during human gestation have provided new detailed information about fetal blood flow in human fetuses (**Fig. 1**).[2,3] A comprehensive summary of the quantitative assessment of the human fetal circulation was recently published.[3,4]

In brief, starting at the level of the placenta, the well-oxygenated blood from branches of the maternal uterine artery flows freely into the placental space in funnel-shaped spurts.[5] Oxygen is then transferred across a concentration gradient from the placental space into vessels within multiple villi that line the fetal side of the placenta. These villi contain capillaries that merge and form the umbilical vein. Umbilical venous blood has an oxygen saturation of 70% to 80%, which is the highest oxygen saturation in the fetal circulation[6] (**Fig. 2**). As the umbilical vein enters the fetus, it splits at the level of the liver with some blood perfusing the hepatic circulation and the remainder entering into the ductus venosus.

The direction of flow of the intrauterine circulation helps to maximize oxygen delivery to the developing brain and heart. Although blood from the ductus venosus and inferior vena cava merges near the fetal heart, blood from each vessel is directed separately within the heart.[3] Poorly oxygenated blood from the inferior vena cava enters the right atrium, merges with the poorly oxygenated superior vena caval blood, and is directed preferentially into the right ventricle. A small portion of the right ventricular

---

Box 1
Unique characteristics of fetal physiology

Right-to-left shunts
  Foramen ovale
  Patent ductus arteriosus

Relative hypoxemic environment

Differential blood flow with ductus venosus flow providing most of left side of heart and inferior vena cava/superior vena cava providing most of right ventricular output; leads to differential in oxygenation in preductal and postductal aortic vessels

High-resistance, low-flow pulmonary circulation

Limited ability to regulate cardiac output (mostly via changes in heart rate)

Pulmonary epithelial cells actively secrete chloride leading to accumulation of fluid within fetal airways

Fetal erythropoiesis occurs in liver until the third trimester when transitions to bone marrow

Fetal hemoglobin, allowing for oxygen uptake in the lower oxygenated placental vascular bed

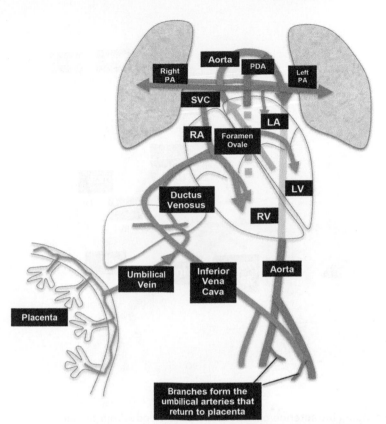

Fig. 1. Fetal circulation. This schematic summarizes the fetal circulation. The placenta provides oxygen and nutrients to the fetus via the umbilical vein (UV). The UV splits at the level of the liver with some blood, perfusing the hepatic circulation and the remainder entering the ductus venosus. Although most of the blood from the ductus venosus is directed across the foramen ovale to the left atrium (LA), the inferior and superior vena caval (SVC) blood preferentially enters the right atrium. Right ventricular (RV) output is directed across the patent ductus arteriosus (PDA) into the descending aorta and left ventricular (LV) output provides blood flow to the preductal vessels supplying the brain, coronary arteries, and upper body. Intrauterine pulmonary blood flow is limited initially because of high pulmonary vascular resistance and the right-to-left shunting across the patent foramen ovale and PDA.

output goes to the lungs via the pulmonary arteries, and the remaining flow is shunted across the ductus arteriosus to the descending aorta. This blood flow in the descending aorta, with an oxygen saturation of 60%, perfuses the abdominal organs and lower body before returning to the low-resistance placenta.

In contrast, better oxygenated blood from the ductus venosus is preferentially directed from the right atrium across the foramen ovale to the left atrium (LA). This right-to-left shunt accounts for approximately 25% of the total cardiac output. This shunted blood then mixes with a small amount of blood from the pulmonary veins before entering the ascending aorta to supply the carotid and coronary arteries. Because most of the source of this blood originated from the better oxygenated ductal venosus blood, the brain and heart receive blood with an oxygen saturation of approximately 65%, slightly higher than the 60% in the postductal aorta.

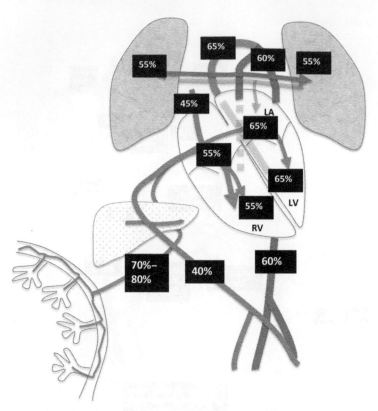

Fig. 2. Estimated intrauterine oxygen saturations. Blood within the umbilical vein has the highest oxygen saturation (70%–80%, estimated Po_2 = 32–35 torr) compared with the rest of the fetal circulation. Because of the preferential shunting of ductus venosus blood into the left atrium (LA), and the poorly oxygenated inferior and superior vena caval blood (40% to 45%, estimated Po_2 = 12–14) preferentially entering the right atrium (RA), the left side of the heart has a slightly higher oxygen saturation (65%, estimated Po_2 = 26–28 torr) compared with the right side of the heart (55%, estimated Po_2 = 20–22 torr). As a result, the left ventricular output to the brain, coronary arteries, and the upper body has a slightly higher oxygen saturation/oxygen content compared with the lower body, which is mostly provided by the right ventricular (RV) output. (*Data from* Kiserud T. Physiology of the fetal circulation. Semin Fetal Neonatal Med 2005;10:493–503; and Freed M. In: Keane J, Lock J, Fyler D, editors. Nadas' Pediatric Cardiology. Philadelphia: Saunders; 2006.)

In addition to the unique cardiac circulation, there are also differences in cardiac function in the fetus compared with the neonate. For example, the inotropic ability of the fetal and neonatal heart is not identical. The contractility of the immature heart is decreased because of lower myofibrillar content per tissue volume. In addition, the relative immaturity of the calcium regulatory mechanism renders the fetal heart intolerant of low calcium levels.[7]

In general, the fetus has a limited ability to adjust cardiac output.[2] In utero, the heart functions at the peak of the Frank–Starling ventricular function curve with increases in preload having a minimal impact on cardiac output. Fetal cardiac output is increased primarily by modulation of the heart rate, with fetal tachycardia leading to an increase in cardiac output and fetal bradycardia corresponding with a lower ventricular output.

However, this mechanism is not ideal, because sympathetic regulation of cardiac function is reduced, with both a decreased number of β-adrenoreceptors and decreased sympathetic innervation.[8]

Pulmonary Development

Lung development occurs in 2 phases: growth followed by maturation.[9] The lung bud septates from the foregut during the first trimester; next, lobar buds subdivide and form bronchopulmonary segments. The gas exchanging portions of the airway are formed during the canalicular phase that occurs during the second trimester. Alveolar ductal development starts at 24 weeks' gestation, and septation of the air sacs begins at 36 weeks' gestation. During both phases of development, distal pulmonary epithelial cells actively secrete a chloride-rich fluid into the bronchial tree.[10] This results in the accumulation of fluid within the fetal airways. Compared with postnatal lungs, the fetus' lungs are hyperexpanded.

Increased intrapulmonary vascular pressures as a result of fluid distension contribute to increased pulmonary vascular resistance.[11] The presence of this airway fluid is critical for stimulating lung development. This idea is supported by data in fetal lambs showing that tracheal ligation, which prevents lung fluid from escaping, leads to faster pulmonary growth and development.[12,13]

Fetal lung fluid contains components that change over the course of gestation. Before birth, the content of fetal lung fluid is altered because of the increased expression of surfactant lipoproteins by type II pneumocytes in response to increasing cortisol levels at the end of the third trimester. These lipoproteins function to lower surface tension in the lungs, allowing for inflation at lower pressures.

As the fetal airways and lung parenchyma develop, so does the pulmonary vasculature. The development of the pulmonary circulation starts by 34 days' gestation in the human fetus. Advances in fetal MRI have allowed more precise examination of the relative blood flow in the human fetus, and recent evidence suggests that pulmonary blood flow increases with gestational age from an initial low of 10% to almost 50% of the combined ventricular output by term gestation.[14]

Because of preferential shunting of deoxygenated blood into the right ventricle, blood reaching the intrauterine pulmonary circulation has an oxygenation saturation of approximately 55%. Fetal hypoxemia decreases pulmonary blood flow, which in turn suppresses the production of nitric oxide and prostaglandin I2.[15] This results in an increased pulmonary vascular resistance at baseline. Any additional fetal hypoxemia as a result of maternal or placental issues leads to lessening of the oxygen delivered to the pulmonary circulation, which increases pulmonary vascular resistance further and activates hypoxia inducible factor-1, triggering vascular remodeling.[16,17]

Much like the cardiovascular system, there are both structural and functional changes in the fetal lungs during gestation. Fetal breathing starts at 10 weeks' gestation and is associated with rapid eye movement sleep. It is inhibited by hypoxemia and stimulated by hyperoxemia.[18] Such breathing movements are important to pulmonary development; cessation of fetal breathing via phrenectomy in fetal sheep leads to pulmonary hypoplasia.[19]

Endocrine Development

Cortisol production increases from 30 to 36 weeks' gestation, and a second peak occurs before spontaneous labor at term gestational age.[18] Elevated cortisol levels lead to activation of thyroid hormone, maturation of hepatic glucose metabolism enzymes, and improved maintenance of euglycemia after delivery. Cortisol levels are lower in the setting of preterm delivery or Cesarean section without labor, and increased with chorioamnionitis.

Hematologic Development

Between 2 and 3 weeks' gestation, the yolk sac initiates fetal erythropoiesis. From 5 weeks' gestation to 6 months' gestation, the liver becomes the primary site of erythropoiesis, followed by the bone marrow thereafter. Relative hypoxemia induces hypoxia-inducible factor-1, which stimulates the fetal kidneys to produce erythropoietin, driving red blood cell production and thereby improving oxygenation of the fetus by increasing the oxygen-carrying capacity.

Another mechanism by which the fetus compensates for the relative hypoxemic environment is by depending on fetal hemoglobin. This unique hemoglobin has a high oxygen affinity, creating a leftward shift in the oxyhemoglobin curve that increases oxygen uptake at the lower oxygenated placental vascular bed. However, given the resultant higher affinity, less oxygen is offloaded to capillary beds in tissues unless local factors modify the oxygen affinity of fetal hemoglobin. For example, fetal acidosis augments delivery of oxygen to tissues by decreasing the affinity of fetal hemoglobin for oxygen.

TRANSITION

Transition to extrauterine life is characterized by changes in circulatory pathways, initiation of ventilation and oxygenation via the lungs instead of the placenta, and many changes in metabolism. These changes are summarized in **Box 2**.

Cardiovascular Changes

With the first postnatal breath, the pulmonary vascular resistance decreases dramatically. This decrease is caused by a combination of increased oxygen exposure as well as ventilation itself.[20] When the umbilical cord is clamped, the low-resistance vascular bed of the placenta is disconnected, leading to an increase in the newborn's systemic vascular resistance. The pressure within the LA then increases because of the increased distal aortic pressure and the greater amount of blood returning to the LA from the lungs. With the left atrial pressure being greater than the right atrial pressure, the flap across the foramen ovale closes.

Box 2
Important physiologic changes during transition to extrauterine life

Increased systemic vascular resistance with separation from the low-resistance placental vasculature

Closure of right-to-left shunts
  Foramen ovale (closes when left atrial pressure greater than right atrial pressure)
  Ductus arteriosus (left-to-right flow within minutes of ventilation, then closure over days)

Rapid lowering of pulmonary vascular resistance with onset of ventilation

Clearance of fluid from airways via active sodium absorption and changes in airway pressure owing to ventilation

Increased metabolic rate leading to higher glucose needs

Increased catecholamine levels to support blood pressure

Most term infants have a reversal of flow across the ductus arteriosus with left-to-right flow occurring within 10 minutes after birth, resulting in greater pulmonary blood flow.[21,22] Serial ultrasonography has demonstrated doubling of LV output and a concomitant increase in stroke volume in the first hour after delivery.[23] During the circulatory transition from fetal to neonatal physiology, systemic vascular resistance has a greater influence on blood pressure than blood flow.[24] The increase in systemic vascular resistance leads to a rapid and transient increase in cerebral blood flow. Increased oxygenation and decreased blood flow leads to closure of the fetal cardiac shunts (**Table 1**). Oxygenation of the ductus arteriosus further leads to increased calcium channel activity resulting in functional closure. Smooth muscle cells of the ductus arteriosus respond to increased oxygen with inhibition of potassium channel activity, also causing ductal constriction.[25]

These events are affected by many factors at birth, including the timing of umbilical cord clamping. Clamping of the umbilical vein before the onset of ventilation removes the primary source of in utero left-sided venous return from the ductus venosus (ie, ductus venosus → right atrium → patent foramen ovale → LA→ LV). This occurs before an increase in pulmonary blood flow, resulting in a period of decreased left ventricular preload and decreased cardiac output that persists until ventilation is established.[26] Delaying cord clamping until the onset of ventilation can prevent this decrease in cardiac output.[27] Theoretically, the umbilical arteries should vasoconstrict before the umbilical vein closes, leading to net blood flow towards the infant. However, in practice this has not always been observed and may depend on the difference in height between the placenta and the infant.

Our understanding of the nuanced cardiovascular changes that occur at birth has been advanced by new, non-invasive method for assessing local perfusion and oxygenation. Near-infrared spectroscopy is a noninvasive monitoring technique that can be used to measure tissue oxygenation index and calculate peripheral blood flow and peripheral oxygen delivery. Using near-infrared spectroscopy to measure cerebral oxygen saturation, term infants experience an increase in cerebral perfusion in the first few minutes of life, corresponding with an increase in blood oxygen content.[28] This increased oxygenation happens faster in the brain than in other tissues.[29] Interestingly, cerebral oxygen saturation is both higher and less variable than abdominal tissue oxygen saturation in preterm infants over the first weeks of life.[30]

Pulmonary Changes

Significant pulmonary changes are triggered at the onset of labor. Surfactant is a mixture of lipids and proteins that reduces the surface tension within airways by forming a monolayer at the liquid–air interface. Surfactant secretion into the fetal lungs is stimulated by labor. Alveolar stretch as a result of initiation of ventilation further increases the secretion of surfactant. These polar molecules function to lower surface tension in the lungs, allowing for inflation at lower pressures.

Table 1
Postnatal mechanisms of cardiac shunt closure

Physiologic Trigger	Effect	Vessel Affected
Increased oxygenation	Constriction	Umbilical artery, ductus arteriosus
	Dilation	Pulmonary artery
Decreased blood flow	Constriction	Umbilical vein, ductus venosus

Clearance of fetal lung fluid also begins before birth, is augmented by labor, and is mostly completed by 2 hours of age. There are multiple mechanisms that assist with this process. During spontaneous labor and immediately after birth, the respiratory epithelium changes from active fluid secretion (with active chloride transport into the intraluminal space) to active fluid absorption (with active sodium transport into the interstitium).[10] The sodium-mediated active absorption process is believed to be initiated even before labor with regulation by increased cortisol and thyroid hormone levels. β-Receptor agonist stimulation promotes this respiratory epithelium transition during spontaneous labor. Increased oxygenation after birth helps to maintain the expression of these sodium-mediated channels.[31] In a rabbit model, fetal airway liquid has also been shown to be cleared postnatally by increases in the transepithelial pressure gradient during inspiration that functions to drive fluid into tissues to where it can be removed by the pulmonary microcirculation and lymphatic vessels.[32] Effective clearance of fetal lung fluid decreases pulmonary vascular resistance, and the increased intravascular fluid volume leads to an increase in the plasma volume during the first few hours of age.[18]

After birth, infants must establish breathing patterns more regular than those of the fetus. Most term and preterm infants breathe spontaneously, unless they have severe hypoxemia, which represses the initiation of breathing.[33] Gas exchange is stabilized by 2 minutes in most babies after vaginal delivery and improvement in heart rate is the best clinical indicator of successful ventilation.[34] Preterm infants have lower lung volumes relative to body weight compared with term infants, and have delayed clearance of fetal lung fluid because of decreased sodium resorption.[35,36] Infants with transient tachypnea of the newborn or surfactant deficiency also have decreased sodium resorption.

As ventilation is initiated, a positive ratio of inspiratory to expiratory volumes results in a functional residual capacity.[37] Preterm infants with lower amounts of surfactant have a lower baseline functional residual capacity. Positive end-expiratory pressure can help preterm infants to establish a more uniform functional residual capacity.[38] Continuous positive airway pressure can help preterm infants to adapt by triggering production and secretion of surfactant.

An observational study of term infants found that oxygen saturation did not reach 90% until an average of 8 minutes after birth in healthy newborns breathing room air, and the postductal saturations remained on average 8% lower than preductal saturations for the first 15 minutes of age.[39,40] Oxygenation has many effects, including relaxation of pulmonary vascular smooth muscle, which is mediated in part by increased cyclic guanosine monophosphate–dependent protein kinase activity.[41]

With the onset of respiration, there are significant changes in pulmonary blood flow. The closure of cardiac shunts changes the circulatory system from a fetal configuration with parallel output from the right and left ventricles contributing to a total cardiac output of 450 mL/kg/min, to a neonatal system where each ventricle has a cardiac output of 400 mL/kg/min.[18] As a result of this increase in right-sided output, pulmonary blood flow increases to 100% in the newborn. Increased pulmonary blood flow causes sheer stress, which in turn reduces pulmonary vascular resistance via increased nitric oxide production.[15]

Pulmonary arterial pressure reaches one-half the systemic arterial pressure by 24 hours of age, attaining adult levels by 2 weeks in most typical infants.[15] Experimental paradigms that allow ventilation without oxygenation show a blunted drop in pulmonary vascular resistance compared with ventilation with the appropriate physiologic increase in oxygen.[20] Endogenous vasoactive agents and their effects are summarized in **Table 2**.

Table 2
Intrauterine and postnatal modulation of pulmonary vascular resistance

Molecule	Synthetic Enzyme	Effect on PVR	Downstream Targets	Activity Pattern
NO	NOS; upregulated by sheer stress	Decrease	Soluble guanylate cyclase generates cGMP; cGMP activates PKG	Expressed early in first trimester; endothelial NOS and neuronal NOS decrease at term whereas iNOS increases
PGI2	COX-1	Decrease	Adenylyl cyclase generates cAMP	Synthesis starts in third trimester and increases after delivery
Bradykinin	—	Decrease	Increases NO, EDRF	—
PDE5	—	Increase	Counteracts NO by degrading cGMP	Increased activity in fetus compared with neonate
Endothelin	Pulmonary endothelium	Increase	Calcium: increases SR release and muscle sensitivity	Increasing levels in second and third trimester, then decreases after birth
Platelet activating factor	PLA$_2$, made in response to hypoxia	Increase	Increased calcium release	Higher in fetus than newborn
Reactive oxygen species	Mitochondria; upregulated by hypoxia; inactivated by SOD and catalase	Increase	Inhibit NO	Catalase expression increases through gestation until 3 mo postnatal[47]

Early in the first trimester, NOS is expressed and stimulates vasodilation.[48] PDE5, which counteracts the downstream effects of nitric oxide, has increased activity in the fetus compared with the neonate. PGI2 synthesis, which lowers PVR, starts in the third trimester in lamb models as a result of an increase in COX-1 expression.[49] Endothelin, produced by the pulmonary endothelium at increasing levels during the second and third trimester and then decreases following delivery, leads to increased PVR via increased calcium flux and sensitivity in vascular smooth muscle cells in fetal pigs.

Abbreviations: cAMP, cyclic adenosine monophosphate; cGMP, cyclic guanosine monophosphate; COX, cyclooxygenase; EDRF, endothelium-derived relaxing factor; iNOS, inducible nitric oxide; NO, nitric oxide; NOS, nitric oxide synthase; PDE5, phosphodiesterase 5; PGI2, prostaglandin I2; PKG, protein kinase G; PLA$_2$, phospholipase A2; PVR, pulmonary vascular resistance; SOD, superoxide dismutase; SR, sarcoplasmic reticulum.

Hematologic Changes

After birth, the production of fetal hemoglobin decreases and there is a concomitant increase in hemoglobin β chain production such that normal levels of adult hemoglobin are achieved by 4 to 6 months of age. Exposure to the increased oxygenation of the extrauterine environment leads to decreased erythropoietin, leading to lower rates of erythropoiesis in the neonate (nadir approximately 1 month) compared with the fetus.

Metabolic Changes

Glucose and amino acids are transported actively to the fetus across the placenta, a process that is stopped by separation from the placental circulation.[42] Generally, smaller mammals have higher metabolic rates. However, the fetus has a low metabolic rate despite a small size, with a metabolic rate similar to that of the pregnant woman. After delivery, there is a progressive increase in metabolic rate, which occurs more slowly in preterm infants.[43] Mitochondrial density increases as the metabolic rate increases.[44]

To maintain blood glucose levels after separation from the placental circulation, the newborn experiences a surge in catecholamine and glucagon levels and a decrease in insulin amounts. Gluconeogenesis and glycogenolysis in the liver ensures stable blood glucose until oral intake volumes improve over the first few days after birth. Ketone bodies and lactate provide additional energy for the brain, with hepatic ketogenesis increasing after the first 12 hours of age.

As with pulmonary changes, many hormonal changes necessary for successful transition to extrauterine life are initiated during the fetal period. Cortisol levels begin to increase at 30 weeks' gestation and peak just after delivery. The combined action of cortisol and thyroid hormone activates sodium channel activity that drives resorption of lung fluid. Stressful deliveries, or Cesarean delivery without labor, can uncover a relative adrenal insufficiency in infants who do not produce an adequate response to the physiologic challenge.

Norepinephrine, epinephrine, and dopamine are released from the neonatal adrenal medulla and other sympathetic nervous system tissues. The importance of catecholamines in adaptation to extrauterine life has been demonstrated using a lamb model. Neonatal lambs who had an adrenalectomy at term had markedly lower levels of epinephrine and norepinephrine, which resulted in lower blood pressures.[45] Birth leads to increased production and release of catecholamines, renin–angiotensin, and vasopressin. These are important for the increase in cardiac output that occurs postnatally, as well as increases in plasma glucose and free fatty acids.[46] Preterm neonates experience a slower increase in catecholamine levels but plateau at serum concentrations higher than those found in term infants. Interestingly, compared with the fetus, term neonates have lower thresholds of catecholamine concentrations necessary to produce changes in blood pressure, serum glucose, and free fatty acids, which are necessary for the transition to the extrauterine environment.

Temperature Regulation

At birth, infants emerge covered in liquid, resulting in potential heat loss via evaporation. If newborns are not held skin to skin or wrapped in a warm blanket, hypothermia can ensue because of conduction, convection, and radiant heat losses. Relative to older children, neonates have a higher body surface area, limited capacity to generate heat via shivering, and decreased subcutaneous fat for insulation. Brown adipose tissue lipolysis triggered by norepinephrine can generate heat, and peripheral vasoconstriction can minimize heat loss.[18] Thyroid hormones surge after birth, possibly in response to the relatively cold extrauterine environment.

SUMMARY

The transition from intrauterine to extrauterine life requires a rapid adaptation of multiple organ systems. Separation from the placental circulation results in increased systemic vascular resistance, whereas the initiation of ventilation lowers pulmonary vascular resistance. These combined factors, with the associated increased oxygenation, result in closures of the foramen ovale, ductus arteriosus, and ductus venosus. A successful transition also requires increased metabolic and endocrine activities to support blood pressure and blood glucose levels. Precise orchestration of these complex physiologic events is necessary to avoid disease relating to birth asphyxia, or failures of the cardiovascular, respiratory, or other organ systems.

REFERENCES

1. Britton JR. The transition to extrauterine life and disorders of transition. Clin Perinatol 1998;25:271–94.
2. Keane JF, Lock JE, Fyler DC. Nadas' pediatric cardiology. 2nd edition. Philadelphia: Saunders; 2006.
3. Kiserud T. Physiology of the fetal circulation. Semin Fetal Neonatal Med 2005;10: 493–503.
4. Freed M. In: Keane J, Lock J, Fyler D, editors. Nadas' Pediatric Cardiology. Philadelphia: Saunders; 2006.
5. Cunningham F, Leveno K, Bloom S, et al. Williams obstetrics. New York: McGraw-Hill Education; 2014.
6. Finnemore A, Groves A. Physiology of the fetal and transitional circulation. Semin Fetal Neonatal Med 2015;20:210–6.
7. Nakanishi T, Okuda H, Kamata K, et al. Development of myocardial contractile system in the fetal rabbit. Pediatr Res 1987;22:201–7.
8. Kim MY, Finch AM, Lumbers ER, et al. Expression of adrenoceptor subtypes in preterm piglet heart is different to term heart. PLoS One 2014;9:e92167.
9. Burri PH. Fetal and postnatal development of the lung. Annu Rev Physiol 1984;46: 617–28.
10. Elias N, O'Brodovich H. Clearance of fluid from airspaces of newborns and infants. Neoreviews 2006;7:e88–94.
11. Swanson JR, Sinkin RA. Transition from fetus to newborn. Pediatr Clin North Am 2015;62:329–43.
12. Alcorn D, Adamson TM, Lambert TF, et al. Morphological effects of chronic tracheal ligation and drainage in the fetal lamb lung. J Anat 1977;123:649–60.
13. Moessinger AC, Harding R, Adamson TM, et al. Role of lung fluid volume in growth and maturation of the fetal sheep lung. J Clin Invest 1990;86:1270–7.
14. Prsa M, Sun L, van Amerom J, et al. Reference ranges of blood flow in the major vessels of the normal human fetal circulation at term by phase-contrast magnetic resonance imaging. Circ Cardiovasc Imaging 2014;7:663–70.
15. Gao Y, Raj JU. Regulation of the pulmonary circulation in the fetus and newborn. Physiol Rev 2010;90:1291–335.
16. van Tuyl M, Liu J, Wang J, et al. Role of oxygen and vascular development in epithelial branching morphogenesis of the developing mouse lung. Am J Physiol Lung Cell Mol Physiol 2005;288:L167–78.

17. Stenmark KR, Fagan KA, Frid MG. Hypoxia-induced pulmonary vascular remodeling: cellular and molecular mechanisms. Circ Res 2006;99:675–91.
18. Hillman NH, Kallapur SG, Jobe AH. Physiology of transition from intrauterine to extrauterine life. Clin Perinatol 2012;39:769–83.
19. Alcorn D, Adamson TM, Maloney JE, et al. Morphological effects of chronic bilateral phrenectomy or vagotomy in the fetal lamb lung. J Anat 1980;130:683–95.
20. Teitel DF, Iwamoto HS, Rudolph AM. Changes in the pulmonary circulation during birth-related events. Pediatr Res 1990;27:372–8.
21. Urlesberger B, Brandner A, Pocivalnik M, et al. A left-to-right shunt via the ductus arteriosus is associated with increased regional cerebral oxygen saturation during neonatal transition. Neonatology 2013;103:259–63.
22. van Vonderen JJ, te Pas AB, Kolster-Bijdevaate C, et al. Non-invasive measurements of ductus arteriosus flow directly after birth. Arch Dis Child Fetal Neonatal Ed 2014;99(5):F408–12.
23. Agata Y, Hiraishi S, Oguchi K, et al. Changes in left ventricular output from fetal to early neonatal life. J Pediatr 1991;119:441–5.
24. Kluckow M, Evans N. Relationship between blood pressure and cardiac output in preterm infants requiring mechanical ventilation. J Pediatr 1996;129:506–12.
25. Weir EK, Obreztchikova M, Vargese A, et al. Mechanisms of oxygen sensing: a key to therapy of pulmonary hypertension and patent ductus arteriosus. Br J Pharmacol 2008;155:300–7.
26. Ersdal HL, Linde J, Mduma E, et al. Neonatal outcome following cord clamping after onset of spontaneous respiration. Pediatrics 2014;134:265–72.
27. Kluckow M, Hooper SB. Using physiology to guide time to cord clamping. Semin Fetal Neonatal Med 2015. http://dx.doi.org/10.1016/j.siny.2015.03.002.
28. Noori S, Wlodaver A, Gottipati V, et al. Transitional changes in cardiac and cerebral hemodynamics in term neonates at birth. J Pediatr 2012;160:943–8.
29. Urlesberger B, Grossauer K, Pocivalnik M, et al. Regional oxygen saturation of the brain and peripheral tissue during birth transition of term infants. J Pediatr 2010;157:740–4.
30. McNeill S, Gatenby JC, McElroy S, et al. Normal cerebral, renal and abdominal regional oxygen saturations using near-infrared spectroscopy in preterm infants. J Perinatol 2011;31:51–7.
31. O'Brodovich HM. Immature epithelial Na+ channel expression is one of the pathogenetic mechanisms leading to human neonatal respiratory distress syndrome. Proc Assoc Am Physicians 1996;108:345–55.
32. Siew ML, Wallace MJ, Allison BJ, et al. The role of lung inflation and sodium transport in airway liquid clearance during lung aeration in newborn rabbits. Pediatr Res 2013;73:443–9.
33. O'Donnell CPF, Kamlin COF, Davis PG, et al. Crying and breathing by extremely preterm infants immediately after birth. J Pediatr 2010;156:846–7.
34. Vento M, Saugstad OD. Resuscitation of the term and preterm infant. Semin Fetal Neonatal Med 2010;15:216–22.
35. Hooper SB, Siew ML, Kitchen MJ, et al. Establishing functional residual capacity in the non-breathing infant. Semin Fetal Neonatal Med 2013;18:336–43.
36. Barker PM, Gowen CW, Lawson EE, et al. Decreased sodium ion absorption across nasal epithelium of very premature infants with respiratory distress syndrome. J Pediatr 1997;130:373–7.
37. Siew ML, Wallace MJ, Kitchen MJ, et al. Inspiration regulates the rate and temporal pattern of lung liquid clearance and lung aeration at birth. J Appl Physiol (1985) 2009;106:1888–95.

38. Siew ML, Te Pas AB, Wallace MJ, et al. Positive end-expiratory pressure enhances development of a functional residual capacity in preterm rabbits ventilated from birth. J Appl Physiol (1985) 2009;106:1487–93.
39. Rabi Y, Yee W, Chen SY, et al. Oxygen saturation trends immediately after birth.
J Pediatr 2006;148:590–4.
40. Mariani G, Dik PB, Ezquer A, et al. Pre-ductal and post-ductal o2 saturation in
healthy term neonates after birth. J Pediatr 2007;150:418–21.
41. Raj U, Shimoda L. EB2002 featured topic. Crit Care 2002;2064:671–7.
42. Platt MW, Deshpande S. Metabolic adaptation at birth. Semin Fetal Neonatal Med
2005;10:341–50.
43. Singer D. Neonatal tolerance to hypoxia: a comparative-physiological approach.
Comp Biochem Physiol A Mol Integr Physiol 1999;123:221–34.
44. Singer D, Mühlfeld C. Perinatal adaptation in mammals: the impact of metabolic
rate. Comp Biochem Physiol A Mol Integr Physiol 2007;148:780–4.
45. Padbury J, Agata Y, Ludlow J, et al. Effect of fetal adrenalectomy on catecholamine release and physiologic adaptation at birth in sheep. J Clin Invest 1987;
80:1096–103.
46. Padbury JF, Ludlow JK, Ervin MG, et al. Thresholds for physiological effects of
plasma catecholamines in fetal sheep. Am J Physiol 1987;252:E530–7.
47. Villamor E, Kessels CG, Fischer MA, et al. Role of superoxide anion on basal and
stimulated nitric oxide activity in neonatal piglet pulmonary vessels. Pediatr Res
2003;54:372–81.
48. Sherman TS, Chen Z, Yuhanna IS, et al. Nitric oxide synthase isoform expression
in the developing lung epithelium. Am J Physiol 1999;276:L383–90.
49. Shaul PW, Pace MC, Chen Z, et al. Developmental changes in prostacyclin synthesis are conserved in cultured pulmonary endothelium and vascular smooth
muscle. Am J Respir Cell Mol Biol 1999;20:113–21.

Pathophysiology of Birth Asphyxia

Matthew A. Rainaldi, MD*, Jeffrey M. Perlman, MB ChB

KEYWORDS

- Neonate • Birth asphyxia • Perinatal • Fetal acidemia
- Hypoxic–ischemic encephalopathy • Cerebral palsy

KEY POINTS

- The pathophysiology of birth asphyxia centers on the interruption of placental blood flow.
- The goal of the fetus is to preserve blood flow to the brain, heart, and adrenal glands during asphyxia.
- Blood flow to noncritical organs is sacrificed to preserve critical organ blood flow.
- Circulatory and noncirculatory adaptive mechanisms allow the fetus to cope with interruption of placental blood flow.
- The most severe consequence of asphyxia is permanent brain injury. Cerebral injury begins with an initial insult and continues during the reperfusion period.

INTRODUCTION

The term asphyxia can be defined as a condition of impaired gas exchange in a subject, which leads to progressive hypoxia, hypercarbia, and acidosis depending on the extent and duration of this interruption. Birth asphyxia, or impaired gas exchange during the perinatal period, does not have precise biochemical criteria. As such, caution must be exercised in labeling a neonate with "asphyxia." Unfortunately, this term is often inappropriately linked with poor neurodevelopmental outcome, commonly referred to as cerebral palsy. Before a potential causal relationship between an acute intrapartum interruption of placental blood flow and a later case of cerebral palsy can be established, the American Congress of Obstetricians and Gynecologists Task Force on Neonatal Encephalopathy and Cerebral Palsy require 4 essential criteria[1]: (1) evidence of a metabolic acidosis in fetal umbilical cord arterial blood obtained at delivery (pH <7.00 and base deficit ≥ 12 mmol/L), (2) early onset of severe or moderate neonatal encephalopathy in infants born at 34 weeks or more of

The authors have nothing to disclose.
Division of Newborn Medicine, Komansky Center for Children's Health, New York Presbyterian Hospital, Weill Cornell Medicine, 525 East 68th Street, N-506, New York, NY 10065, USA
* Corresponding author.
E-mail address: Mar9198@med.cornell.edu

gestation, (3) cerebral palsy of the spastic quadriplegic or dyskinetic type, and (4) exclusion of other identifiable etiologies such as trauma, coagulation disorders, infectious conditions, or genetic disorders.

Asphyxia may occur before, during, or after delivery. Its pathophysiology is extremely complex and can be a result of factors related to the mother, the placenta, and/or the fetus and neonate. This section focuses predominantly on the interruption of placental blood flow and the fetal adaptive mechanisms that occur around the time of birth.

The goals of this article are to (1) review the fetal and neonatal circulations and how transition can be disrupted with asphyxia, (2) describe the adaptive responses, both circulatory and noncirculatory that are protective against asphyxia, (3) review the biochemical processes regulating gas exchange in the placenta, and (4) define the mechanisms of cell death after asphyxia and discuss pathologic brain injury as it relates to the asphyxial insult.

NORMAL FETAL CIRCULATION

The human fetus exists in a hypoxemic, but not a pathologically hypoxic state. A number of remarkable mechanisms allow the fetus to thrive under these conditions. Oxygen diffuses readily from the maternal to fetal circulation to bind high-affinity fetal hemoglobin. This blood from the placenta returns through the umbilical vein to the fetus and the majority enters the ductus venosus. The blood has a Po_2 of approximately 40 to 50 mm Hg[2] before joining less oxygenated blood from the inferior vena cava en route to the right atrium. Interestingly, the more oxygenated blood from the umbilical vein is directed through the foramen ovale to the left side of the heart. This blood goes on to exit the left ventricle via the aorta to the carotid and coronary arteries.[3] Thus, the fetus preferentially supplies more oxygenated blood to the brain and heart. Less oxygenated blood from the inferior vena cava remains in the right side of the heart to exit via the pulmonary trunk. The majority of this blood bypasses the lungs via the ductus arteriosus[3] and enters the aorta distal to the carotid and coronary pathways. This mixture of blood has a Po_2 of 15 to 25 mm Hg,[3] and a portion travels out the umbilical arteries to the placenta.

Additional factors unique to the fetus ensure adequate oxygen delivery to meet tissue demand. Hemoglobin levels are higher in the fetus compared with adults and children.[4] Fetal hemoglobin has a high affinity for oxygen and shifts the oxygen–hemoglobin dissociation curve to the left. This facilitates transfer of oxygen from the mother to the fetus across a smaller concentration gradient. These factors increase the oxygen-carrying capacity of fetal blood. The rate of tissue perfusion is higher in the fetus than the adult.[3] Thus, increased delivery of blood counteracts relatively low oxygen saturation. Additionally, the fetus expends less energy on thermoregulation and respiratory effort than the neonate.

CIRCULATORY CHANGES DURING LABOR AND NEONATAL TRANSITION

Uterine contractions lead to decreased uterine arterial blood flow[5] and decreased flow into the intervillous spaces. Transplacental gas exchange may be impaired transiently,[6] but this is generally inconsequential during normal labor.[7] When the fetal side of the circulation is examined, uterine contractions do not seem to affect umbilical blood flow. This was shown by Malcus and colleagues,[8] who measured umbilical artery flow velocity waveforms via Doppler ultrasonography and found no differences before or during contractions. However, it was noted that fetuses with an arterial pH of 7.1 or less were more likely to have increased resistance to arterial flow during contractions.

Significant circulatory changes occur with the transition to ex utero life. Many of these changes happen simultaneously. In an infant that cries immediately after birth, the lungs rapidly expand and pulmonary vascular resistance drops. Pulmonary blood flow increases significantly. Right-to-left shunting at the ductus arteriosus decreases and eventually reverses as pulmonary artery pressure decreases below systemic blood pressure. Increases in Pao_2 stimulate ductal closure. The pulmonary venous system then returns more blood to the left atrium than in fetal life. Left atrial pressure exceeding right atrial pressure causes the foramen ovale to functionally close. In the systemic circulation, the low resistance placenta is removed from the circulation when the umbilical cord is clamped. An increase in systemic vascular resistance leads to an increase in systemic blood pressure, aiding in reversal of the ductal shunt. An adult circulation pattern is established.

CAUSES OF PERINATAL ASPHYXIA

Impaired gas exchange can occur before, during, or after delivery. This process, including recovery, may be entirely isolated to fetal life. It may occur during labor and delivery, and result in abnormal circulatory transition. Asphyxia may also develop in the immediate neonatal period if an infant cannot support his or her own gas exchange without the placenta.[3]

During fetal life as well as labor and delivery, interruption of the placental blood flow is the most common final pathway leading to asphyxia. Factors leading to interruption of blood flow come in many forms (**Table 1**). Maternal diseases such as diabetes, hypertension, or preeclampsia may alter placental vasculature and decrease blood flow. Hypotension in the mother can be translated to the fetal circulation (eg, medication effect, maternal disease, spinal anesthesia, etc). Placental factors such as abruption, fetomaternal hemorrhage, or inflammation may compromise blood flow. Chorioamnionitis and funisitis are strongly linked to placental compromise and asphyxia.[9] The umbilical cord may be compressed extrinsically, as is seen with a nuchal cord or cord prolapse. Factors solely related to the neonate may also be responsible for asphyxia. For example, congenital airway anomalies may not allow for adequate pulmonary gas exchange once the placental circulation ceases. Neurologically abnormal neonates may not have appropriate respiratory drive to effectively ventilate. This may be intrinsic to the neonate (ie, central nervous system anomaly, spinal cord injury) or owing to extrinsic effects of medications.

Table 1
Selected causes of perinatal asphyxia

Maternal	Placental/Umbilical Cord	Neonatal
Diabetes mellitus	Placental abruption	Airway anomalies
Hypertension	Fetomaternal hemorrhage	Neurologic disorders
Preeclampsia	Umbilical cord compression (prolapse, nuchal cord, knot, etc)	Severe cardiopulmonary disease
Hypotension/shock	Infection/inflammation	Severe circulatory compromise (blood loss)
Uterine rupture	Velamentous cord insertion	Infection
Severe anemia	—	Medication effect
Infection	—	—

ADAPTIVE MECHANISMS AFTER ASPHYXIA

The disruption of placental blood flow initiates important adaptive mechanisms in the fetus that are both circulatory and noncirculatory in nature. Circulatory changes involve redistribution of cardiac output and "centralization" of blood flow to vital organs. Noncirculatory responses aim to preserve cell viability. With a severe or prolonged interruption of placental blood flow, these adaptations are overwhelmed, increasing the risk of end-organ injury.

Circulatory Changes After Asphyxia

When placental blood flow is compromised, the fetus aims to redistribute cardiac output to protect more vital organs (eg, brain, myocardium, and adrenal glands). Known as the "diving reflex," this alteration of blood flow is at the expense of decreased flow to less vital organs, such as the kidney, intestine, skin, and muscle. A number of factors contribute to this reflex. Hypoxemia is sensed by carotid artery chemoreceptors, leading to catecholamine release.[10] This surge of catecholamines, in turn, causes peripheral vasoconstriction and centralization of blood flow. Hypoxemia also causes constriction of the pulmonary vasculature, with a resultant decrease in pulmonary blood flow, left atrial blood return, and left atrial pressure.[11,12] Right-to-left shunting across the foramen ovale increases in an effort to deliver even more oxygenated blood to the left heart (preferentially directed to the brain and myocardium). In addition, adaptive mechanisms within the cerebral circulation facilitate this process. Thus, cerebral vascular resistance decreases in the presence of hypoxemia. Experimental studies indicate that resistance can decrease by as much as 50%, increasing cerebral blood flow, and compensating for decreased blood oxygen content during initial asphyxia.[13–15]

Preservation of critical organ blood flow comes at the expense of decreased flow to "noncritical" organs (**Fig. 1**). When systemic blood pressure drops low enough, compensatory mechanisms fail. This critical threshold is at a point below which the cerebral circulation can no longer dilate to maintain flow.[16] Cerebral oxygen delivery is superseded by demand and brain injury occurs.

Although the diving reflex represents the ideal pathway to preserve critical organ function, not all neonates seem to exhibit these protective adaptive mechanisms consistently.[17,18] Phelan and colleagues[18] described 14 cases of hypoxic–ischemic encephalopathy (HIE) in which multiorgan dysfunction did not occur. All of these infants developed cerebral palsy. It was postulated that the mechanisms contributing to asphyxia in these cases did not allow sufficient time to centralize fetal blood flow (eg, uterine rupture, prolonged fetal heart rate deceleration). Studies in both humans and animals have suggested that intermittent asphyxia for less than 1 hour is unlikely to lead to brain injury, but severe "total" asphyxia can cause brain injury much sooner.[19–21] The adaptations of the diving reflex may be overwhelmed in extreme cases. Shah and colleagues[17] reviewed records of infants with HIE for a 10-year period. They found no differences when comparing multiorgan dysfunction of infants with severe adverse outcome to those with good outcome, suggesting a variable activation of the diving reflex.

Respiratory Responses to Asphyxia

In addition to the cardiovascular changes that occur with asphyxia, characteristic changes in breathing patterns occur. Critical to understanding the relationship between respiratory and circulatory changes is the work of Dawes and colleagues.[22] Using rhesus monkeys, these investigators initiated asphyxia by ligating the umbilical cord and covering the head with a small bag of warm saline. A characteristic series of changes

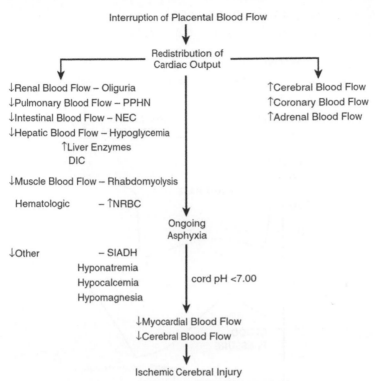

Fig. 1. Adaptive mechanisms and systemic consequences of interruption of placental blood flow. DIC, disseminated intravascular coagulation; NEC, necrotizing enterocolitis; NRBC, nucleated red blood cells; PPHN, persistent pulmonary hypertension of the newborn; SIADH, syndrome of inappropriate antidiuretic hormone release.

were seen. Within 30 seconds of total asphyxia, a brief period of rapid rhythmic respiratory effort occurred. This culminated in apnea (primary) and bradycardia, which lasted for approximately 30 to 60 seconds (**Fig. 2**). The animal then began to have gasping respirations, but spontaneous regular respiration could be induced via prompt physical stimulation. If no intervention was performed, the gasping lasted for approximately 4 minutes. It gradually became weaker until a terminal "last gasp" occurred. This was deemed secondary apnea and, unless resuscitation was initiated, death followed.

Noncirculatory Responses to Asphyxia

Several biologic factors aid in preserving critical organ viability during and after asphyxia. The cerebral metabolic rate is lower in the fetus versus the term infant or adult, creating a more favorable ratio of energy supply and demand.[23] Additionally, the neonatal brain has the capacity to use alternate energy sources when needed.[24] In situations of relative oxygen and glucose depletion, energy substrates such as lactate and ketones become critical for cerebral metabolism.[23,25] The fetal and neonatal myocardium is more resistant to hypoxia–ischemia than the adult myocardium.[26] In addition to the brain and heart, protective effects of fetal hemoglobin may also allow for a greater tolerance to a hypoxic environment.[27] Importantly, at low oxygen tensions (ie, below a "crossover Po_2"), a left-shifted fetal hemoglobin–oxygen dissociation curve may be advantageous in delivering more oxygen to tissues.[28–30] During acute acidosis, the affinity of oxygen for hemoglobin immediately decreases via the Bohr effect.[28] This

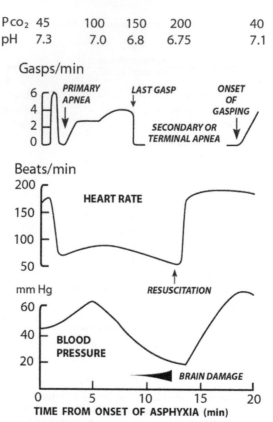

Fig. 2. Relationship between respiration, heart rate, blood pressure, and acidosis in rhesus monkeys during asphyxia and resuscitation. (*Adapted from* Dawes G, Jacobson H, Mott JC, et al. The treatment of asphyxiated, mature foetal lambs and rhesus monkeys with intravenous glucose and sodium carbonate. J Physiol 1963;169(1):174.)

decrease allows for an easier unloading of oxygen to tissues during acidosis, as is seen in perinatal asphyxia.

IMPAIRED GAS EXCHANGE AND ACIDOSIS

Diminished oxygen and carbon dioxide gas exchange across the placenta is the hallmark of perinatal asphyxia. Both gases move down a partial pressure gradient via simple diffusion. Impaired exchange of each gas contributes to acidosis.

As stated, the fetus is able to thrive at relatively low oxygen tensions. The maternal uterine artery delivers oxygenated blood to the placenta via spiral arteries. This blood enters the relatively large intervillous space (mixing with deoxygenated blood) and interfaces with chorionic villi containing fetal vessels. Oxygen is transported via simple diffusion in a passive, non–energy-dependent manner. The principal factors that dictate placental oxygen transfer are shown in **Table 2**. When fetal oxygen demand exceeds placental oxygen delivery, cells resort to anaerobic respiration to combat energy needs. Via the anaerobic pathway, lactic acid accumulates, and pH decreases.

Carbon dioxide is produced by the fetus and transported in the blood in 3 forms: (1) in the red blood cell as bicarbonate, (2) by hemoglobin as carbamate, and (3) as

Table 2
Major factors affecting placental oxygen transfer

Factor	Components
Placental membrane diffusing capacity	Surface area, thickness, oxygen solubility, diffusivity of tissues
Maternal arterial P_{O_2}	Inspired P_{O_2}, alveolar ventilation, mixed venous P_{O_2}, pulmonary blood flow, pulmonary diffusing capacity
Fetal arterial P_{O_2}	Maternal arterial P_{O_2}, maternal placental Hb flow, placental diffusing capacity, umbilical venous P_{O_2}, fetal O_2 consumption, fetal peripheral blood flow
Maternal and fetal Hb-O_2 affinities (P_{50})	pH, temperature, P_{CO_2}, 2,3-diphosphoglycerate concentration, CO concentration
Maternal placental blood flow	Arterial pressure, placental resistance to blood flow, venous pressure
Fetal placental blood flow	Umbilical artery blood pressure, umbilical venous blood pressure, placental resistance to blood flow
Spatial relationship between maternal and fetal blood flow	Vascular architecture
Amount of CO_2 exchange	—

Abbreviations: CO, carbon monoxide; Hb, hemoglobin.
Adapted from Longo LD, Hill EP, Power GG. Theoretical analysis of factors affecting placental O 2 transfer. Am J Physiol 1972;222(3):730–9.

dissolved gas. Although dissolved CO_2 gas accounts for a smaller proportion of blood CO_2 content than bicarbonate and carbamate, it is responsible for the majority of placental transfer.[31] In fact, CO_2 diffuses quite quickly, approximately 20 times faster than oxygen. Because of this, carbon dioxide transfer is predominantly dependent on blood flow, that is, intact uteroplacental and fetoplacental circulations.[31] CO_2 moves from a higher fetal to a lower maternal concentration and is ultimately eliminated by the maternal lungs. As such, the maternal pH is slightly higher (approximately 0.1 units) than the fetal pH. Two interesting phenomena, the Bohr and Haldane effects, aid in gas exchange across the placenta. The Bohr effect refers to the enhanced oxygen transfer as influenced by pH and P_{CO_2}. As maternal blood accepts CO_2 and becomes more acidotic, its oxygen–hemoglobin dissociation curve shifts to the right. This decreases oxygen affinity and facilitates unloading of oxygen. At the same time, the fetal circulation loses CO_2 and becomes more alkalotic, shifting the curve to the left, and promoting oxygen uptake. The Haldane effect refers to a complementary process by which CO_2 transport by hemoglobin is influenced by oxygen. Binding of oxygen to hemoglobin increases unloading of CO_2 on the fetal side. Thus, more fetal CO_2 becomes available in the placenta for transport to the maternal circulation. Analogously, when hemoglobin is deoxygenated, greater amounts of CO_2 can bind, which assists maternal circulation in CO_2 removal.

Fetal acidemia, or accumulation of acid occurs via 3 pathways: (1) excess carbon dioxide and in turn carbonic acid, (2) excess noncarbonic or metabolic acid (eg, lactic, uric, or keto acids), or (3) both carbonic and noncarbonic acids.[19,32] As stated, carbon dioxide quickly diffuses across the placenta and is excreted by the maternal lungs.[33] Thus, alterations in fetal pH owing to carbon dioxide accumulation can occur and resolve quickly. In contrast, noncarbonic acids only slowly diffuse across the placenta into the maternal circulation. The primary noncarbonic acid, lactic acid, accumulates as a result of oxygen deprivation and anaerobic glycolysis and does so more slowly than carbonic acid. This process results in a more sustained acidemia, the degree of which may relate to both the severity and duration of the hypoxic–ischemic insult.[19]

Because metabolic acids diffuse slowly into the maternal circulation for excretion by the maternal kidneys, some degree of acidemia may be seen in maternal conditions, such as diabetes, preeclampsia, and chronic hypertension, which may result in a more acidic pH in the umbilical artery not necessarily owing to fetal asphyxia.

The degree of acidosis or umbilical arterial pH that best defines asphyxia remains imprecise. Traditionally, asphyxia was defined as a cord umbilical arterial pH of less than 7.20.[34] Severe fetal acidemia, or an umbilical arterial pH of less than 7.00 reflects a degree of acidemia where the risk of adverse neurologic sequelae is increased.[34,35] However, even with this degree of acidemia, the likelihood of subsequent brain injury remains low. The majority of these infants (>60%) have an uneventful delivery, remain in the well nursery, and are discharged home without complication.[36] Even when infants with severe fetal acidemia are admitted to intensive care (usually because of respiratory difficulties) about 80% to 90% exhibit a benign neurologic course and it is only a small percentage present with encephalopathy.[37–39] In 1 study, 8 of 47 infants (12%) with severe fetal acidemia admitted to the intensive care unit developed HIE, including seizures.[37] In this study, infants with seizures were 234 times more likely to require cardiopulmonary resuscitation in the delivery room versus those without seizures.[37] Therefore, the presence of severe fetal acidemia, although a distinct marker of stress, does not equate necessarily with the inability of the fetus to maintain cerebral perfusion. However, when severe acidemia is seen in the context of a bradycardic neonate requiring intensive delivery room resuscitation, a significant intrapartum insult is more likely. It is in this case that cerebral perfusion and oxygen delivery were compromised. The resistance of the brain to asphyxia, even when profound, is extraordinary and is in part based on the ability of the fetus to adapt to interruption of placental blood flow to preserve cerebral perfusion and oxygen delivery (as described previously).

NEURONAL CELL DEATH AFTER ASPHYXIA

When compensatory mechanisms are overwhelmed and cerebral blood flow can no longer meet demand, a cascade of biochemical events begins. These events are complex, interrelated, and ultimately lead to cell death without intervention. This section focuses on the cellular pathophysiology of hypoxic–ischemic brain injury, as is seen with asphyxia.

In the asphyxiated fetus or neonate, oxygen delivery is reduced, anaerobic glycolysis takes over, and high-energy phosphate compounds decrease (ie, adenosine triphosphate and phosphocreatinine). Lactic acid accumulates and membrane ion pumps fail (Na^+/K^+ adenosine triphosphatase and Na^+/Ca^{2+} exchanger). With membrane pump failure, sodium and water influx into cells, leading to cell swelling. Calcium also flows into cells, which initiates release of excitatory amino acids such as glutamate into the extracellular space. This overexcitation leads to more calcium influx, fostering an excitotoxic cycle.[40] Further consequences include formation of free radicals, production of nitric oxide, and lipid peroxidation of cell membranes (**Fig. 3**).

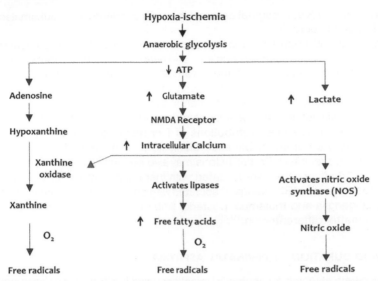

Fig. 3. Potential biochemical mechanisms of hypoxic–ischemic brain injury. ATP, adenosine triphosphate.

The endpoint of cell death is described classically to occur via necrosis or apoptosis (programmed cell death). Necrosis is defined by cell swelling, disruption of organelles, and loss of phospholipid membrane integrity with cell lysis. It represents a rapid and severe breakdown of cellular function that occurs with the primary hypoxic–ischemic insult.[41] After resuscitation, cerebral perfusion and oxygenation are restored, along with partial restoration of energy sources. However, there is a subsequent progressive decrease in high-energy phosphates 24 to 48 hours later, that is, a secondary energy failure.[42]

During secondary energy failure, reperfusion injury occurs owing to extended reactions from the primary insult. This injury is characterized by inflammation, generation of reactive oxygen species and free radicals, and importantly cell death via apoptosis.[43] When apoptotic pathways are initiated, adenosine triphosphate is used to actively dismantle cells into consumable components.[41] Cells shrink, chromatin condenses, and nuclei become pyknotic. Apoptosis may be induced through caspase-dependent or gene transcription (caspase-independent) processes.[40] Caspase-3 is the most abundant effector caspase in the developing brain[44] and there is a direct correlation between the activation of caspase-3 and the degree of injury after hypoxia–ischemia.[45] Because of its delayed nature, apoptosis has become an enticing target for potential therapies for HIE.[46] Recently, hybrid forms of neuronal death have gained attention, filling in the gaps between necrosis and apoptosis along a continuum of cell death.[41]

PATHOLOGIC BRAIN INJURY AFTER PERINATAL ASPHYXIA

Brain injury after asphyxia is hypoxic–ischemic in nature and occurs in characteristic locations on MRI or at autopsy. The injured region can vary depending on the type and duration of insult, gestational age, and whether the infant was treated with hypothermia.[47,48] The classic patterns of neuropathologic injury from HIE include (1) selective neuronal necrosis, (2) parasagittal cerebral injury, (3) periventricular leukomalacia, and (4) focal ischemic necrosis.

Selective neuronal necrosis is the most common type of brain injury. It generally has 3 patterns: diffuse, cortical–deep nuclear, and deep nuclear–brain stem. Parasagittal cerebral injury occurs in the end-arterial watershed area of the parietooccipital cortex and subcortical white matter. Periventricular leukomalacia refers to a classic white matter necrosis and gliosis of preterm infants, although it can be identified in term infants after hypoxia–ischemia. Focal ischemic necrosis pertains to arterial stroke and can be identified in vascular distributions of 1 or more cerebral arteries. Heterogeneous patterns are common, because elements of more than 1 of these patterns are frequently appreciated. Partial lesions may also be found, as described in a recent study where 10 infants that were treated with therapeutic hypothermia had isolated hippocampal injury.[48] MRI findings associated with poor outcome include involvement of the basal ganglia and thalamus, posterior limb of the internal capsule, and loss of gray–white matter differentiation.[19,49]

TIMING AND DURATION OF PERINATAL ASPHYXIA

The precise time at which an asphyxial event occurred is often a focus of intense scrutiny by the obstetrician, neonatologist, and parents. This may be obvious in cases with profound sentinel events, that is, change in fetal heart rate tracing (absent variability or decelerations), uterine rupture, placental abruption, cord prolapse, or trauma. But, in some cases, this remains elusive. In this sense, the asphyxial insult can be classified as acute or subacute.

A classic example of an acute asphyxial insult is that of a "megacode," where a full resuscitation occurs.[50] An abrupt change in fetal heart rate may have been appreciated, and the neonate presented with poor Apgar scores and severe acidosis. Renal and other end-organ dysfunction is often seen along with encephalopathy.

A subset of asphyxiated infants may not present with significant circulatory collapse at birth. In these cases, the insult likely occurred in a subacute fashion, allowing the fetus to "self-resuscitate" in utero. Labor is often uncomplicated and the neonate does not require serious intervention at delivery. As a result, severe acidemia is not apparent, but encephalopathy may be present. Some of these infants may go unrecognized initially, then develop a syndrome of encephalopathy and seizures within 12 to 24 hours.[51] A distinctly different presentation was described in a recent study of term infants treated with hypothermia. Seven infants with subacute insults based on intrapartum characteristics presented with more severe encephalopathy at birth and were less likely to require intensive resuscitation as compared with 26 with acute insults (eg, uterine rupture).[52] With either presentation systemic organ injury is common, particularly renal dysfunction, along with evidence of brain injury on MRI. In these cases, timing of the injury is often difficult. Subtle clues from the maternal history may be valuable (ie, decreased fetal movement), as well as characteristic MRI findings. Injury on MRI may evolve throughout the reperfusion period and the interpretation of an MRI should take this into account.[53] For instance, diffusion and metabolic changes worsen until day 4 or 5 and then begin to normalize.[54]

Certain injury patterns can offer suggestions as to the duration of asphyxia. The most severe and prolonged insults often result in diffuse neuronal injury.[19] Moderate to severe prolonged insults tend to lead to cortical and deep nuclear (basal ganglia and thalamic) neuronal injury (**Fig. 4**). Hypoxia–ischemia that is severe and abrupt predominantly causes deep nuclear–brain stem injury.

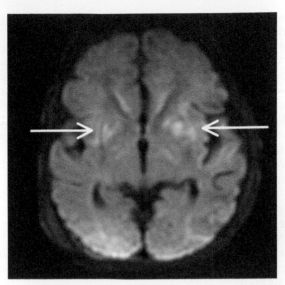

Fig. 4. Diffusion-weighted MRI (axial) image showing basal ganglia injury (*arrows*).

SUMMARY

The fetal circulation is remarkable in its ability to adequately deliver oxygen in a hypoxemic environment. The pathophysiology of perinatal asphyxia centers around the interruption of placental blood flow. Although there are many adaptive mechanisms that aim to prevent adverse consequences of asphyxia, these mechanisms can be overwhelmed. When compensatory mechanisms can no longer keep up with blood flow demand, acidosis and ultimately cell death occur. A comprehensive understanding of the pathophysiology of asphyxia is crucial to effective management of these infants.

REFERENCES

1. American Congress of Obstetricians and Gynecologists (ACOG). Committee Opinion. Number 326. Inappropriate use of the terms fetal distress and birth asphyxia. Obstet Gynecol 2005;106:1469–70.
2. Nicolaides K, Economides D, Soothill P. Blood gases, pH, and lactate in appropriate-and small-for-gestational-age fetuses. Am J Obstet Gynecol 1989; 161(4):996–1001.
3. Martin RJ, Fanaroff AA, Walsh MC. Fanaroff and Martin's neonatal-perinatal medicine: diseases of the fetus and infant. 9th edition. Philadelphia: Saunders/Elsevier; 2011.
4. Walker J, Turnbull EN. Haemoglobin and red cells in the human foetus and their relation to the oxygen content of the blood in the vessels of the umbilical cord. Lancet 1953;262(6781):312–8.
5. Li H, Gudmundsson S, Olofsson P. Clinical significance of uterine artery blood flow velocity waveforms during provoked uterine contractions in high-risk pregnancy. Ultrasound Obstet Gynecol 2004;24(4):429–34.
6. Boylan PC, Parisi VM. Fetal acid–base balance. In: Creasy RK, Resnik R, editors. Maternal–Fetal Medicine. 3rd edition. Philadelphia: Saunders; 1994. p. 349–58.
7. Stuart B, Drumm J, Fitzgerald D, et al. Fetal blood velocity waveforms in uncomplicated labour. BJOG 1981;88(9):865–9.

8. Malcus P, Gudmundsson S, Marsal K, et al. Umbilical artery Doppler velocimetry as a labor admission test. Obstet Gynecol 1991;77(1):10–6.
9. Mir IN, Johnson-Welch SF, Nelson DB, et al. Placental pathology is associated with severity of neonatal encephalopathy and adverse developmental outcomes following hypothermia. Am J Obstet Gynecol 2015;213(6):849.e1-7.
10. Kara T, Narkiewicz K, Somers VK. Chemoreflexes–physiology and clinical implications. Acta Physiol Scand 2003;177(3):377–84.
11. Rudolph AM, Heymann MA. The circulation of the fetus in utero methods for studying distribution of blood flow, cardiac output and organ blood flow. Circ Res 1967;21(2):163–84.
12. Rudolph A, Yuan S. Response of the pulmonary vasculature to hypoxia and H+ ion concentration changes. J Clin Invest 1966;45(3):399.
13. Koehler RC, Jones M, Traystman RJ. Cerebral circulatory response to carbon monoxide and hypoxic hypoxia in the lamb. Am J Physiol 1982;243(1):H27–32.
14. Jones M, Sheldon RE, Peeters LL, et al. Regulation of cerebral blood flow in the ovine fetus. Am J Physiol 1978;235(2):H162–6.
15. Ashwal S, Dale PS, Longo LD. Regional cerebral blood flow: studies in the fetal lamb during hypoxia, hypercapnia, addosis, and hypotension. Pediatr Res 1984;18(12):1309–16.
16. Block BS, Schlafer DH, Wentworth RA, et al. Intrauterine asphyxia and the breakdown of physiologic circulatory compensation in fetal sheep. Am J Obstet Gynecol 1990;162(5):1325–31.
17. Shah P, Riphagen S, Beyene J, et al. Multiorgan dysfunction in infants with post-asphyxial hypoxic-ischaemic encephalopathy. Arch Dis Child Fetal Neonatal Ed 2004;89(2):F152–5.
18. Phelan JP, Alen MO, Korst L, et al. Intrapartum fetal asphyxial brain injury with absent multiorgan system dysfunction. J Matern Fetal Med 1998;7(1):19–22.
19. Volpe JJ. Neurology of the newborn. 5th edition. Philadelphia: Saunders/Elsevier; 2008.
20. Low JA, Galbraith R, Muir D, et al. Factors associated with motor and cognitive deficits in children after intrapartum fetal hypoxia. Am J Obstet Gynecol 1984; 148(5):533.
21. Pasternak JF, Gorey MT. The syndrome of acute near-total intrauterine asphyxia in the term infant. Pediatr Neurol 1998;18(5):391–8.
22. Dawes G, Jacobson H, Mott JC, et al. The treatment of asphyxiated, mature foetal lambs and rhesus monkeys with intravenous glucose and sodium carbonate. J Physiol 1963;169(1):167–84.
23. Cremer JE. Substrate utilization and brain development. J Cereb Blood Flow Metab 1982;2(4):394–407.
24. Vannucci RC, Yager JY. Glucose, lactic acid, and perinatal hypoxic-ischemic brain damage. Pediatr Neurol 1992;8(1):3–12.
25. Yager JY, Heitjan DF, Towfighi J, et al. Effect of insulin-induced and fasting hypoglycemia on perinatal hypoxic-ischemic brain damage. Pediatr Res 1992;31(2): 138–42.
26. Dawes G, Mott JC, Shelley HJ. The importance of cardiac glycogen for the maintenance of life in foetal lambs and new-born animals during anoxia. J Physiol 1959;146(3):516–38.
27. Oski FA. The unique fetal red cell and its function. E. Mead Johnson Award address. Pediatrics 1973;51(3):494–500.
28. Wimberley P. A review of oxygen and delivery in the neonate. Scand J Clin Lab Invest 1982;160(Suppl):114–8.

29. Aberman A. Crossover PO2, a measure of the variable effect of increased P50 on mixed venous PO2 1. Am Rev Respir Dis 1977;115(1):173–5.
30. Woodson RD. Physiological significance of oxygen dissociation curve shifts. Crit Care Med 1979;7(9):368–73.
31. Cowett RM. Principles of perinatal-neonatal metabolism. New York: Springer Science & Business Media; 2012.
32. Wyka KA, Mathews PJ, Rutkowski JA. Foundations of respiratory care. Clifton Park, NY: Delmar Publishing; 2011.
33. Thorp JA, Rushing RS. Umbilical cord blood gas analysis. Obstet Gynecol Clin North Am 1999;26(4):695–709.
34. Goldaber K, Gilstrap L III, Leveno K, et al. Pathologic fetal acidemia. Obstet Gynecol 1991;78(6):1103–7.
35. Sehdev HM, Stamilio DM, Macones GA, et al. Predictive factors for neonatal morbidity in neonates with an umbilical arterial cord pH less than 7.00. Am J Obstet Gynecol 1997;177(5):1030–4.
36. King TA, Jackson GL, Josey AS, et al. The effect of profound umbilical artery acidemia in term neonates admitted to a newborn nursery. J Pediatr 1998; 132(4):624–9.
37. Perlman JM, Risser R. Severe fetal acidemia: neonatal neurologic features and short-term outcome. Pediatr Neurol 1993;9(4):277–82.
38. Goodwin TM, Belai I, Hernandez P, et al. Asphyxial complications in the term newborn with severe umbilical acidemia. Am J Obstet Gynecol 1992;167(6): 1506–12.
39. Fee SC, Malee K, Deddish R, et al. Severe acidosis and subsequent neurologic status. Am J Obstet Gynecol 1990;162(3):802–6.
40. Calvert JW, Zhang JH. Pathophysiology of an hypoxic–ischemic insult during the perinatal period. Neurol Res 2005;27(3):246–60.
41. Northington FJ, Chavez-Valdez R, Martin LJ. Neuronal cell death in neonatal hypoxia-ischemia. Ann Neurol 2011;69(5):743–58.
42. Vannucci RC, Towfighi J, Vannucci SJ. Secondary energy failure after cerebral hypoxia-ischemia in the immature rat. J Cereb Blood Flow Metab 2004;24(10): 1090–7.
43. Vannucci RC. Hypoxic-ischemic encephalopathy. Am J Perinatol 2000;17(3): 113–20.
44. Sakahira H, Enari M, Nagata S. Cleavage of CAD inhibitor in CAD activation and DNA degradation during apoptosis. Nature 1998;391(6662):96–9.
45. Zhu C, Wang X, Xu F, et al. The influence of age on apoptotic and other mechanisms of cell death after cerebral hypoxia-ischemia. Cell Death Differ 2005;12(2): 162–76.
46. Dixon BJ, Reis C, Ho WM, et al. Neuroprotective strategies after neonatal hypoxic ischemic encephalopathy. Int J Mol Sci 2015;16(9):22368–401.
47. Sie LT, van der Knaap MS, Oosting J, et al. MR patterns of hypoxic-ischemic brain damage after prenatal, perinatal or postnatal asphyxia. Neuropediatrics 2000; 31(3):128–36.
48. Kasdorf E, Engel M, Heier L, et al. Therapeutic hypothermia in neonates and selective hippocampal injury on diffusion-weighted magnetic resonance imaging. Pediatr Neurol 2014;51(1):104–8.
49. Rutherford MA, Pennock JM, Counsell SJ, et al. Abnormal magnetic resonance signal in the internal capsule predicts poor neurodevelopmental outcome in infants with hypoxic-ischemic encephalopathy. Pediatrics 1998;102(2):323–8.

50. Wyckoff MH, Aziz K, Escobedo MB, et al. Part 13: neonatal resuscitation: 2015 American Heart Association guidelines update for cardiopulmonary resuscitation and emergency cardiovascular care. Circulation 2015;132(18 Suppl 2):S543–60.
51. Perlman JM. Intrapartum asphyxia and cerebral palsy: is there a link? Clin Perinatol 2006;33(2):335–53.
52. Kasdorf E, Grunebaum A, Perlman JM. Subacute hypoxia-ischemia and the timing of injury in treatment with therapeutic hypothermia. Pediatr Neurol 2015; 53(5):417–21.
53. Rutherford M, Counsell S, Allsop J, et al. Diffusion-weighted magnetic resonance imaging in term perinatal brain injury: a comparison with site of lesion and time from birth. Pediatrics 2004;114(4):1004–14.
54. Barkovich A, Miller S, Bartha A, et al. MR imaging, MR spectroscopy, and diffusion tensor imaging of sequential studies in neonates with encephalopathy. AJNR Am J Neuroradiol 2006;27(3):533–47.

Perinatal Asphyxia from the Obstetric Standpoint
Diagnosis and Interventions

Christina A. Herrera, MD[a,b,*], Robert M. Silver, MD[a,b]

KEYWORDS

- Perinatal asphyxia • Cerebral palsy • Neonatal encephalopathy
- Hypoxic ischemic encephalopathy • Birth asphyxia

KEY POINTS

- Perinatal asphyxia refers to deprivation of oxygen severe enough to cause neonatal encephalopathy as a result of events surrounding birth.
- Perinatal (birth) asphyxia is often interchangeably used with terms that describe the neonatal sequelae, such as hypoxic-ischemic encephalopathy and cerebral palsy.
- Apgar scores, umbilical cord gas pH, base deficit, lactate, and neuroimaging can aid in determination of the timing of injury.
- Emergent obstetric complications, such as umbilical cord prolapse, placental abruption, or uterine rupture, are associated with the highest risk for intrapartum-associated perinatal asphyxia.
- Screening modalities, such as ultrasound and antenatal testing, can aid in prediction of a compromised fetus but are most useful in the setting of chronic maternal/fetal conditions.

INTRODUCTION

Balancing the safety of the mother and fetus is a major challenge for clinicians, particularly when the risks and benefits are not equivalent. For instance, a vaginal delivery is almost always safer for the mother but may not be optimal for the fetus. Complications during delivery can lead to poor neonatal outcomes in otherwise normal fetuses. Birth asphyxia is a general term for neonatal encephalopathy resulting from events during labor and delivery. Although some cases of asphyxia are preventable, our ability to predict those fetuses at risk remains poor.[1]

Disclosures: The authors have no disclosures.
[a] Department of Obstetrics and Gynecology, University of Utah, Salt Lake City, UT 84132, USA;
[b] Department of Maternal Fetal Medicine, Intermountain Healthcare, 121 Cottonwood Street, Murray, UT 84157, USA
* Corresponding author. Division of Maternal Fetal Medicine, Department of Obstetrics and Gynecology, University of Utah, 30 North Medical Drive, Room 2B200, Salt Lake City, UT 84132.
E-mail address: Christina.Herrera@hsc.utah.edu

Clin Perinatol 43 (2016) 423–438
http://dx.doi.org/10.1016/j.clp.2016.04.003
0095-5108/16/$ – see front matter Published by Elsevier Inc.
perinatology.theclinics.com

Perinatal (birth) asphyxia is a general term referring to neonatal encephalopathy related to events during birth. It is often interchangeably used with terms describing the neonatal sequelae such as hypoxic-ischemic encephalopathy and cerebral palsy (CP). Asphyxia refers to a deprivation of oxygen long enough to cause neurologic injury. Neonatal encephalopathy is a clinical syndrome of neurologic dysfunction manifested by abnormal level of consciousness or seizures, difficulty maintaining respiration, and depression of tone and reflexes.[2] The likelihood that the encephalopathy incurred as a result of birth increases when specific criteria are met.

The American College of Obstetrics and Gynecology (ACOG) gave this opinion:

Intrapartum asphyxia implies to fetal hypercarbia and hypoxemia, which, if prolonged, will result in metabolic acidemia. Because the intrapartum disruption of uterine or fetal blood flow is rarely, if ever, absolute, asphyxia is an imprecise, general term. Descriptions such as hypercarbia, hypoxia, and metabolic, respiratory, or lactic acidemia are more precise for immediate assessment of the newborn infant and retrospective assessment of intrapartum management.[3]

Perinatal asphyxia with acute hypoxia-ischemia may result in neonatal signs, which are temporally proximal to delivery. The Apgar score, umbilical cord gas, neuroimaging, and multiorgan dysfunction can be used to help determine whether the injury is consistent with a peripartum event (**Table 1**).[2]

Other factors can help distinguish timing of injury resulting from an acute event. For instance, severe obstetric complications, such as uterine rupture, abruptio placentae, umbilical cord prolapse, or fetal exsanguination, are strong risk factors for birth asphyxia. Additionally, progression from a normal, category I (**Fig. 1**) fetal heart rate pattern to a category III (see **Fig. 3**) pattern is suggestive of a hypoxic-ischemic intrapartum event.[4] Importantly, there should be no evidence of other causes, such as maternal/fetal infection, fetal anomalies, aneuploidy, or genetic syndromes, which may affect neurodevelopment or cause aberrant fetal growth. Lastly, CP of the spastic quadriplegic or dyskinetic type (as opposed to other subtypes) is more suggestive of perinatal injury.

INTRAPARTUM SCREENING AND DIAGNOSIS

Intrapartum electronic fetal heart monitoring (EFM) during labor was designed to prevent perinatal asphyxia. Unfortunately, despite the use of EFM, CP rates have not decreased over the past 3 decades.[5] A 3-tier fetal heart rate interpretation system was proposed by the National Institutes of Child Health and Development (NICHD) in 2008 and is still widely used today.[6] Category I tracings represent a normal fetal heart rate pattern. Category II tracings are indeterminate and require further evaluation. Intervention depends on the clinical situation. Category III tracings are abnormal and warrant prompt evaluation, intervention, and consideration of urgent delivery (see

Table 1 Neonatal signs of perinatal asphyxia	
Apgar score	Less than 5 at 5 and 10 min of life
Umbilical arterial cord gas	Less than 7.0 and/or base deficit $\geq$12 mmol/L
Neuroimaging[a]	Deep nuclear gray matter or watershed cortical injury
Organ dysfunction	Multisystem organ failure
CP	Spastic quadriplegic or dyskinetic type

[a] MRI is the most sensitive test.

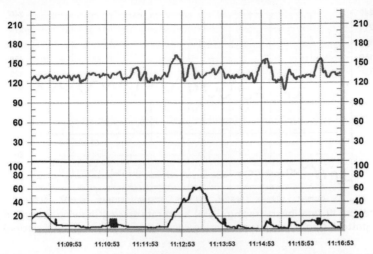

Fig. 1. Category I fetal heart tracing. Fetal heart rate tracing showing normal baseline, moderate variability, and accelerations (*red tracing*). One contraction is noted (*blue tracing*).

Fig. 1; Figs. 2 and **3**). The presence of fetal heart rate accelerations and/or moderate variability is a strong predictor of a nonacidotic fetus.[4]

Because of the low prevalence of target conditions (fetal death, CP) and mediocre validity, the positive predictive value of EFM is near zero.[1] A Cochrane review of 13 trials assessing the effectiveness of continuous EFM during labor showed that the intervention was associated with a reduced risk of neonatal seizures but no difference in neonatal mortality or CP. Furthermore, EFM significantly increased the rate of cesarean deliveries and operative vaginal deliveries.[7] One study attempted to estimate the

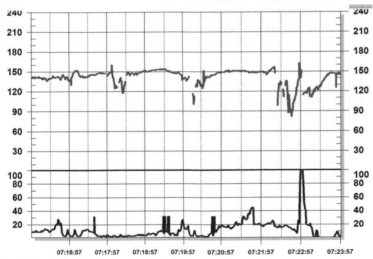

Fig. 2. Category II fetal heart tracing. Fetal heart rate tracing showing variable decelerations with moderate variability (*red tracing*). Uterine contractions are noted and coincident with decelerations (*blue tracing*).

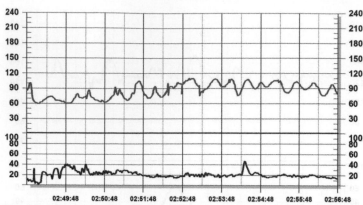

Fig. 3. Category III fetal heart tracing. Fetal heart rate tracing showing bradycardia and a sinusoidal pattern (*red tracing*) with uterine contraction monitoring (*blue tracing*).

accuracy of EFM in predicting neonatal encephalopathy requiring whole-body hypothermia therapy. The investigators discovered that the fetal heart tracing during the last hour before delivery was poorly predictive of neonatal encephalopathy requiring whole-body cooling treatment.[8] It may be that specific characteristics of a fetal tracing rather than the NICHD categorization better predicts fetal acidemia. One study determined that 4 EFM features best predicated fetal acidemia including: repetitive prolonged decelerations, baseline tachycardia, repetitive variable decelerations, and repetitive late decelerations.[9]

Fetal scalp stimulation is one strategy to assess intrapartum fetal status, which can aid in predicting a nonacidotic fetus with an indeterminate tracing. The fetal head is stimulated during digital examination. Normal fetuses have a sympathetic nervous system–mediated increase in the heart rate (acceleration) indicating an intact nervous system and, thus, reassuring fetal status. A positive fetal scalp stimulation (acceleration of 15 beats per minute for 15 seconds or more) reliably predicts a fetal pH of at least 7.20 at that moment.[10] Many experts acknowledge the limitations of EFM in determination of fetal status and advocate for alternative strategies such as scalp stimulation before concluding that operative delivery is necessary for nonreassuring fetal status.[11]

Lastly, fetal electrocardiogram analysis of the ST segment (STAN) monitoring is used in European countries in addition to conventional EFM. A recent controlled trial performed in the United States by the Maternal Fetal Medicine Unit Network randomized 11,108 women to conventional EFM versus conventional EFM with STAN. The investigators concluded that the addition of STAN monitoring did not result in improvement in perinatal morbidity, mortality, or operative delivery rates.[12] Accordingly, STAN is not currently recommended.

ANTEPARTUM SCREENING AND DIAGNOSIS

Antenatal fetal testing was designed to prevent the risk of intrauterine injury or death in pregnancies at high risk. For instance, women with comorbid medical conditions, such as diabetes, hypertension, or complicated pregnancies such as monochorionic multi-fetal gestations, may benefit from testing. Each of these conditions is associated with an increased risk of stillbirth, neonatal death, and encephalopathy. In theory, such testing can identify at-risk pregnancies and allow for expedited delivery before irreversible injury to the fetus from hypoxia. This concept is very attractive, and rates of adverse outcomes associated with hypertension and diabetes have decreased with increased use of antenatal testing.[13] Nonetheless, few data are available proving efficacy of antenatal testing for most conditions. For example, intrahepatic cholestasis of pregnancy may increase the risk of stillbirth[14]; but fetal death is thought to be acute rather than chronic and, thus, may not be predicted by antenatal testing. Antepartum testing is designed to identify placental insufficiency from chronic conditions. Because stillbirth due to intrahepatic cholestasis may be due to direct effects on fetal myocardium, rather than placental function, antenatal testing may not be useful.

The NICHD attempted to identify gaps in evidence to guide the clinical application of antenatal testing. They noted important questions that remain unanswered, including the gestational age at which to initiate testing, testing frequency, and more targeted or specific testing for each underlying pathology.[15]

The contraction stress test (CST), nonstress test (NST), biophysical profile (BPP), and modified BPP comprise the most commonly used antenatal testing modalities. The BPP (**Table 2**) consists of an NST combined with real-time ultrasonography. When normal, these tests are highly reassuring with a low false-negative rate, defined as the risk of stillbirth within 7 days of a normal test (**Table 3**). The negative predictive value (the odds that a negative/normal test is truly negative) is 99.8% for the NST and greater than 99.9% for the CST, BPP, and modified BPP.[16] Thus, a normal test result is highly reassuring. However, the low false-negative rate of these tests depends on appropriate clinical response to an acute change in maternal or fetal status. In other words, a recent normal test should not preclude further evaluation in the setting of deterioration in clinical status. For instance, worsening maternal hypertension, acute bleeding, or decreased fetal movement warrant further evaluation and testing.

In most centers, testing is performed via NST one to 2 times per week with or without a modified BPP (NST with fluid assessment). Whether to perform testing once or twice a week remains controversial. One study attempted to answer this question and found that increasing testing frequency to twice a week improved stillbirth rates from 6.1 per 1000 to 1.9 per 1000.[17]

Obstetric ultrasound to screen for signs of placental insufficiency is one of the most reliable methods of identifying pregnancies at risk for adverse outcomes. Placental insufficiency occurs when the placenta is unable to provide adequate blood flow

Table 2
The biophysical profile scoring and management

NST[a]	Reactive: 2 Points Nonreactive: 0 Points	Management
Fetal breathing movement	At least one episode of breathing movement for 30 s: 2 points	10 out of 10 or 8 out of 10 → normal test
Fetal movement	3 or more discrete body movements: 2 points	6 out of 10 → equivocal test, should be repeated within 24 h
Fetal tone	1 or more flexion/extension movements of extremity or hand: 2 points	4 out of 10 → abnormal test, should prompt delivery if >32 wk; if <32 wk, individualize based on provider judgment
Amniotic fluid volume	Deepest vertical pocket of at least 2 cm: 2 points	2 out of 10 → abnormal test, deliver immediately

Duration of test 30 minutes.
[a] May be omitted without compromising the validity of the test if all other components normal.

Table 3 Antepartum fetal testing modalities		
Test	False-Negative Rate[a]	False-Positive Rate
CST (oxytocin challenge test)	0.04	35–65
NST	0.2–0.65	55–90
BPP	0.07–0.08	40–50
Modified BPP	0.08	60

[a] Defined as stillbirth within 7 days of a normal test.[15]

(oxygen) to support the growing fetus. It may be due to abnormal placental development, placental damage, decreased uterine blood flow, or a combination of these factors. Signs of placental insufficiency include fetal growth restriction, oligohydramnios, and abnormal umbilical cord Doppler velocimetry. With placental insufficiency, the most common form of growth restriction is asymmetric, with normal growth of the head (head sparing) and development of a small abdominal circumference due to lack of subcutaneous fat. Oligohydramnios, or abnormally low amniotic fluid, results from increased placental vascular resistance leading to decreased perfusion of the fetal kidneys and, thus, decreased urine production. Fetal growth restriction is associated with a significantly increased risk of stillbirth; at estimated fetal weights less than the 10th percentile, the risk of fetal death is 1.5%; at weights less than the fifth percentile, the risk is 2.5%.[18] Furthermore, growth restriction is associated with an increased risk of CP (odds ratio [OR] 4.81, confidence interval [CI] 2.7–8.5).[19]

Screening for placental insufficiency is indicated for pregnancies in which fetal compromise is suspected from maternal disease, fetal chromosomal or structural anomalies, or complicated pregnancies, such as multifetal gestations. However, some cases of placental insufficiency are idiopathic without risk factors. Detecting such cases is difficult, but clinical assessment of uterine growth is one method of monitoring appropriate fetal growth. Fundal height measurement is typically performed after 24 weeks' gestation, and a discrepancy between the fundal height (in centimeters) and the gestational age of greater than 3 cm warrants further evaluation with ultrasound for fetal growth.[18] Caution is advised in women with obesity or uterine fibroids, which may preclude accurate measurement of fundal height.

Umbilical artery Doppler velocimetry is a noninvasive technique used to assess placental vascular resistance (blood from the fetus to the mother). Among pregnancies complicated by growth restriction, absent or reversed end diastolic flow (**Fig. 4**) is

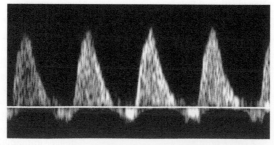

Fig. 4. Umbilical artery Doppler reversed end diastolic flow. Peaks above the line represent systolic flow; peaks below the line represent diastolic flow, which is reversed from its normal forward (above the line) flow.

associated with an increased risk of fetal demise.[20] One randomized controlled trial aimed to determine the utility of Doppler velocimetry compared with cardiotocography (NST) and found that, with Doppler monitoring, no stillbirths occurred in 214 pregnancies (a negative predictive value of 100%).[20] Also, Doppler led to less frequent monitoring and fewer antenatal admissions.[21] Despite the proven benefit in growth-restricted fetuses, Doppler velocimetry has not been shown to improve perinatal outcomes or to be predictive of adverse outcomes in normally grown fetuses.[18] Thus, its role remains uncertain in pregnancies with normal fetal growth.[16]

Fetal movement counting is another method commonly used to assess fetal status. The practice involves a woman quantifying the movements she feels in a given period of time. Unfortunately, studies to date are insufficient to show benefit (reduction in stillbirth risk); furthermore, it may cause harm because of increased anxiety.[22] Additionally, there is little evidence to guide management of decreased fetal movement that can result from a variety of causes, including maternal perception, obesity, smoking, or anterior placenta location.[23] Management often involves further antenatal testing at the expense of cost, time, and maternal stress as well as the potential for false-positive results leading to iatrogenic preterm birth. Nonetheless, some experts strongly advocate fetal kick counts as an important strategy to reduce stillbirth and asphyxia risk. The choice to do movement counting should be at the discretion of the patients, provider, and clinical situation.

Maternal biochemical screens have been proposed as a method to screen for and predict fetal growth restriction. Elevated alpha fetal protein, human chorionic gonadotropin, and inhibin A or low unconjugated estriol are associated with fetal growth restriction; the presence of 2 or more abnormal markers increases the risk. However, the sensitivity of biochemical screening is quite poor (most <50%) and the positive predictive values are dismal. Accordingly, results should be interpreted with caution in context with the clinical scenario.[24] Abnormal biomarkers may prompt increased pregnancy surveillance with obstetric ultrasounds and/or antenatal testing, although utility is uncertain.

POSTPARTUM SCREENING AND DIAGNOSIS

Post hoc examinations to consider after delivery include placental histologic examination and umbilical cord gas analysis with lactate. Placentas may be abnormal in women with placental insufficiency. Findings may include placental infarction, chorionic villitis, chronic chorioamnionitis, membrane necrosis, increased nucleated red blood cells, increased syncytial knotting, increased villous maturation, fetal thrombosis, and distal villus hypoplasia.[25] Certain placental lesions are also strongly associated with stillbirth, including acute inflammation, retroplacental hematomas, and thrombotic lesions.[26] Although some of these histologic findings are more associated with chronic causes, findings such as acute inflammation or acute thrombosis/hematoma formation may identify more acute causes.

As previously mentioned, umbilical cord arterial gas pH and base excess should be obtained because values less than 7 and greater than 12, respectively, are associated with birth asphyxia. Umbilical cord lactate levels may also aid in identifying a temporal cause. Two studies recently assessed the best predictor of neonatal morbidity and perinatal asphyxia. They found that lactate performed better than pH and base deficit.[27,28] However, the investigators warn that lactate levels are not yet standardized and most neonatal hypothermic cooling protocols use base deficit criteria.

OBSTETRIC RISK FACTORS
Bleeding in Pregnancy

Vaginal bleeding during pregnancy is often due to placenta previa or placental abruption. Placental abruption complicates 3 to 10 in 1000 pregnancies[29] and is defined as bleeding at the placental-decidual interface, or placental separation, before delivery. Depending on severity, placental abruption can lead to catastrophic maternal/fetal outcomes due to acute blood loss and decreased fetal blood flow. In one case-control study, moderate to severe vaginal bleeding was associated with an increased risk of neonatal encephalopathy (adjusted OR 3.57, 95% CI 1.30–9.85).[30] Another investigation noted that placental abruption was one of the strongest risk factors (along with umbilical cord prolapse and uterine rupture) for neonatal encephalopathy requiring whole-body cooling (OR 17, 95% CI 7–44).[31]

The incidences of placenta previa and placenta accreta (**Figs. 5** and **6**) are 1 in 200 and 1 in 500, respectively.[32] Placenta previa refers to a placenta overlying the cervical os, whereas placenta accreta spectrum denotes an abnormally adherent placenta with varied levels of myometrial invasion. Placenta previa and accreta have been associated with a small increase in risk of perinatal asphyxia due to severe hemorrhage.[9,10] However, studies to date are low powered; definitive conclusions cannot be made about the link between previa and perinatal asphyxia.[5,33]

It is difficult to imply primary causation of asphyxia from antepartum bleeding alone. Most often, bleeding occurs along with an underlying cause or risk factor. For instance, placental abruption is usually associated with antecedent maternal hypertension, substance abuse, uterine overdistention, trauma, or ruptured membranes. Thus, bleeding during pregnancy is often the result of (sometimes long-standing) underlying conditions antedating clinical bleeding. Importantly, intervention during labor may not impact such cases.[2]

Emergent Obstetric Complications

Emergent obstetric complications, which may precipitate maternal/fetal hemorrhage and loss of blood flow (and oxygen) to the fetus, are associated with the highest

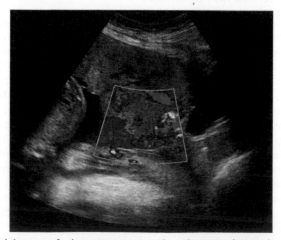

Fig. 5. Ultrasound image of placenta accreta. The placenta shows the typical tornado-shaped vascular lacunae with increased, disorganized, turbulent flow represented by color Doppler.

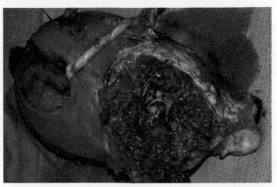

Fig. 6. Gross image of placenta accreta. The placenta is seen invading the lower uterine segment. The umbilical cord is protruding through the high vertical hysterotomy made to avoid the placenta during delivery.

risk of asphyxia.[31,34] Conditions such as uterine rupture, umbilical cord prolapse, massive placental abruption, and vasa previa (**Fig. 7**) portend the greatest risk because of acute fetal exsanguination or hypoxia.[31] Vasa previa refers to fetal blood vessels traversing membranes overlying the cervical os. When labor occurs (cervical dilation or ruptured membranes), acute fetal exsanguination can occur. Uterine rupture is an uncommon consequence of a trial of labor after cesarean section. This complication may be associated with neonatal asphyxia, low Apgar scores, and the need for mechanical ventilation.[35] These catastrophic events are usually not preventable and may or may not be predictable. Importantly, they only account for about 12% of cases of perinatal asphyxia that require infant cooling.[31] In contrast, most infants

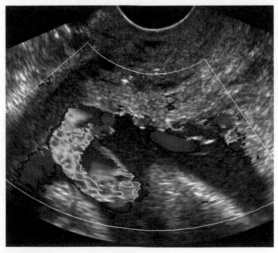

Fig. 7. Ultrasound image of vasa previa. The vessel seen to the right in the image shows a vasa previa overlying the cervix contained within membranes of a low-lying placenta.

with hypoxia and ischemia have nonspecific antecedents more properly designated as associations rather than causes.

Delivery Complications

Delivery complications, such as shoulder dystocia and other difficult or (prolonged) deliveries, for example, abdominal wall dystocia, are also associated with an increased risk of asphyxia.[36] This risk is primarily due to a lack of fetal oxygenation during uterine contractions, cord compression, and maternal expulsive efforts proximal to delivery. Importantly, prolonged second stage of labor without dystocia at delivery has not been associated with adverse neonatal outcomes. Hence, the second stage of labor should not be terminated for duration alone.[37]

Maternal Medical Conditions

Placental insufficiency is one of the most common causes of abnormal fetal heart rate tracings and can result in asphyxia, especially in the setting of uterine contractions. Placental insufficiency is often associated with underlying maternal conditions, such as hypertension, renal disease, or diabetes.

Maternal thyroid disease, obesity, and age of 35 years or older also have been implicated as associations with perinatal asphyxia.[2,30] Poorly controlled hyperthyroidism and hypothyroidism can be associated with fetal growth restriction, preterm birth, low birth rate, and hypertensive disorders of pregnancy.[38,39] In addition, inadequately treated hypothyroidism can result in childhood cognitive and neurodevelopmental impairment.[40] However, there does not seem to be an increased risk of perinatal asphyxia in pregnancies strictly due to thyroid disease. Similarly, advanced maternal age (older than 35 years) is associated with an increased risk of stillbirth[41]; but the risk of perinatal asphyxia is not increased over younger-aged women in the absence of additional maternal comorbidities. Lastly, obesity is an important risk factor for perinatal asphyxia. In a Swedish cohort of term infants, the risk of an Apgar score of 0 to 3 at 5 minutes increased with increasing maternal body mass index (BMI) to a 3-fold increase with morbid obesity, with a BMI greater than 40 (OR 3.41, CI 1.91–6.09).[42] The mechanism for asphyxial events is unclear. Theories include increased inflammation due to adipokines, insulin resistance, and fatty acids, which may lead to lipotoxicity resulting in oxidative stress and endothelial dysfunction in maternal and placental tissues.

Intra-Amniotic Infection

Intra-amniotic infection (IAI) or chorioamnionitis refers to maternal/fetal infection during labor usually caused by ascending microbial invasion from the vagina. Features of the syndrome include maternal fever, tachycardia, elevated white blood cell count, foul-smelling amniotic fluid, uterine tenderness, or fetal tachycardia.[43] Two or more criteria are required for the diagnosis of IAI. Intrapartum fever alone and IAI increase the risk of neonatal encephalopathy by 3.1 fold and 5.4 fold, respectively. In addition, both intrapartum fever alone and IAI increase the risk of CP.[44,45]

INTERVENTIONS

Antenatal testing, ultrasound, and EFM are all modalities for interrogating antepartum fetal status. When abnormal, these tests may prompt further evaluation or delivery. If there is concern for preterm birth, corticosteroids for fetal lung maturity, tocolytic medications to delay labor, and magnesium sulfate for fetal neuroprotection should be considered, depending on the clinical situation.

Intrapartum resuscitative measures may effectively improve category II to III tracings. These measures include the following: lateral positioning, maternal oxygen, fluid bolus, reduction of uterine contractions, discontinuation of induction agents, tocolytic medication, and amnioinfusion.[46] Unfortunately, in some cases, a category II to III tracing persists despite these measures, warranting further intervention. It is important to note recent controversy in the literature regarding maternal oxygen use during labor. A lack of data showing benefit, or improvement in fetal oxygenation and neonatal outcomes, as well as evidence showing potential harm has caused some experts to refute the practice, citing need for further research in the form of randomized trials before continuing its use.[47,48] Nonetheless, maternal oxygen use for nonreassuring tracings fetal heart tracings remains standard among many hospital protocols and is mentioned in the ACOG practice bulletin algorithm for resuscitation of nonreassuring tracings (an article that predated recent literature.)[46]

Expeditious delivery can be lifesaving for the fetus and, depending on the circumstance, may decrease the risk of perinatal asphyxia. For patients who are remote from delivery, cesarean delivery can be urgently performed. One study analyzed the effects of a protocol to shorten the decision-to-delivery interval and found a mean decrease of about 10 minutes and lower neonatal rates of pH less than 7.1 and Apgar less than 7 at 5 mintues.[49] For patients proximal to delivery (complete cervical dilation), operative vaginal delivery should be considered and can decrease exposure to intrauterine insults.[50,51]

Because of the possible need for operative vaginal or abdominal delivery, obstetric and anesthesia providers should remain readily available. This requirement is of utmost importance in high-risk labor circumstances, such as a trial of labor after cesarean section, because of the risk of uterine rupture. Other unpredictable events can also occur without warning. Umbilical cord prolapse is most common after rupture of membranes with the fetus in a noncephalic presentation. Having a well-practiced, standardized, emergency response (often termed *obstetric code*) for a labor and delivery unit enables prompt intervention and assembly of appropriate obstetric, anesthesia, and pediatric teams. Likewise, hospital protocols can aid in standardizing safe care for all mothers in these high-risk situations. The ACOG suggests that hospitals and birthing centers are the safest setting for deliveries[52] and recommends that patients be informed of the 2-fold increased risk of perinatal mortality with out-of-hospital births.[53]

STRATEGIES TO REDUCE RISK

Screening high-risk pregnancies is one of the most effective ways of attenuating the risk of perinatal asphyxia (**Box 1**). Women with chronic hypertension, diabetes, thrombophilia, renal disease, or autoimmune disease are at risk of placental insufficiency; thus, serial ultrasounds should be performed with early delivery as indicated by screening.

The routine anatomy ultrasound in the midtrimester (around 20 weeks) is an optimal time to exclude abnormal placentation, such as placenta previa, accreta, or vasa previa. Women with any of these high-risk conditions are typically delivered via cesarean in the early term (37–39 weeks) or late preterm (34–37 weeks) stage. Additionally, women with a history of prior cesarean delivery should be counseled about the risk of uterine rupture and importance of delivery in a hospital

---

Box 1
Strategies to reduce the risk of perinatal asphyxia

Antepartum

1. Screen for high-risk pregnancy conditions
2. Monitor with serial ultrasound assessments, including Doppler velocimetry if indicated
3. Antenatal fetal testing
4. Consider fetal movement counting

Intrapartum

1. Safe labor conditions, including protocols for trial of labor after cesarean
2. Electronic fetal monitoring
3. Intrauterine resuscitation
4. Fetal scalp stimulation
5. Operative delivery

Postpartum

1. Umbilical cord blood gas ± lactate
2. Placental pathology examination

---

setting with continuous monitoring and 24-hour obstetric and anesthesia services available.

As previously noted, most perinatal asphyxia cases are not caused by labor events or predicted by obstetric interventions. For the uncommon intrapartum events that may cause asphyxia, providers must be hypervigilant to recognize the condition, intervene appropriately, and expedite safe delivery for the mother and fetus.

SUMMARY

Perinatal asphyxia refers to neonatal encephalopathy caused by events surrounding birth. Because the terminology is nonspecific and because intrapartum asphyxia is rarely absolute, more precise descriptive terms, such as *metabolic* or *respiratory acidosis*, should be considered. Most perinatal asphyxia cases are caused by conditions unrelated to labor. When asphyxia occurs from an intrapartum event, it is usually due to an obstetric emergency. For these uncommon emergencies, prompt intervention and delivery are imperative for decreasing the likelihood of neonatal encephalopathy. Our ability to predict intrapartum asphyxia remains poor. Strategies such as screening high-risk pregnancies, scalp stimulation for indeterminate fetal heart tracings, intrauterine resuscitation, and expeditious delivery may aid in the diagnosis and prevention of perinatal asphyxia.

Future research should focus on diagnostic methods for predicting metabolic acidosis before it occurs and appropriate interventions for management. The Human Placenta Project sponsored by the NICHD is currently focused on such efforts. Determining appropriate timing of antenatal testing and proving the efficacy of testing in certain high-risk populations is another top priority.

Best practices box

What changes in current practice are likely to improve outcomes?
Vigilance of at-risk pregnancies and appropriate timely intervention are key to risk reduction.

Is there a clinical algorithm?
Screening high-risk pregnancies with ultrasound, antenatal testing when indicated, and appropriate timing of delivery can aid in improving neonatal outcomes.

Although there is no clinical algorithm that fits every patient alike, safe labor conditions, fetal heart rate monitoring, intrauterine resuscitation, scalp stimulation, and operative delivery are the most valuable interventions for perinatal asphyxia prevention.

Rating for the strength of the evidence: II

Summary statement
Most cases of perinatal asphyxia are associated with underlying chronic maternal and fetal conditions. Of intrapartum causes, obstetric emergencies are the most common. Safe labor conditions, fetal heart rate monitoring, intrauterine resuscitation, scalp stimulation, and operative delivery are the most valuable tools to aid in prevention of asphyxia.

REFERENCES

1. Grimes DA, Peipert JF. Electronic fetal monitoring as a public health screening program: the arithmetic of failure. Obstet Gynecol 2010;116(6):1397–400.
2. Executive summary: neonatal encephalopathy and neurologic outcome, second edition. Report of the American College of Obstetricians and Gynecologists' Task Force on Neonatal Encephalopathy. Obstet Gynecol 2014;123(4):896–901.
3. Committee on Obstetric Practice, ACOG, American Academy of Pediatrics, Committee on Fetus and Newborn, ACOG. ACOG Committee Opinion. Number 333, May 2006 (replaces No. 174, July 1996): The Apgar score. Obstet Gynecol 2006; 107(5):1209–12.
4. American College of Obstetricians and Gynecologists. ACOG practice bulletin No. 106: intrapartum fetal heart rate monitoring: nomenclature, interpretation, and general management principles. Obstet Gynecol 2009;114(1):192–202.
5. Nelson KB, Ellenberg JH. Obstetric complications as risk factors for cerebral palsy or seizure disorders. JAMA 1984;251(14):1843–8.
6. Macones GA, Hankins GDV, Spong CY, et al. The 2008 National Institute of Child Health and Human Development workshop report on electronic fetal monitoring: update on definitions, interpretation, and research guidelines. J Obstet Gynecol Neonatal Nurs 2008;37(5):510–5.
7. Alfirevic Z, Devane D, Gyte GML. Continuous cardiotocography (CTG) as a form of electronic fetal monitoring (EFM) for fetal assessment during labour. Cochrane Database Syst Rev 2013;(5):CD006066.
8. Graham EM, Adami RR, McKenney SL, et al. Diagnostic accuracy of fetal heart rate monitoring in the identification of neonatal encephalopathy. Obstet Gynecol 2014;124(3):507–13.
9. Cahill AG, Roehl KA, Odibo AO, et al. Association and prediction of neonatal acidemia. Am J Obstet Gynecol 2012;207(3):206.e1–8.
10. Elimian A, Figueroa R, Tejani N. Intrapartum assessment of fetal well-being: a comparison of scalp stimulation with scalp blood pH sampling. Obstet Gynecol 1997;89(3):373–6.

11. Cahill AG, Spain J. Intrapartum fetal monitoring. Clin Obstet Gynecol 2015;58(2): 263–8.
12. Belfort MA, Saade GR, Thom E, et al. A randomized trial of intrapartum fetal ECG ST-segment analysis. N Engl J Med 2015;373(7):632–41.
13. Landon MB, Gabbe SG. Antepartum fetal surveillance in gestational diabetes mellitus. Diabetes 1985;34(Suppl 2):50–4.
14. Williamson C, Miragoli M, Sheikh Abdul Kadir S, et al. Bile acid signaling in fetal tissues: implications for intrahepatic cholestasis of pregnancy. Dig Dis 2011; 29(1):58–61.
15. Signore C, Freeman RK, Spong CY. Antenatal testing-a reevaluation: executive summary of a Eunice Kennedy Shriver National Institute of Child Health and Human Development workshop. Obstet Gynecol 2009;113(3):687–701.
16. Practice bulletin no. 145: antepartum fetal surveillance. Obstet Gynecol 2014; 124(1):182–92.
17. Boehm FH, Salyer S, Shah DM, et al. Improved outcome of twice weekly non-stress testing. Obstet Gynecol 1986;67(4):566–8.
18. American College of Obstetricians and Gynecologists. ACOG practice bulletin no. 134: fetal growth restriction. Obstet Gynecol 2013;121(5):1122–33.
19. Blair EM, Nelson KB. Fetal growth restriction and risk of cerebral palsy in single-tons born after at least 35 weeks' gestation. Am J Obstet Gynecol 2015;212(4): 520.e1–7.
20. Karsdorp VH, van Vugt JM, van Geijn HP, et al. Clinical significance of absent or reversed end diastolic velocity waveforms in umbilical artery. Lancet 1994; 344(8938):1664–8.
21. Almström H, Axelsson O, Cnattingius S, et al. Comparison of umbilical-artery velocimetry and cardiotocography for surveillance of small-for-gestational-age fetuses. Lancet 1992;340(8825):936–40.
22. Mangesi L, Hofmeyr GJ. Fetal movement counting for assessment of fetal well-being. Cochrane Database Syst Rev 2007;(1):CD004909.
23. Hofmeyr GJ, Novikova N. Management of reported decreased fetal movements for improving pregnancy outcomes. Cochrane Database Syst Rev 2012;(4):CD009148.
24. Savasan ZA, Gonçalves LF, Bahado-Singh RO. Second- and third-trimester biochemical and ultrasound markers predictive of ischemic placental disease. Semin Perinatol 2014;38(3):167–76.
25. Veerbeek JHW, Nikkels PGJ, Torrance HL, et al. Placental pathology in early intrauterine growth restriction associated with maternal hypertension. Placenta 2014;35(9):696–701.
26. Pinar H, Goldenberg RL, Koch MA, et al. Placental findings in singleton stillbirths. Obstet Gynecol 2014;123(2 Pt 1):325–36.
27. Knutzen L, Svirko E, Impey L. The significance of base deficit in acidemic term neonates. Am J Obstet Gynecol 2015;213(3):373.e1–7.
28. Tuuli MG, Stout MJ, Shanks A, et al. Umbilical cord arterial lactate compared with pH for predicting neonatal morbidity at term. Obstet Gynecol 2014;124(4):756–61.
29. Ananth CV, Keyes KM, Hamilton A, et al. An international contrast of rates of placental abruption: an age-period-cohort analysis. PLoS One 2015;10(5):e0125246.
30. Badawi N, Kurinczuk JJ, Keogh JM, et al. Antepartum risk factors for newborn encephalopathy: the Western Australian case-control study. BMJ 1998;317(7172): 1549–53.
31. Nelson DB, Lucke AM, McIntire DD, et al. Obstetric antecedents to body-cooling treatment of the newborn infant. Am J Obstet Gynecol 2014;211(2):155.e1–6.

32. Silver RM. Abnormal placentation: placenta previa, vasa previa, and placenta accreta. Obstet Gynecol 2015;126(3):654–68.

33. Furuta K, Tokunaga S, Furukawa S, et al. Acute and massive bleeding from placenta previa and infants' brain damage. Early Hum Dev 2014;90(9):455–8.

34. Wayock CP, Meserole RL, Saria S, et al. Perinatal risk factors for severe injury in neonates treated with whole-body hypothermia for encephalopathy. Am J Obstet Gynecol 2014;211(1):41.e1–8.

35. Kieser KE, Baskett TF. A 10-year population-based study of uterine rupture. Obstet Gynecol 2002;100(4):749–53.

36. MacKenzie IZ, Shah M, Lean K, et al. Management of shoulder dystocia: trends in incidence and maternal and neonatal morbidity. Obstet Gynecol 2007;110(5): 1059–68.

37. Rouse DJ, Weiner SJ, Bloom SL, et al. Second-stage labor duration in nulliparous women: relationship to maternal and perinatal outcomes. Am J Obstet Gynecol 2009;201(4):357.e1–7.

38. Leung AS, Millar LK, Koonings PP, et al. Perinatal outcome in hypothyroid pregnancies. Obstet Gynecol 1993;81(3):349–53.

39. Kriplani A, Buckshee K, Bhargava VL, et al. Maternal and perinatal outcome in thyrotoxicosis complicating pregnancy. Eur J Obstet Gynecol Reprod Biol 1994;54(3):159–63.

40. Haddow JE, Palomaki GE, Allan WC, et al. Maternal thyroid deficiency during pregnancy and subsequent neuropsychological development of the child. N Engl J Med 1999;341(8):549–55.

41. Fretts RC, Schmittdiel J, McLean FH, et al. Increased maternal age and the risk of fetal death. N Engl J Med 1995;333(15):953–7.

42. Persson M, Johansson S, Villamor E, et al. Maternal overweight and obesity and risks of severe birth-asphyxia-related complications in term infants: a population-based cohort study in Sweden. PLoS Med 2014;11(5):e1001648.

43. Tita ATN, Andrews WW. Diagnosis and management of clinical chorioamnionitis. Clin Perinatol 2010;37(2):339–54.

44. Blume HK, Li CI, Loch CM, et al. Intrapartum fever and chorioamnionitis as risks for encephalopathy in term newborns: a case-control study. Dev Med Child Neurol 2008;50(1):19–24.

45. Grether JK, Nelson KB. Maternal infection and cerebral palsy in infants of normal birth weight. JAMA 1997;278(3):207–11.

46. American College of Obstetricians and Gynecologists. Practice bulletin no. 116: management of intrapartum fetal heart rate tracings. Obstet Gynecol 2010; 116(5):1232–40.

47. Hamel MS, Anderson BL, Rouse DJ. Oxygen for intrauterine resuscitation: of unproved benefit and potentially harmful. Am J Obstet Gynecol 2014; 211(2):124–7.

48. Hamel MS, Hughes BL, Rouse DJ. Whither oxygen for intrauterine resuscitation? Am J Obstet Gynecol 2015;212(4):461–2.

49. Weiner E, Bar J, Fainstein N, et al. The effect of a program to shorten the decision-to-delivery interval for emergent cesarean section on maternal and neonatal outcome. Am J Obstet Gynecol 2014;210(3):224.e1–6.

50. Practice bulletin No. 154: operative vaginal delivery. Obstet Gynecol 2015;126(5): e56–65.

51. Leung WC, Lam HSW, Lam KW, et al. Unexpected reduction in the incidence of birth trauma and birth asphyxia related to instrumental deliveries during the study period: was this the Hawthorne effect? BJOG 2003;110(3):319–22.

52. ACOG Committee on Obstetric Practice. ACOG committee opinion No. 476: planned home birth. Obstet Gynecol 2011;117(2 Pt 1):425–8.
53. Snowden JM, Tilden EL, Snyder J, et al. Planned out-of-hospital birth and birth outcomes. N Engl J Med 2015;373(27):2642–53.

Stillbirths
The Hidden Birth Asphyxia — US and Global Perspectives

Robert L. Goldenberg, MD[a],*, Margo S. Harrison, MD[a],
Elizabeth M. McClure, PhD[b]

KEYWORDS

- Stillbirth • Intrapartum asphyxia • High-income countries
- Low-income and middle-income countries

KEY POINTS

- Stillbirths occur 10 times more commonly in low-income countries than in high-income countries (HICs).
- More than half of the stillbirths in low-income countries occur in the intrapartum period.
- Most intrapartum stillbirths are due to intrapartum asphyxia.
- The final common pathway for obstetric conditions that lead to stillbirth, such as abruption, preeclampsia, and obstructed labor, is asphyxia.
- In HICs, placental lesions, such as necrosis, thrombosis, and fibrosis, are associated with a majority of stillbirths.

OVERVIEW AND DEFINITIONS

This article explores the relationship between fetal asphyxia and stillbirth, demonstrating that a large proportion of stillbirths, especially in low-income and middle-income countries (LMICs), is due to intrauterine fetal asphyxia. Fetal asphyxia is an intrauterine condition of impaired placental blood gas exchange leading to progressive fetal hypoxemia and hypercapnia with metabolic acidosis.[1] Adverse clinical outcomes of fetal asphyxia include stillbirth, neonatal death, and, in surviving children, both short-term and long-term neurologic impairment, including cerebral palsy and mental retardation.[2,3] Possible causes of fetal asphyxia include maternal hypotension, poor placental perfusion, uterine tetany, and compression of the umbilical cord.[4,5]

Disclosure: The authors declare no conflicts of interest.
a Department of Obstetrics and Gynecology, Columbia University, 622 West 168th Street, PH 16-66, New York, NY 10032, USA; b Research Triangle Institute, Social, Statistical and Environmental Health Sciences, 3040 Cornwallis Road, Research Triangle Park, NC 27709, USA
* Corresponding author.
E-mail address: Rlg88@columbia.edu

Clin Perinatol 43 (2016) 439–453
http://dx.doi.org/10.1016/j.clp.2016.04.004
0095-5108/16/$ – see front matter © 2016 Elsevier Inc. All rights reserved.

Stillbirths are defined as fetal deaths occurring in utero in which a baby is born with no signs of life, including movement, breathing, or the presence of a heartbeat.[6] To distinguish stillbirth from spontaneous abortion, countries use different lower gestational age cutoffs, ranging from 20 weeks in most US states to 28 weeks in many LMICs.[7,8] In cases when the gestational age unknown, the inclusion criteria may be defined by birth weight or a fetal length measurement.[9] For international comparisons, to define stillbirth, the World Health Organization and many investigators recommend a lower gestational age cutoff of 28 weeks.[10]

Because of poor vital statistics systems, especially in the countries where the stillbirth rates are highest, estimates of stillbirth prevalence are often inexact.[8] Nevertheless, often attained using survey data and modeling, stillbirth prevalence estimates are available for most countries but only for stillbirths at 28 weeks or more (late stillbirths). Reasonably reliable data for 20 to 27 week stillbirths (early stillbirths) are only available for some HICs, such as the United States and Australia, where approximately half of all stillbirths occur from 20 to 27 weeks.[11–14] In some European countries, where 22 and 24 weeks are used as the lower gestational age cutoffs for defining a stillbirth, approximately a third of stillbirths occur at less than 28 weeks.[11] Thus, if the proportion of early versus late stillbirths in HICs is applied to LMICs, there may be twice as many stillbirths worldwide each year than those estimated to occur at greater than or equal to 28 weeks. Because an estimated 3 million third-trimester or late stillbirths are reported globally each year,[8,15] worldwide, up to 6 million stillbirths at 20 weeks or more likely occur each year.

An estimated 98% of all stillbirths now occur in LMICs with few occurring in HICs.[7,8] Comparing third-trimester rates, countries, such as Norway, Sweden, and Japan, have stillbirth rates approaching 2 per 1000 births, with most HICs having rates below 5 per 1000 births.[7] The US third-trimester stillbirth rate is approximately 3 per 1000 births.[13] Conversely, third-trimester stillbirth rates in LMICs in sub-Saharan Africa and south Asia may approach 40 per 1000 births or more.[15] The worldwide average for third-trimester stillbirths is now approximately 20 per 1000 births.[7] The difference in stillbirth rates between HICs and LMICs is due predominately to differences in quality of care, although certain risk factors, such as infection, likely play a role.[15,16]

STILLBIRTH HISTORY IN HIGH-INCOME COUNTRIES

In HICs, stillbirth rates have fallen precipitously, from approximately 40 to 50 to under 5 per 1000 births over the past 70 years.[17,18] Reasons for the decline are not well documented or easy to determine but include screening for and/or prevention and treatment of syphilis, diabetes, Rh disease, obstructed labor, and preeclampsia.[19–24] Probably contributing to the decline, but with little evidence in the literature, is the reduction in stillbirths associated with uterine hyperstimulation, which occurs in the setting of aggressive attempts at labor induction or augmentation. Folic acid food fortification has reduced some congenital anomaly–associated stillbirths,[25] as has ultrasound screening for anomalies followed by pregnancy termination prior to 20 weeks.[24] Fetal monitoring for distress both in the antepartum and intrapartum periods along with the availability of rapid delivery for fetuses in distress or with conditions, such as placental abruption or eclampsia, usually by cesarean section, also contributed to lower stillbirth rates.[22] Screening for delivery of fetuses with fetal growth restriction, postdate status, placenta previa, and many other maternal and fetal conditions has also led to a reduction in stillbirths.[26] Better maternal nutrition, education, and overall improved health have likely had a smaller but still important role in stillbirth reduction. Because of the many interventions introduced over the years, and the many conditions they affect, the specific reductions in stillbirth associated with any specific intervention can at best be estimated. For many of those conditions, however, in which large reductions in stillbirth have occurred, much of the reduction is associated with decreases in fetal asphyxia.

CAUSE OF DEATH IN STILLBIRTHS IN LOW-INCOME COUNTRIES

This discussion focuses on clinical causes of fetal death, although it is clear that many other factors, such as low levels of maternal education; drug, alcohol, and tobacco use; and poor nutritional status — including malnutrition and obesity, may influence the stillbirth risk. Among the most common causes in LMICs, and thus worldwide, are obstructed labor, placental abruption, and preeclampsia/eclampsia.[8] Fetal growth restriction is commonly associated with stillbirth, but whether it is causal or simply a marker for another underlying condition, such as poor placental circulation, is a matter of debate.[27,28] Fetal distress, commonly diagnosed by alterations in the fetal heart rate, is thought to occur secondary to poor fetal oxygenation and may be associated with each of the potential causes already discussed but may present spontaneously without another maternal or fetal condition present.[28] Infants in the breech or other abnormal positions and those from multiple births also have substantially higher risk of stillbirth than singleton vertex infants and the cause of death is often fetal distress or one of the maternal conditions discussed previously.[29–31]

Another important cause of stillbirth, especially in LMICs, is infection. Many different organisms have caused a stillbirth and extensive reviews regarding the types of infection, the organisms involved, the types of transmission, and mechanisms of death have been published.[16,32–34] In endemic areas, malaria and syphilis are common causes of stillbirth, but in these areas and elsewhere, bacterial and viral maternal infections are often linked to stillbirth. Maternal obesity and diabetes also are risk factors for or are causal for some stillbirths.[35] In a literature review the authors performed on stillbirths in sub-Saharan Africa, the prevalence of many of the maternal and fetal conditions associated with stillbirth, the stillbirth case fatality rates associated with those conditions, and the percent of all stillbirths associated with those conditions were estimated (**Table 1**). Although obstructed labor, preeclamsia/eclampsia, fetal distress, and placental abruption led the list, no condition was responsible for more than 15% of all stillbirths. As in HICs, some proportion of stillbirths is associated with uterine hyperstimulation during induction or augmentation of labor.[36] Although stillbirths from this cause have mostly been eliminated in HICs due to fetal monitoring and rapid access to cesarean section, in LMICs where fetal heart rate monitoring is not available, stillbirths from this cause may be common but data to evaluate this issue are not available.

STILLBIRTH CAUSE OF DEATH CLASSIFICATION

Classifying causes of death in stillbirths has been an ongoing source of controversy for many years.[37–39] There are now more than 50 stillbirth cause of death classification systems described in the literature.[6,38,40] Few of these, if any, are widely used and they often have differing goals and characteristics. Some systems are clinically based, whereas others require extensive laboratory testing. Some try to define a primary cause, others consider underlying causes, and some try to define degree of certainty about the cause of death. Conditions that are considered important causes of stillbirth in some systems are not even considered in others. In part, the proliferation of classification systems is explained by the difficulty in diagnosing a specific cause of stillbirth. When a maternal or neonatal death occurs, the events usually can be

Condition	Prevalence of Maternal and Fetal Conditions Associated with Stillbirth (%)	Case Fatality Rates Resulting in a Stillbirth Associated with Various Conditions (%)	Proportion of all Stillbirths Associated with the Condition (%)
Obstructed labor	4.0	14	15
Preeclampsia/eclampsia	5	8	14
De novo fetal distress	2.3	18	12
Abruption	0.9	33	10
Syphilis	5.5	6	10
Intrauterine growth restriction	9	3.2	10
Congenital anomalies	1	18	5
Cord accident	1	12	4
Malaria in pregnancy	30	0.6	4
Ruptured uterus	0.2	50	3
Diabetes	5	1.2	2
Breech	2.2	1.4	1
Multiple births	1.3	2.3	1
Previa	0.3	11	1
Other or unknown	—	—	8
			100

Table 1
Stillbirth in sub-Saharan Africa

observed and the pathway to death is often apparent. Stillbirths occur within the uterus and the events leading to the death are often hidden from view.

A useful consideration in classifying stillbirths is whether they occurred prior to labor or were intrapartum.[41–43] In many low-income areas, it is often unknown when the fetus died. Because signs of maceration begin to appear about 12 hours after fetal death, whether the fetus showed signs of maceration is often used to distinguish an antepartum from an intrapartum demise.[44] Stillbirths are also classified by cause of death, by birth weight, by gestational age, and by whether an anomaly was present. These characteristics often help determine whether the stillbirth was likely due to asphyxia or some other cause.

INTRAPARTUM VERSUS ANTEPARTUM STILLBIRTHS

It is important to distinguish intrapartum from antepartum stillbirths because the interventions to prevent their occurrence — or at least the timing of those interventions — are different. Intrapartum stillbirths, which represent between 50% and 70% of all stillbirths in LMICs, are nearly always caused by asphyxia and can be substantially reduced by monitoring the fetus during labor and providing a cesarean section when distress is discovered.[44] Other intrapartum interventions that contribute to a reduction in intrapartum stillbirths include not overstimulating contractions during induction or augmentation of labor, preventing seizures in women with preeclampsia, and maintaining maternal blood pressure in cases of dehydration or hemorrhage.[45–48] Because labor is generally of short duration, vigilance during this time may not require extensive resources. In a study done in 5 LMIC hospitals, with fetal viability on admission determined by a Doptone assessment of the fetal heartbeat, approximately half of all stillbirths occurred after admission to the hospital.[44] Of the in-hospital stillbirths, most occurred in term nonanomalous fetuses. The cause of death was likely asphyxia. In the authors' judgment, a majority of these deaths were preventable.

On the other hand, the antepartum period lasts for months and a fetal death could occur at any point during this time. The causes of antepartum stillbirths are more varied then those that occur during labor. Because of the length of the antepartum period and the variable causes, preventing antepartum stillbirth has proved more difficult than preventing intrapartum stillbirth. That said, a majority of antepartum stillbirths are also caused by asphyxia. Conditions that cause intrapartum stillbirths also lead to asphyxia in the antepartum period with the exception of conditions that are labor dependent, such as uterine hyperstimulation and prolonged/obstructed labor. Fetal growth restriction due to placental insufficiency likely plays a more important role in these deaths, as does preeclampsia.[49,50]

ASPHYXIA AS A CAUSE OF STILLBIRTH

For neonatal deaths, asphyxia as a cause is often diagnosed in infants who fail to initiate or maintain spontaneous respirations.[45] This cause of death is confirmed by low Apgar scores and in HICs, in many cases, by a low umbilical cord pH or other abnormal cord blood gas measurements.[1] These parameters are not generally not available in LMICs to confirm asphyxia as a cause of death. With a stillbirth, the death is not generally observed, so the cause of stillbirth is often based on limited information. In most cases, to accurately determine cause of stillbirth, a thorough placental and postmortem examination is recommended.[6] In most of the world, however, placental histologic examinations are not performed and fetal autopsies are not available. Even when placenta histology and fetal autopsies are available, determining a specific cause of stillbirth is difficult.[37,51] There are few if any pathognomonic findings on placental examination or even autopsy that prove that a death was caused by asphyxia. Instead, a diagnosis usually rests on a combination of clinical history and the presence of various placental lesions and autopsy findings.[52,53] Absence of evidence of other stillbirth causes, such as congenital anomalies or infection, often leads to asphyxia assigned as the likely cause of death.

The characteristics of stillbirths vary by location and especially differ between HICs and LMICs. As stated previously, most stillbirths in HICs occur in the preterm period and half occur between 20 and 28 weeks.[7] In LMICs, most stillbirths seem to occur either at term or late in the preterm period. The mean birth weight of stillbirths in HICs is close to 1000 g whereas it averages approximately 2500 g in LMICs.[53] In HICs, approximately 15% of the small number of stillbirths are associated with a major congenital anomaly, whereas in LMICs, congenital anomalies are associated with a lower percentage of a larger number of stillbirths.[54] Thus, congenital anomalies seem to occur in approximately the same percentage of all births in both HICs and LMICs but represent a larger proportion of stillbirths in HICs. Currently, intrapartum stillbirths are rare in HIC whereas in LMICs, 50% to 70% of all stillbirths occur during labor. Thus, a typical stillbirth in LMICs is near-term or at-term weight greater than 2500 g and occurs intrapartum and free of congenital anomalies. These stillbirths are frequently associated with an asphyxial event.

Overall, asphyxia is rarely listed as the cause of stillbirth. Many of the conditions associated with stillbirth cause stillbirth by asphyxiation associated with some decrease in oxygenated blood reaching the fetus. Thus, prolonged, obstructed labor; placental abruption; preeclampsia/eclampsia; fetal distress; and many deaths associated with breech and multiple births are caused by fetal asphyxia. Those stillbirths associated with postdates and fetal growth restriction also are most likely due to fetal asphyxia as are stillbirths due to cord accidents. Thus, the authors argue that nearly all stillbirths, with the exception of some stillbirths caused by congenital anomalies and direct fetal infections, are likely caused by fetal asphyxia. As discussed previously, in LMICs, up to 70% of all stillbirths occur at term, during labor, and are free of congenital anomalies. These stillbirths are almost certainly due to an asphyxic event. In fact, various investigators have recommended using the term, intrapartum event, to describe these cases because proving asphyxia as a cause of death in individual cases is often difficult if not impossible.[45]

To illustrate the problem of isolating asphyxia as a cause of stillbirth, both malaria and syphilis kill some fetuses by producing placental infiltrates and reducing fetal oxygenation.[55] Fetal death may occur without direct infection of the fetus. Maternal parvovirus infection during pregnancy is a well-known cause of stillbirth, with the death most often due to depletion of fetal red cells and hypoxemia. Similarly, fetuses that die as a result of Rh sensitization or fetal-maternal hemorrhage also die from a severe anemia and thus a hypoxic death. Maternal sickle cell anemia causes fetal death because of poor placental blood flow. In those pregnancies complicated by antiphospholipid syndrome or systemic lupus erythematosus, placental disease followed by asphyxia is often reported as the cause of fetal death.[56] Why stillbirths occur more frequently when the mother has diabetes is unknown, but some authorities suspect that a significant proportion of these stillbirths are associated with fetal asphyxia.[57] Thus, even conditions associated with stillbirth that initially may not be considered a cause of poor fetal oxygenation, in fact, may cause stillbirth via that mechanism.

Proving that a fetus died because of asphyxia is complicated and nearly always accompanied by some degree of uncertainty. No lesions discoverable by the placental examination or the fetal autopsy are pathognomonic for asphyxia in that it describes a symptom or sign that indicates almost beyond doubt the specific cause of the stillbirth. More commonly, asphyxia as a cause of fetal death is determined by the clinical conditions and events preceding the demise. In most studies, asphyxia is not listed as a cause of stillbirth. Instead, the clinical conditions leading to asphyxia are listed as the cause or underlying cause. **Box 1** lists the maternal and fetal clinical conditions generally associated with or causal for stillbirth in LMICs and indicates those likely causing fetal death by asphyxia.

GESTATIONAL AGE AND ASPHYXIA

Another issue in relating asphyxia to stillbirths involves infants born preterm.[58] Among live births, even in HICs, it is difficult to distinguish asphyxia from respiratory distress syndrome in preterm infants with respiratory problems at birth, although cord gases may help. In stillbirths, however, respiratory distress syndrome is not a consideration, and immature lungs or apnea cannot be a cause of death. Thus, if the mother or fetus has one of the conditions commonly associated with asphyxia in term infants, and there is no evidence of an anomaly or infection, the preterm fetus/stillbirth likely died an asphyxic death. **Fig. 1** presents an algorithm used by the Global Network for Women's and Children's Health Research to assign cause of death for stillbirths.[42] In this classification system, gestational age is not a factor in the cause of death assignment.

DISTINGUISHING A STILLBIRTH FROM AN EARLY NEONATAL DEATH

A clear source of confusion in many LMICs is distinguishing a stillbirth from an early neonatal death.[59] Because many of the birth attendants in LMICs are unskilled and

---

Box 1
Conditions associated with stillbirth and those likely causing fetal death by asphyxia

Maternal

Prolonged obstructed labor[a]

Preeclampsia/eclampsia[a]

Placental abruption[a]

Placenta previa[a]

Postdates[a]

Diabetes

Syphilis

Malaria

Many other bacterial, viral, and protozoan infections

Fetal

Fetal growth restriction[a]

Fetal distress[a]

Umbilical cord prolapse[a]

Rh disease[a]

Multiple fetuses[a]

Abnormal lie[a]

Congenital anomalies

[a] When a stillbirth occurs, usually caused by asphyxia.

---

most cannot use a stethoscope to listen for heart tones before the delivery or once the baby is born, whether a fetus or motionless newborn is living or dead is often unknown.[60] It seems that many depressed but living fetuses with a possible heartbeat have been in the past - and even now are - classified as stillbirths. An area where this distinction becomes important is in the evaluation of newborn resuscitation programs in LMICs.[61] Several of these studies have shown reductions in the stillbirth rate associated with resuscitation, with little impact on neonatal mortality. The authors' interpretation of these data is that because an unskilled attendant attended the delivery, or even because the one skilled attendant mostly focused on the mother, no one listened for heart tones and many of these infants were labeled a stillbirth. Now, in many locations, with increased focus on the newborn with attempts at resuscitation, many of these infants show signs of life and even survive. Thus, the stillbirth rate seems to fall. Because the neonatal mortality rate in these resuscitated infants is high, the neonatal mortality rate may not fall and may even increase.

MECHANISM OF DEATH

In HICs, there is a wide variation in the percent of stillbirths with the cause attributed to asphyxia.

In part, these variations occur because in many cases, the death is attributed to the associated clinical condition, not the mechanism of death, or because the classification system requires placental or autopsy pathologic proof of asphyxia, which often does not exist. An interesting approach was undertaken by a Dutch group, which

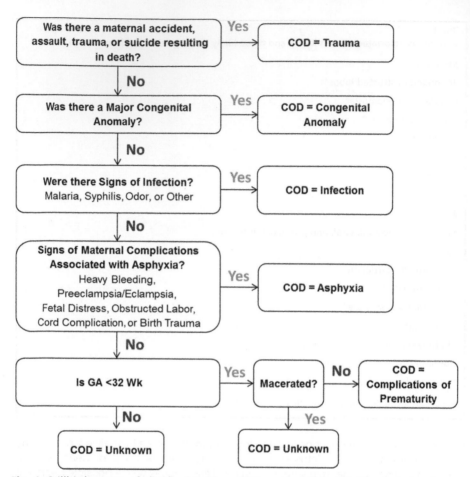

Fig. 1. Stillbirth cause of death algorithm. COD, cause of death; GA, gestational age. (*From* McClure EM, Bose CL, Garces A, et al. Global network for women's and children's health research: a system for low-resource areas to determine probable causes of stillbirth, neonatal and maternal death. Matern Health Neonatol Perinatol 2015;1:11.)

examined the placentas of a large number of stillbirths. Overall, they found evidence of a placental lesion associated with poor placental blood flow and, therefore, fetal asphyxia, in 65% of the stillbirth cases.[62] The most common condition causing stillbirth was labeled "placental bed pathology," in which inadequate spiral artery remodeling and/or spiral artery pathology leads to uteroplacental vascular insufficiency associated with placental infarction, necrosis, and abruption. In a study performed by the National Institute of Child Health and Development Stillbirth Collaborative Research Network in the United States, in which all stillbirth placentas were compared with both gestational age-matched as well as term-matched controls, several placental lesions were significantly more common in the stillbirth placentas. Many of these lesions are associated with decreased placental blood flow and include infarction, necrosis, and fibrosis as well as evidence of abruption.[51] Clinically, this condition is often referred to as placental insufficiency, or placental ischemic disease, a situation in which the placenta cannot provide sufficient oxygen and nutrients to the developing fetus. **Box 2** shows the most common umbilical cord and placental lesions

---

Box 2
Umbilical cord and placental conditions and lesions associated with fetal asphyxia

Umbilical cord conditions and lesions

Umbilical cord prolapse

True knots

Strangulation due to long cord

Furcate insertion

Velamentous insertion

Neoplasms of the umbilical cord

Placental parenchymal lesions

Abruptio placenta

Thrombohematoma

Massive fibrin deposition involving the basal plate (maternal floor infarction)

Perivillous fibrin deposition

Infarction

Nonspecific chronic villitis and intervillositis

Chronic histiocytic intervillositis

Fetal vascular thrombosis

Neoplasms involving the entire placental parenchyma

Complications of multiple gestation

Twin-twin transfusion syndrome (advanced stage)

Twin reversed arterial perfusion sequence

Strangulation due to umbilical cord entanglement (monoamnionic-monochorionic gestations)

---

significantly associated with stillbirth. These types of data support the hypothesis that there is a strong association between umbilical cord and placental lesions causing decreased placental blood flow leading to fetal asphyxia and stillbirth.

As described previously, in LMICs where most stillbirths occur, there is general agreement about the most common clinical conditions associated with stillbirth. At the top of the list is prolonged and obstructed labor, followed by placental abruption, preeclampsia/eclampsia, fetal distress, fetal growth restriction, and post-date status. Multiple births, abnormal presentations, and cord accidents are also on the list. What these conditions have in common is that most of the fetal and neonatal deaths associated with these conditions are caused by diminished placental or fetal blood flow, and fetal asphyxia is the final common pathway leading to death. There is virtually no literature from LMICs describing placental histology in those stillbirths.

PREVENTION OF ISCHEMIC PLACENTAL DISEASE

As described previously, poor placentation may manifest itself as preeclampsia, fetal growth restriction, or perinatal death. The underlying cause is a deficiency in tropho-blast invasion of the spiral arteries, associated with placental inflammation and oxidative stress. Therapies, such as prenatal maternal corticosteroids and magnesium sulfate, can prevent some of the adverse neonatal outcomes, but there is currently no consensus on the treatment of poor placentation itself or prevention of the placental conditions leading to stillbirth. Instead, management relies on identifying the consequences of poor placentation in the mother and fetus, with elective preterm delivery to minimize mortality and morbidity. Low-dose aspirin, especially when given at less than 16 weeks, has been shown in several studies to reduce the incidence of fetal growth restriction and preeclampsia — precursors of stillbirth — and is recommended by many authorities for use in women at risk for those conditions. Several other promising therapies are currently under investigation as a treatment of poor placentation, to improve fetal growth, and to prevent adverse fetal and neonatal outcomes.[49,50] These include maternal nitric oxide donors, sildenafil citrate, vascular endothelial growth factor gene therapy, hydrogen sulfide donors, and statins to address the underlying pathology. Except for aspirin, however, none of the other therapies has been recommended for routine clinical use.

REDUCING STILLBIRTH CAUSED BY ASPHYXIA IN HIGH-INCOME COUNTRIES

In HICs, where stillbirths are one-tenth as common as in LMICs, the conditions associated with asphyxic stillbirth are generally similar to those in LMICs. The major difference is that in HICs, appropriate obstetric treatment generally occurs before the asphyxia becomes severe or the fetus dies. Fetal death from obstructed labor, for example, occurs only rarely because women having prolonged labor are generally delivered by cesarean section prior to the development of severe fetal distress. Women with a placental abruption are usually delivered prior to fetal death. Women with preeclampsia/eclampsia and intrauterine fetal growth restriction are usually carefully monitored for fetal complications and fetal distress and are delivered prior to fetal death. It is now rare for even low-risk pregnancies to be allowed to continue past term, so the stillbirths previously seen in postdate pregnancies and due to fetal asphyxia now rarely occur. Fetuses of multiple pregnancies and abnormal lies are monitored carefully and frequently delivered by cesarean section, thereby averting potential fetal asphyxia and a stillbirth. And in the United States and many other HICs, most fetuses in labor, whether considered high risk or not, are monitored electronically for heart rate patterns consistent with fetal distress; those with perceived distress are delivered by cesarean section. The few stillbirths currently due to asphyxia in labor in HICs occur because of delayed care or because the fetus is thought to be too immature to survive, even if delivered alive. Thus in HICs, although a few asphyxia-related stillbirths in labor still occur, they are usually due to an acute obstetric event, such as a placental abruption or an eclamptic seizure, in which fetal death occurs before adequate medical care could be provided or because inadequate attention is paid by the caregivers to the maternal or fetal condition. Improving quality of obstetric care is likely to reduce asphyxia-related stillbirths and much of the related disparities in stillbirth rates in HICs.

In HICs, most of the stillbirths now occur in preterm fetuses prior to the onset of labor. Attempts to prevent stillbirths prior to labor involve monitoring the pregnancy for risk factors, such as fetal growth restriction and maternal preeclampsia. These pregnancies are often monitored with various tests, such as contraction stress or nonstress tests, biophysical profiles, amniotic fluid volume, Doppler flow assessments, and fetal movement counting.[24–26] A decision to deliver is generally based on the perceived severity of the distress and the gestational age of the fetus.

REDUCING STILLBIRTH CAUSED BY ASPHYXIA IN LOW-INCOME AND MIDDLE-INCOME COUNTRIES

Substantially reducing stillbirths in LMICs requires focusing on the large proportion of stillbirths caused by asphyxia.[63–66] These stillbirths occur in conjunction with prolonged/obstructed labor; antepartum hemorrhage, including placental abruption and previa; preeclampsia/eclampsia; fetal growth restriction; postdates; fetal distress; cord accidents; and abnormal presentations and multiple births. Most of these conditions do not cause stillbirth in settings with high-quality obstetric care. Although in this article it is not appropriate to review the management of each condition, certain common approaches almost certainly are associated with large reductions in stillbirth. First, these conditions must be recognized or diagnosed by the mother and her caregiver. Without this crucial step, none of the following interventions occur. On recognition of the maternal condition associated with stillbirth, the mother must be cared for in a facility that can effectively manage the maternal condition and monitor the fetus.[63] For those mothers not scheduled to deliver in such a facility, timely transport is a requirement. Because far and away the most appropriate intervention for a fetus at risk of stillbirth is delivery by induction of labor or more often by cesarean section, a facility must have these capabilities and a staff with sufficient skills to choose and carry out the appropriate interventions. Qualified staffing and availability of cesarean section must be available 24 hours a day and 7 days a week, a situation not often seen in many LMIC hospitals.[66] Both the 2011 and 2015 *Lancet* "Stillbirth Series" estimated various interventions and their impact on stillbirths. Above all, appropriate hospital-based obstetric care during labor and delivery stood out as the most effective way to prevent stillbirths in LMICs.[7,8,67,68]

This is not to say that a reduction in asphyxic stillbirths comes free of cost. Infants delivered prematurely because of concern about risk of stillbirth may suffer all the complications of infants born prematurely after a spontaneous birth. Concern about stillbirth prompts much monitoring and delivery by cesarean section, and although cesarean sections are safe operations in HICs, in LMICs a greater number of women who undergo a cesarean section die with complications of the surgery, and many others who live have life-threatening complications. Some have lifelong complications from the surgery, including urogenital fistulae. Women with a cesarean section in a first pregnancy also are highly likely to be delivered by cesarean section in future pregnancies and in those pregnancies may suffer uterine scar dehiscence and placental accreta, increasing the risk of subsequent stillbirths and other maternal, fetal, and neonatal complications. Unfortunately, the tests used to predict stillbirth, such as contraction stress tests or Doppler-flow analyses, all have high false-positive rates. Thus, although acting on these tests prevents some stillbirths, many mothers and babies are subjected to risks of surgery and early delivery, not necessarily of benefit to either. The optimal rate of cesarean section to reduce stillbirth has been estimated at 10% to 15%.[69] It is not clear if the cesarean section rates of 30% or more, currently seen in many HICs and middle-income countries, contributes to additional reductions in stillbirths compared with the stillbirth rates that could be achieved with a lower cesarean section rate. The goal, therefore, should be to do just the right amount of fetal monitoring and cesarean sections to reduce asphyxia-related stillbirths and neonatal deaths, and no more. Getting to the right balance has proved an illusory goal.

SUMMARY

In summary, most stillbirths occur in LMICs and most of these are in term or near-term fetuses free of congenital anomalies. Half or more occur during the intrapartum period. Most stillbirths in LMICs are associated with conditions, such as prolonged or obstructed labor, placental abruption, and preeclampsia, which cause the fetal death by asphyxiation. With appropriate facility-based obstetric care, as generally occurs in HICs, nearly all of these stillbirths would be preventable.

Best practices

What is the current practice?

This is a review of the relationship of intrauterine asphyxia to stillbirth in both HICs and in LMICs. The review emphasizes that a majority of stillbirths in both locations, but especially in low-income countries, are due to intrauterine asphyxia often occurring during labor. In many areas, the obstetric conditions leading to intrauterine asphyxia are not identified, the woman and fetus are not monitored appropriately, and delivery is not performed expeditiously.

What changes in current practice are likely to improve outcomes?

In all locations, the conditions leading to intrauterine asphyxia, such as prolonged labor, preeclampsia, placental abruption, and many others, need to be identified appropriately, and the fetus then monitored for asphyxia. When fetal distress is discovered, a timely delivery, often by cesarean section, needs to be performed.

REFERENCES

1. Low JA. Intrapartum fetal asphyxia: definition, diagnosis, and classification. Am J Obstet Gynecol 1997;176:957–9.
2. Dilenge ME, Majnemer A, Shevell MI. Long-term developmental outcome of asphyxiated term neonates. J Child Neurol 2001;16:781–92.
3. Ellenberg JH, Nelson KB. The association of cerebral palsy with birth asphyxia: a definitional quagmire. Dev Med Child Neurol 2013;55:210–6.
4. Laughon SK, Berghella V, Reddy UM, et al. Neonatal and maternal outcomes with prolonged second stage of labor. Obstet Gynecol 2014;124:57–67.
5. Buchmann EJ, Pattinson RC. Babies who die from labour-related intrapartum hypoxia: a confidential enquiry in South African public hospitals. Trop Doct 2006;36:8–10.
6. Reddy UM, Goldenberg RL, Silver R, et al. Stillbirth Classification: developing an international consensus for research: executive summary of NICHD Development Workshop. Obstet Gynecol 2009;114:901–14.
7. Cousens S, Blencowe H, Stanton C, et al. National, regional, and worldwide estimates of stillbirth rates in 2009 with trends since 1995: a systematic analysis. Lancet 2011;377:1319–30.
8. Lawn JE, Blencoe H, Pattinson R, et al, and the Lancet Stillbirth Series Steering Committee. Stillbirths: when, where and why? How to make the data count. Lancet 2011;377:1448–63.
9. Aminu M, Unkels R, Mdegela M, et al. Causes of and factors associated with stillbirth in low- and middle-income countries: a systematic literature review. BJOG 2014;121(Suppl 4):141–53.
10. Moxon SG, Ruysen H, Kerber KJ, et al. Count every newborn; a measurement improvement roadmap for coverage data. BMC Pregnancy Childbirth 2015; 15(Suppl 2):S8.
11. Flenady V, Wojcieszek AM, Middleton P, et al. Stillbirths: recall to action in high-income countries. Lancet 2016;387:691–702.
12. Sarfraz AA, Samuelsen SO, Eskild A. Changes in fetal death during 40 years-different trends for different gestational ages: a population-based study in Norway. BJOG 2011;118:488–94.

13. Gregory EC, MacDorman MF, Martin JA. Trends in fetal and perinatal mortality in the United States, 2006-2012. NCHS Data Brief 2014;169:1–8.

14. Copper RL, Goldenberg RL, DuBard MB, et al. Risk factors for fetal death in white, black and Hispanic women. Obstet Gynecol 1994;84:490–5.

15. McClure EM, Pasha O, Goudar SS, et al, Global Network Investigators. Epidemiology of stillbirth in low-middle income countries: a Global Network Study. Acta Obstet Gynecol Scand 2011;90:1379–85.

16. Goldenberg RL, McClure EM, Saleem S, et al. Infection-related stillbirths. Lancet 2010;375:1482–90.

17. Vallgårda S. Why did the stillbirth rate decline in Denmark after 1940? Popul Stud (Camb) 2010;64:117–30.

18. Eriksson AW, Fellman J. Factors influencing the stillbirth rates in single and multiple births in Sweden, 1869 to 1967. Twin Res Hum Genet 2006;9:591–6.

19. Goldenberg RL, McClure EM, Macguire ER, et al. Lessons for low-income regions following the reduction in hypertension-related maternal mortality in high-income countries. Int J Gynaecol Obstet 2011;113:91–5.

20. Sparling FP. Diagnosis and management of syphilis. N Engl J Med 1971;284:642–53.

21. Tovey GH, Valaes T. Prevention of stillbirth in Rh haemolytic disease. Lancet 1959;2:521–4.

22. Chamberlain G, Williams AS. Antenatal care in South Wales 1934-1962. Soc Hist Med 1995;8:480–8.

23. Pakzad M, Saling E. Perinatal mortality of infants with signs of foetal distress before the introduction of the newer methods of obstetrical surveillance. Ger Med Mon 1969;14:499–500.

24. Smith GC, Yu CK, Papageorghiou AT, et al, Fetal Medicine Foundation Second Trimester Screening Group. Maternal uterine artery doppler flow velocimetry and the risk of stillbirth. Obstet Gynecol 2007;109:144–51.

25. Yakoob MY, Menezes EV, Soomro T, et al. Reducing stillbirths: behavioural and nutritional interventions before and during pregnancy. BMC Pregnancy Childbirth 2009;9:S3.

26. Yakoob MY, Ali MA, Ali MU, et al. The effect of providing skilled birth attendance and emergency obstetric care in preventing stillbirths. BMC Public Health 2011;11(Suppl 3):S7.

27. Gardosi J, Giddings S, Clifford S, et al. Association between reduced stillbirth rates in England and regional uptake of accreditation training in customised fetal growth assessment. BMJ Open 2013;3:e003942.

28. Bukowski R, Hansen NI, Willinger M, et al. Fetal growth and risk of stillbirth: a population-based case-control study. PLoS Med 2014;11:e1001633.

29. Vogel JP, Souza JP, Gülmezoglu AM. Patterns and outcomes of induction of labour in Africa and Asia: a secondary analysis of the WHO global survey on maternal and neonatal health. PLoS One 2013;8:e65612.

30. Kayem G, Combaud V, Lorthe E, et al. Mortality and morbidity in early preterm breech singletons: impact of a policy of planned vaginal delivery. Eur J Obstet Gynecol Reprod Biol 2015;192:61–5.

31. Albrechtsen S, Rasmussen S, Irgens LM. Secular trends in peri- and neonatal mortality in breech presentation; Norway 1967-1994. Acta Obstet Gynecol Scand 2000;79:508–12.

32. Chi BH, Wang L, Read JR, et al. Predictors of stillbirth in sub-Saharan Africa. Obstet Gynecol 2007;110:989–97.

33. Engmann C, Matendo R, Kinoshita R, et al. A Prospective survey of stillbirth and early neonatal mortality rates in a rural region of Central Africa. Int J Gynaecol Obstet 2009;105:112–7.
34. McClure EM, Goldenberg RL. Infectious causes of stillbirth. Semin Fetal Neonatal Med 2009;14:182–9.
35. Mission JF, Marshall NE, Caughey AB. Pregnancy risks associated with obesity. Obstet Gynecol Clin North Am 2015;42:335–53.
36. Shah S, Van den Bergh R, Prinsloo JR, et al. Unregulated usage of labour-inducing medication in a region of Pakistan with poor drug regulatory control: characteristics and risk patterns. Int Health 2016;8:89–95.
37. Dudley DJ, Goldenberg RL, Conway D, et al, for the Stillbirth Collaborative Research Network. A new system for determining the causes of stillbirth. Obstet Gynecol 2010;116:254–60.
38. Flenady V, Frøen JF, Pinar H, et al. An evaluation of classification systems for stillbirth. BMC Pregnancy Childbirth 2009;9:24.
39. Stillbirth Collaborative Research Network Writing Group. Causes of death among stillbirths. JAMA 2011;306:2459–68.
40. Gardosi J, Pattinson RC. Classification of stillbirth: a global approach. In: Facchinetti F, Decker G, Barnciani D, et al, editors. Stillbirth: understanding and management. London: Informa Healthcare; 2010. p. 114–7.
41. Engmann C, Jehan I, Ditekemena J, et al. An alternative strategy for perinatal verbal autopsy coding: single versus multiple coders. Trop Med Int Health 2011;16:18–29.
42. McClure EM, Bose CL, Garces A, et al. Global network for women's and children's health research: a system for low-resource areas to determine probable causes of stillbirth, neonatal and maternal death. Matern Health Neonatol Perinatol 2015;1:11.
43. Goldenberg RL, McClure EM, Bann CM. The relationship of intrapartum and antepartum stillbirth rates to measures of obstetric care in developed and developing countries. Acta Obstet Gynecol Scand 2007;86:1303–9.
44. Goldenberg RL, McClure EM, Kodkany B, et al. A multi-country study of the "intrapartum stillbirth and early neonatal death indicator" in hospitals in low-resource settings. Int J Gynaecol Obstet 2013;122:230–3.
45. Lawn JE, Lee AC, Kinney M, et al. Two million intrapartum-related stillbirths and neonatal deaths: where, why, and what can be done? Int J Gynaecol Obstet 2009;107(Suppl):S5–19.
46. Harmon QE, Huang L, Umbach DM, et al. Risk of fetal death with preeclampsia. Obstet Gynecol 2015;125:628–35.
47. Ersdal HL, Mduma E, Svensen E, et al. Birth asphyxia: a major cause of early neonatal mortality in a Tanzanian rural hospital. Pediatrics 2012;129:e1238–43.
48. Goldenberg RL, McClure EM. Reducing intrapartum stillbirths and intrapartum-related neonatal deaths. Int J Gynaecol Obstet 2009;107:S1.
49. Friedman AM, Cleary KL. Prediction and prevention of ischemic placental disease. Semin Perinatol 2014;38:177–82.
50. Spencer RN, Carr DJ, David AL. Treatment of poor placentation and the prevention of associated adverse outcomes – what does the future hold? Prenat Diagn 2014;34:677–84.
51. Pinar H, Goldenberg RL, Koch MA, et al. Placental findings in singleton stillbirths. Obstet Gynecol 2014;123(2 Pt 1):325–36.
52. Clark RB. Definition of fetal asphyxia. Am J Obstet Gynecol 1990;163(4 Pt 1):1364.

53. McClure EM, Saleem S, Goudar SS, et al. Stillbirth rates in low-middle income countries 2010-2013: a population-based, multi-country study from the Global Network. Reprod Health 2015;12(Suppl 2):S7.

54. Frey HA, Odibo AO, Dicke JM, et al. Stillbirth risk among fetuses with ultrasound-detected isolated congenital anomalies. Obstet Gynecol 2014;124:91–8.

55. McClure EM, Dudley DJ, Reddy UM, et al. Infectious causes of stillbirth: a clinical perspective. Clin Obstet Gynecol 2010;53:635–45.

56. Liu LC, Wang YC, Yu MH, et al. Major risk factors for stillbirth in different trimesters of pregnancy –a systematic review. Taiwan J Obstet Gynecol 2014;53:141–5.

57. Jovanovič L, Liang Y, Weng W, et al. Trends in the incidence of diabetes, its clinical sequelae, and associated costs in pregnancy. Diabetes Metab Res Rev 2015;31:707–16.

58. Lawn JE, Gravett MG, Nunes TM, et al. Global report on preterm birth and stillbirth (1 of 7): definitions, description of the burden and opportunities to improve data. BMC Pregnancy Childbirth 2010;10(Suppl 1):S1.

59. Goldenberg RL, McClure EM, Jobe AH, et al. Stillbirths and neonatal mortality as outcomes. Int J Gynaecol Obstet 2013;123:252–3.

60. Garces A, McClure EM, Chomba E, et al. Home birth attendants in low income countries: who are they and what do they do? BMC Pregnancy Childbirth 2012;12:34.

61. Goudar SS, Somannavar MS, Clark R, et al. Stillbirth and newborn mortality in India after helping babies breathe training. Pediatrics 2013;131:e344–52.

62. Korteweg FJ, Erwich JJ, Holm JP, et al. Diverse placental pathologies as the main causes of fetal death. Obstet Gynecol 2009;114:809–17.

63. Bhutta ZA, Das JK, Bahl R, et al. Can available interventions end preventable deaths in mothers, newborn babies, and stillbirths, and at what cost? Lancet 2014;384:347–70.

64. McClure EM, Saleem S, Pasha O, et al. Stillbirth in developing countries: a review of causes, risk factors and prevention strategies. J Matern Fetal Neonatal Med 2008;21:1–8.

65. Hinderaker SG, Olsen BE, Bergsjø PB, et al. Avoidable stillbirths and neonatal deaths in rural Tanzania. BJOG 2003;110:616–23.

66. Hussein J, Goodburn EA, Damisoni H, et al. Monitoring obstetric services: putting the 'UN Guidelines' into practice in Malawi: 3 years on. Int J Gynaecol Obstet 2001;75:63–73.

67. Lawn JE, Blencowe H, Waiswa P, et al, Lancet Ending Preventable Stillbirths Series study group, Lancet Stillbirth Epidemiology investigator group. Stillbirths: rates, risk factors, and acceleration towards 2030. Lancet 2016;387:587–603.

68. Pattinson R, Kerber K, Buchmann E, et al, Lancet's Stillbirths Series steering committee. Stillbirths: how can health systems deliver for mothers and babies? Lancet 2011;377:1610–23.

69. McClure EM, Goldenberg RL, Bann CM. Maternal mortality, stillbirth and measures of obstetric care in developing and developed countries. Int J Gynaecol Obstet 2007;96:139–46.

Novel Approaches to Neonatal Resuscitation and the Impact on Birth Asphyxia

CrossMark

Arjan B. Te Pas, MD, PhD[a],*, Kristina Sobotka, PhD[b],
Stuart B. Hooper, PhD[c]

KEYWORDS

- Asphyxia • Resuscitation • Sustained inflation • Oxygen • Cord clamping
- Cardiac compressions

KEY POINTS

- In neonatal asphyxia at birth, effective and timely resuscitative measures are vital to avoid prolonging the hypoxic and ischemic insult.
- Adequate lung aeration is the key to a prompt restoration of heart rate and cardiac function, for which a sustained inflation can be helpful in achieving this.
- Hyperoxia needs to be avoided, and the extra oxygen that may be needed to restore cardiac function and spontaneous breathing needs to be titrated based on measured oxygen saturations.
- When ventilation is given effectively, cardiac compression is seldom needed.

INTRODUCTION

Birth asphyxia accounts for a quarter of neonatal deaths worldwide[1]; although 5% to 10% of newborns require some assistance at birth, only approximately 1% of infants need more extensive resuscitative measures.[2,3] If newborns are asphyxic, these measures should be initiated in a timely and effective manner to avoid prolonging the hypoxic and ischemic insults, which may cause permanent injury. Most asphyxiated infants only require assistance in the form of effective ventilation to restore breathing and improve circulatory function. Although a small proportion of infants will need cardiac resuscitation (chest compression and adrenaline) in most of these cases, it is likely

Disclosure Statement: The authors have nothing to disclose.
[a] Division of Neonatology, Department of Pediatrics, Leiden University Medical Centre, J6-S, PO Box 9600, Leiden 2300 RC, The Netherlands; [b] Institute of Neuroscience and Physiology, The Sahlgrenska Academy, University of Gothenburg, Box 432, Göteborg 405 30, Sweden; [c] The Ritchie Centre, MIMR-PHI Institute of Medical Research, Monash Institute of Medical Research, Monash University, 27-31 Wright Street, Clayton, Melbourne, Victoria 3168, Australia
* Corresponding author.
E-mail address: a.b.te_pas@lumc.nl

Clin Perinatol 43 (2016) 455–467
http://dx.doi.org/10.1016/j.clp.2016.04.005
0095-5108/16/$ – see front matter © 2016 Elsevier Inc. All rights reserved.

perinatology.theclinics.com

that the bradycardia only persists when the ventilation is inadequate.[4] For this reason, the emphasis on neonatal resuscitation is on administering effective ventilation.

With regard to resuscitation procedures, caregivers are guided by the international consensus on science that informs resuscitation guidelines every 5 years. These guidelines were largely based on dogma; but more recently, recognition that the first few minutes after birth are critical for determining neonatal outcomes has prompted renewed interest in studies performed in infants at birth. Most new data are derived from experimental studies, as it is very difficult or impractical to perform clinical trials because of the infrequent occurrence of birth asphyxia and the unpredictable need for extensive resuscitation. In this article, the authors review the current knowledge on the physiologic responses to asphyxia and the novel approaches for resuscitation.

PATHOPHYSIOLOGY OF PERINATAL ASPHYXIA

Asphyxia is a mixture of hypoxia, hypercapnia, and a combination of both respiratory and metabolic acidosis caused by a reduction in respiratory gas exchange as well as the ensuing metabolic stress response.[5] Perinatal asphyxia can result from multiple complications, including disruption of blood flow through the placenta, placental detachment, compression of the umbilical cord, prolonged labour,[5] and failure of the newborn to initiate pulmonary gas exchange after birth.[6]

Although adults respond to hypoxia/asphyxia with tachycardia and an increase in respiratory drive, the fetal response is very different as it induces apnea and brady-cardia.[6] Our current understanding of the cardiorespiratory responses to birth asphyxia is primarily based on animal experiments conducted in the 1960s, which usually involved placing a water-filled bag over the newborn's head after delivery (**Fig. 1**).[7–9] With the onset of asphyxia, the first sign of compromise is cessation of respiratory efforts, commonly referred to as primary apnea, which is accompanied by a profound bradycardia (see **Fig. 1**; **Fig. 2**). This bradycardia is rapid in onset, mediated by vagal inputs, and is most strongly initiated by both hypoxia and acidosis in the fetus. Primary apnea is followed by a period of irregular gasping, which culminates in secondary or terminal apnea that eventually results in cardiac arrest if the compromise continues. Although the bradycardic response to asphyxia is immediate, arterial blood pressure tends to initially increase before gradually decreasing because of myocardial energy failure caused by the hypoxia (see **Fig. 1**). If ventilation of the lungs occurs before the blood pressure decreases to less than a critical level, both heart rate (HR) and blood pressure are rapidly restored but of concern can cause a rebound tachycardia and hypertension.[5,6,10,11]

The pathophysiology of fetal asphyxia has been well documented by animal studies; but the interpretation of these data has been overextrapolated, and the experimental context in which the data were collected has been overlooked. As a result, it is widely assumed that all bradycardic infants at birth are asphyxic and that reoxygenation is the key to birth asphyxia and perinatal resuscitation. Although oxygen is important, this is clearly an inaccurate assumption as a high proportion of normal term infants, considered normoxic, have a HR less than 100 within the first minute after birth.[12] Clearly there are other factors influencing HRs at birth, one of which is the timing of umbilical cord clamping (UCC).[13,14]

As the placenta receives a large proportion of fetal cardiac output (30%–50%), umbilical venous return provides a large proportion of preload for the fetal heart, particularly the left ventricle. In contrast to adults, fetal pulmonary blood flow (PBF) is low and so pulmonary venous return provides only a small proportion of left ventricular preload, with the majority coming from umbilical venous return.[15] This umbilical venous return

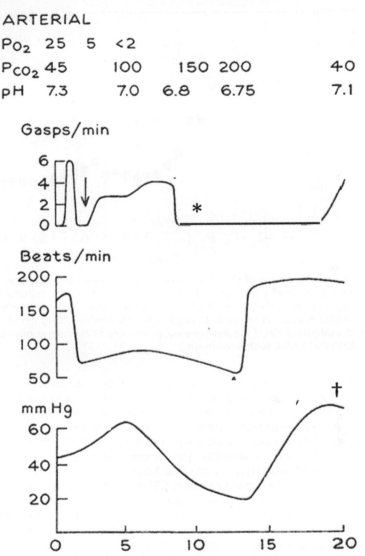

ARTERIAL

P_{O_2}	25	5	<2				
P_{CO_2}	45		100	150	200		40
pH	7.3		7.0	6.8	6.75		7.1

Fig. 1. Changes of breathing, heart rate, and blood pressure set out against time from onset of asphyxia (minutes) in rhesus monkeys during asphyxia and on resuscitation by positive pressure ventilation. The top panel represents breathing (gasp) rate in breaths, the middle panel the heart rate, and the bottom panel the blood pressure. After onset of asphyxia, respiratory efforts will cease (primary apnea, *arrow*) together with an acute vagal induced bradycardia. The primary apnea is followed by irregular gasping that, if sustained, will ultimately lead to a secondary or terminal apnea (*asterisk*). The arterial blood pressure tends to initially increase before gradually decreasing because of myocardial energy failure caused by the hypoxia. A rebound tachycardia and hypertension occurs when ventilation restores heart rate and blood pressure (*dagger*). (*Adapted from* Dawes GS. Birth asphyxia, resuscitation and brain damage in foetal and neonatal physiology. 1st edition. Chicago: Year Book Medical Publishers; 1968.)

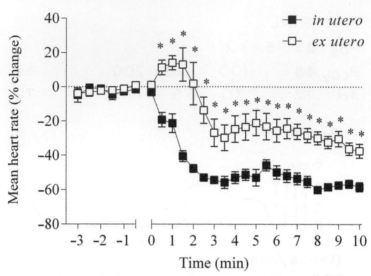

Fig. 2. Mean (standard error of the mean) heart rate, expressed as percentage of control, measured before and after umbilical cord clamping in near-term lambs. Following umbilical cord clamping, the lambs either remained in utero (*closed squares*) or were ex utero (*open squares*). *P<0.05 in utero vs ex utero. (*From* Sobotka KS, Morley C, Ong T et al. Circulatory responses to asphyxia differ if the asphyxia occurs in utero or ex utero in near-term lambs. PLoS One 2014;9:e112264; with permission.)

flows via the ductus venosus, inferior vena cava, and foramen ovale. As a result, UCC causes an immediate cessation of umbilical venous return and a loss of preload for the left ventricle, which is not restored until PBF increases following lung aeration.[14] UCC also causes a sudden increase in peripheral vascular resistance due to the loss of the low resistance placental vascular bed, which increases arterial pressures (by ~30%) and the afterload on the left ventricle. The combined effect of a decrease in preload and an increase in afterload is a marked reduction in cardiac output, which is reflected by both a decrease in HR and stroke volume. This reduction likely explains the brady-cardia in normoxic infants in the absence of asphyxia at birth.[12] Delaying UCC until after the lungs have aerated and PBF has increased mitigates all of these effects of UCC, including the effect on HR,[14,16] because, on UCC, pulmonary venous return can imme-diately replace umbilical venous return as the primary source of preload for the left ventricle, thereby avoiding the reduction in cardiac output. These experiments have been performed in nonasphyxiated preterm lambs, but so far no data are available regarding the effects of delayed cord clamping in an asphyxiated model.

Apart from the effect of UCC, the fetal/newborn HR response to asphyxia also de-pends on whether the asphyxia is initiated in utero, with water surrounding the face, or ex utero. When the asphyxia occurs ex utero, vagal-mediated bradycardia is blunted, resulting in significantly higher HRs, despite similar levels of asphyxia (see **Fig. 2**).[17] As the in utero response can be duplicated ex utero by placing a water-filled bag over the newborn's head, it is highly likely that a diving reflex–type response contributes to the bradycardia.[17] It is important to note that the early studies of Dawes and colleagues[7] involved placing a water-filled bag over the newborn's head to prevent ventilation, and most other studies have been conducted in utero (see **Fig. 1**).

In view of more recent findings, it is now clear that the sequence of cardiorespiratory events that guide current resuscitation practices require further clarification. Indeed, although oxygenation is important, it is not the only defining factor, as other factors, such as the timing of UCC in relation to lung aeration and the supply of preload to the left ventricle, are also important. This point is exemplified by the recent finding that aeration of the newborn rabbit lung with 100% nitrogen increases both PBF and HR, with the latter most likely being secondary to the increase in pulmonary venous return.[18] It was speculated that this global increase in PBF is likely to be a vagal response to the lung aeration.[18] The rapid accumulation of liquid in the interstitial tissue may possibly activate J-receptors.[19] These receptors, located within the alveolar walls, are known to respond to fluid accumulation and signal via vagal C-fibers to cause global pulmonary vasodilatation.[20]

This study highlights the role of lung aeration and increasing PBF to increase or sustain cardiac output at birth, which also applies to asphyxic infants at birth. Although myocardial energy production is severely reduced during asphyxia, if the cord is clamped and the lungs are unaerated, cardiac output is also restricted by a lack of preload. Logically, therefore, ventilation is the key. It not only supplies oxygen but it also stimulates a decrease in pulmonary vascular resistance to enable pulmonary venous return to increase with the restoration of myocardial function.

UPPER AIRWAY SUCTIONING AT BIRTH

Following the recommendation that suctioning of vigorous infants with meconium-stained amniotic fluid should be avoided, the recent guidelines have now also abandoned routine intubation for tracheal suction in nonvigorous infants with meconium-stained amniotic fluid.[2] In a recent experiment with asphyxiated lambs and meconium aspiration, the onset of resuscitation was considerably delayed. Tracheal suctioning improved ventilation and oxygenation, but the pulmonary vascular resistance remained elevated.[21] In a recent small trial of term nonvigorous infants born through meconium-stained amniotic fluid, infants were randomized to endotracheal suctioning and no suctioning. No significant differences were observed between the groups in meconium aspiration syndrome, its severity, and complications, mortality, and neurodevelopmental outcome.[22] Although the benefit of routine suctioning is still unknown and a larger study is needed, the International Liaison Committee on Resuscitation (ILCOR) has emphasized the need to avoid possible harm caused by suctioning and a delay in appropriate ventilation and oxygenation.

VENTILATION AT BIRTH

Although international guidelines recommend how lung inflation in term asphyxiated infants can be initially established,[2] there is a lack of evidence to support any initial ventilation strategy. There are no clinical trials available on depressed term infants evaluating the effect of ventilation, although there are numerous animal studies. In animals, an initial sustained inflation (SI) can improve lung liquid clearance and aeration when enough inflation pressure is given for a sufficient time.[23,24] As liquid is more viscous than air, the resistance to moving lung liquid through the airways and into the alveoli is markedly greater than air (~100 times), thereby requiring a longer period of time for any given inflation pressure. Preterm rabbit studies using phase contrast x-ray imaging have shown that an SI of 10 to 20 seconds produces larger functional residual capacity (FRC) and more homogenous lung aeration than intermittent positive pressure ventilation (iPPV), if combined with a positive end-expiratory pressure at the end of the SI.[23,25] Although some beneficial effects of an SI have been demonstrated in preterm infants,[26–28] no trials have been performed in term infants. However, Vyas and colleagues[29] described the physiologic response of term asphyxiated infants to an initial SI of 5 seconds. The initial volume given with the SI was twice the volume reached during standard resuscitation, and an SI always led to the formation of FRC.[29]

Klingenberg and colleagues[30] compared the effect of an initial 30-second SI with iPPV in near-term asphyxiated lambs and found that an SI markedly increased HR and blood pressure recovery, resulting in better oxygenation and lung compliance when compared with iPPV (**Fig. 3**). However, the rebound tachycardia and hypertension that followed the asphyxia caused higher cerebral blood flows, which could increase the risk for hemorrhage in asphyxiated infants who are unable autoregulate.[30,31] Nevertheless, the increase in HR in asphyxic lambs could be

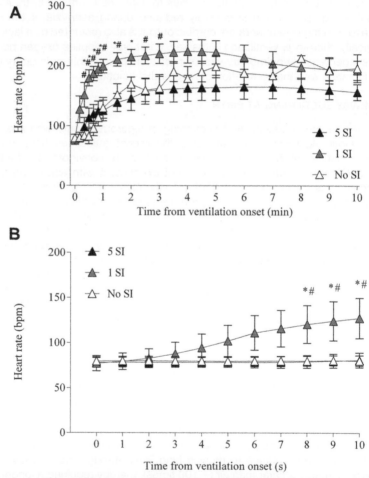

Fig. 3. Recovery in HR, following a period of severe asphyxia, in response to ventilation with a single 30-second inflation (*grey triangles*), iPPV using inflation and deflation times of times of 0.5 seconds (*open triangles*), and five 3-second inflations (*closed triangles*). With each strategy, the peak inflation pressure was 35 cm H_2O. The HR changes are displayed over the first 10 minutes (*A*) and over the first 10 seconds (*B*). bpm, beats per minute. Data are mean (SD). *$P<0.05$ 5 × 3s SI vs 30 s SI; #$P<0.05$ 30 s SI vs No SI. (*From* Klingenberg C, Sobotka KS, Ong T, et al. Effect of sustained inflation duration; resuscitation of near-term asphyxiated lambs. Arch Dis Child Fetal Neonatal Ed 2013;98:F224; with permission.)

detected within 5 seconds of initiating the SI, raising the question of whether an increase in oxygenation or lung aeration and an increase in PBF was the predominant factor leading to the increase in HR.[30]

To answer this question, these studies were repeated using a 30-second SI and gases with differing oxygen content.[31] Asphyxiated, bradycardic lambs did not increase HR or PBF, unless oxygen (O_2) was present in the gas, although a gas mixture with 5% O_2 was found to be almost as effective as air. Although increasing the O_2 content from 5% to 21% improved the HR recovery, no further improvement was found by increasing the O_2 to 100% (**Fig. 4**).[31] This finding likely indicates that, once aerated, O_2 exchange is not a significant limiting factor in the mature near-term lung and that only a small amount of oxygen is needed in the inhaled gas to increase PBF and myocardial energetics. This increase in PBF and myocardial energetics is likely to result from a direct effect of increasing oxygen levels on both the myocardium and the pulmonary vasculature as well as the effect of lung aeration (irrespective of inspired oxygen level) on PBF. The rapid increase in PBF, which increases pulmonary venous return and left atrial filling, may then further contribute to the increase in HR by increasing left ventricular preload.

The recent studies have provided new insights into the circulatory transition of asphyxiated infants at birth, but there are likely to be several mechanisms working both independently and collectively to sustain cardiac output after birth. Although the interacting mechanisms are complex, they can be summarized by the suggestion that during a low-risk birth, without signs of asphyxia, only lung aeration is needed to increase PBF and HR; but in severely asphyxiated infants, when the myocardium is deprived of oxygen, oxygen is also required in the inhaled gas mixture.

OXYGEN USE

It seems obvious that the hypoxia, which is responsible for the apnea and myocardial function failure, needs to be reversed at birth as quickly as possible. Until 2010, it was recommended to resuscitate all asphyxiated infants using 100% oxygen. However, much research in oxidative stress over the last 20 years has led to increased

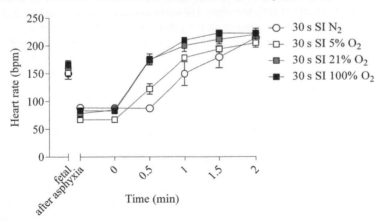

Fig. 4. Recovery in HR, following a period of severe asphyxia, in response to ventilation with a single 30-second inflation using a gas mixture of 100% nitrogen (N_2) (*open circles*), 5% oxygen (*open squares*), 21% oxygen (*grey squares*), and 100% oxygen (*closed squares*). bpm, beats per minute. (*From* Sobotka KS, Ong T, Polglase GR, et al. The effect of oxygen content during an initial sustained inflation on heart rate in asphyxiated near-term lambs. Arch Dis Child Fetal Neonatal Ed 2015;100:F337–43.)

concerns with the use of oxygen in asphyxiated infants at birth. The use of 100% oxygen, which was titrated based on the infants color, can easily lead to hyperoxia, resulting in oxygen toxicity. This toxicity leads to upregulation of inflammatory cytokines,[32] release of highly reactive free radicals (oxidative stress),[33] and increased pulmonary vascular reactivity.[34] High oxygenation levels should be avoided, as the antioxidant defense mechanisms in newborns are immature and oxidative stress can easily lead to cell structural damage in a variety of organs, including the brain.[35]

The hypoxia and hypercapnia associated with asphyxia induces potent cerebral vasodilation and peripheral vasoconstriction to redirect cardiac output to the brain. This response is an autoregulatory response that develops early in gestation, ensuring that as the blood oxygen content decreases, cerebral blood flow increases to sustain oxygen delivery to the brain.[36] On the other hand, although increased oxygenation normally results in a reduction in cerebral blood flow, this autoregulatory response is relatively slow. Sobotka and colleagues[31] observed that the cerebral blood flow was much higher in asphyxiated lambs resuscitated with 100% oxygen when compared with air. It was speculated that the cerebral circulation following asphyxia is mostly pressure passive and not sensitive to arterial oxygen levels, which increases the risk of hyperoxia-induced brain injury.[31] Rapid reperfusion and increase in blood oxygen content exposes the brain to increased oxidative stress, increased blood-brain barrier permeability, and hemorrhage.[37]

Meta-analysis of clinical studies has compared the use of 100% versus 21% oxygen during resuscitation of asphyxiated infants at birth. Although one has demonstrated a reduction in mortality and a trend toward a reduction in hypoxic ischemic encephalopathy when 21% was used,[38] a more recent meta-analysis could detect no differences in the long-term follow-up.[39] Since 2010, the guidelines from the Neonatal Resuscitation Program and ILCOR recommend that initial resuscitation of term infants should be started with room air; but if bradycardia (<60 beats per minute) persists, oxygen should be increased to 100% while performing chest compressions.[2] It is also recommended to use a pulse oximeter such that supplementary oxygen may be administered and titrated to achieve a preductal oxygen saturation approximating the interquartile range of the available normograms.[2] It should be emphasized that most trials were performed before pulse oximetry was introduced in the delivery room, and 100% oxygen was given and either not titrated or titrated based on a judgment of the infant's color. No trials have been performed in asphyxiated term infants comparing starting with 100% oxygen versus 21% oxygen and titration of content guided by oxygen saturation.

Hypoxia is a potent inhibitor of fetal breathing maneuver prenatally because of direct inhibitory neural input into the respiratory center from a region located in the upper lateral pons.[40] The hypoxic sensitivity is still low in newborns shortly after birth; to initiate breathing, the oxygen levels need to be restored.[41] On the other hand, hyperoxia could also inhibit the chemoreceptors, as a delay in onset of breathing was observed in asphyxiated animals resuscitated with 100% oxygen.[42] Although this delay is also clinically observed in human studies,[33,43] it can be very difficult to observe spontaneous breathing and the first breath can easily be missed.

Based on the current available data, the authors suggest that asphyxiated infants should be initially resuscitated without extra oxygen; but when cardiac compressions are needed or if despite adequate ventilation bradycardia persists, oxygen should be increased to 100%. In all cases the extra oxygen should be titrated based on the infant's measured oxygen saturations, and reductions in fraction of inspired oxygen (FIO_2) should commence before normal saturations are reached to avoid hyperoxia; preferably FIO_2 can be decreased as the HR increases.

CARDIAC COMPRESSIONS

Adequate ventilation restores myocardiac failure in most asphyxiated infants, and the need for cardiac compressions and adrenaline is rare.[4] It has been estimated that chest compressions have been given to 8 in 10,000 term and near-term infants per year.[44,45] Perlman and Riser[4] suggested that, in two-thirds of the cases, chest compressions and adrenaline were given because of persisting bradycardia due to inadequate ventilation. This finding emphasizes the fact that, in most cases, spontaneous circulation is restored by adequate ventilation alone. However, when ventilation is not sufficient, chest compressions can increase coronary perfusion pressure and pump blood systemically until the myocardium becomes sufficiently oxygenated to restore function. Nevertheless, appropriate ventilation is still required to get oxygen into the infant's circulation.

High rates of mortality and neurodevelopmental impairment have been reported when infants received cardiac compressions or adrenaline.[46] Although this most likely reflects the severity of asphyxia and the infant's poor clinical condition at birth, it has been questioned whether improving cardiac resuscitation could improve this poor outcome. Much effort has been taken in performing animal and manikin studies to investigate several factors of cardiac compressions (ratio, rate, depth, chest recoil, technique, adrenaline dose).[47] However, the effectiveness of different approaches is very limited as most of the data are derived from adult, manikin, and animal models that do not resemble the transition of an asphyxiated infant. The current guidelines recommend a ratio of 3 chest compressions to 1 inflation to achieve 120 events per minute, using a 2-thumbs technique. The optimal depth of one-third of the anterior-posterior chest diameter is best reached when using a 3:1 ratio as compared with higher ratios.[48] Recently it was demonstrated in a newborn piglet model that cardiac compressions not synchronized with ventilation led to similar tidal volume and oxygen delivery when compared with synchronized.[49] This finding is reassuring, as in clinical practice most caregivers do not comply with synchronized cardiopulmonary resuscitation.[50] In addition, applying an SI without interrupting cardiac compressions improved hemodynamics, minute ventilation, and survival when compared with a 3:1 ratio.[51]

SUMMARY

In the last decade, research studies have greatly improved our understanding of the problems encountered by infants during transition and how to improve resuscitation of asphyxiated infants. It is necessary for every caregiver to keep abreast with this rapid change in knowledge to comprehend modern resuscitation practices. Alternative ways for ventilation, oxygenation, and chest compressions have been investigated in mostly experimental studies and have challenged the current resuscitative practices. Although it is difficult to perform studies in the delivery room, there is a need for clinical trials to fill the gap in human data regarding resuscitation of asphyxiated infants.

Best practices box

What is the current practice?

In perinatal asphyxia, prompt resuscitative measures are vital to avoid further hypoxia and ischemia. Most asphyxiated infants need ventilation at birth; cardiac compressions are seldom needed.

What changes in current practice are likely to improve outcomes?

Aiming for an effective ventilation strategy will lead to adequate lung aeration, which is the key to prompt restoration of HR and cardiac function.

No benefits have been shown in suctioning, and it can delay appropriate ventilation.

Avoid immediate cord clamping.

Avoid hyperoxia, but extra oxygen may be needed to restore cardiac function and spontaneous breathing.

Major recommendations

Make sure that resuscitative measures are timely started in asphyxiated apneic infants at birth.

Make sure that ventilation is appropriate and lung aeration is achieved. An initial SI can be helpful in this.

Do not delay ventilation for routine suctioning when there is meconium stained amniotic fluid (MSAF).

Titrate oxygen on measured oxygen saturations; restore hypoxia, but avoid hyperoxia.

When ventilation is effectively given, cardiac compressions are seldom needed.

Summary statement

Adequate lung aeration is the key for prompt restoration of cardiac function, hypoxia, and ischemia in perinatal asphyxia.

REFERENCES

1. Black RE, Cousens S, Johnson HL, et al. Global, regional, and national causes of child mortality in 2008: a systematic analysis. Lancet 2010;375:1969–87.
2. Wyllie J, Perlman JM, Kattwinkel J, et al. Part 7: neonatal resuscitation: 2015 international consensus on cardiopulmonary resuscitation and emergency cardiovascular care science with treatment recommendations. Resuscitation 2015;95: e169–201.
3. Kattwinkel J. Textbook of neonatal resuscitation. 4th edition. Elk Grove Village, IL: American Academy of Pediatrics and American Heart Association; 2000.
4. Perlman JM, Risser R. Cardiopulmonary resuscitation in the delivery room. Associated clinical events. Arch Pediatr Adolesc Med 1995;149:20–5.
5. Wall SN, Lee AC, Carlo W, et al. Reducing intrapartum-related neonatal deaths in low- and middle-income countries-what works? Semin Perinatol 2010;34:395–407.
6. Boyle DW, Szyld EG, Field D. Ventilation strategies in the depressed term infant. Semin Fetal Neonatal Med 2008;13:392–400.
7. Dawes GS, Jacobson HN, Mott JC, et al. The treatment of asphyxiated, mature foetal lambs and rhesus monkeys with intravenous glucose and sodium carbonate. J Physiol 1963;169:167–84.
8. Adamson K Jr, Behrman R, Dawes GS, et al. Resuscitation by positive pressure ventilation and tris-hydroxymethylaminomethane of rhesus monkeys asphyxiated at birth. J Pediatr 1964;65:807–18.

9. Dawes GS, Hibbard E, Windle WF. The effect of akali and glucose infusion on permanent brain damage in rhesus monkeys asphyxiated at birth. J Pediatr 1964;65:801–6.
10. Bennet L, Peebles DM, Edwards AD, et al. The cerebral hemodynamic response to asphyxia and hypoxia in the near-term fetal sheep as measured by near infrared spectroscopy. Pediatr Res 1998;44:951–7.
11. Ley D, Oskarsson G, Bellander M, et al. Different responses of myocardial and cerebral blood flow to cord occlusion in exteriorized fetal sheep. Pediatr Res 2004;55:568–75.
12. Dawson JA, Kamlin CO, Wong C, et al. Changes in heart rate in the first minutes after birth. Arch Dis Child Fetal Neonatal Ed 2010;95:F177–81.
13. Smit M, Dawson JA, Ganzeboom A, et al. Pulse oximetry in newborns with delayed cord clamping and immediate skin-to-skin contact. Arch Dis Child Fetal Neonatal Ed 2014;99:F309–14.
14. Bhatt S, Alison BJ, Wallace EM, et al. Delaying cord clamping until ventilation onset improves cardiovascular function at birth in preterm lambs. J Physiol 2013;591:2113–26.
15. Rudolph AM. Fetal and neonatal pulmonary circulation. Annu Rev Physiol 1979; 41:383–95.
16. Polglase GR, Dawson JA, Kluckow M, et al. Ventilation onset prior to umbilical cord clamping (physiological-based cord clamping) improves systemic and cerebral oxygenation in preterm lambs. PLoS One 2015;10:e0117504.
17. Sobotka KS, Morley C, Ong T, et al. Circulatory responses to asphyxia differ if the asphyxia occurs in utero or ex utero in near-term lambs. PLoS One 2014;9:e112264.
18. Lang JA, Pearson JT, Binder-Heschl C, et al. Increase in pulmonary blood flow at birth; role of oxygen and lung aeration. J Physiol 2015;594(5):1389–98.
19. Siew ML, Wallace MJ, Allison BJ, et al. The role of lung inflation and sodium transport in airway liquid clearance during lung aeration in newborn rabbits. Pediatr Res 2013;73:443–9.
20. Paintal AS. Mechanism of stimulation of type J pulmonary receptors. J Physiol 1969;203:511–32.
21. Lakshminrusimha S, Mathew B, Nair J, et al. Tracheal suctioning improves gas exchange but not hemodynamics in asphyxiated lambs with meconium aspiration. Pediatr Res 2015;77:347–55.
22. Chettri S, Adhisivam B, Bhat BV. Endotracheal suction for nonvigorous neonates born through meconium stained amniotic fluid: a randomized controlled trial. J Pediatr 2015;166:1208–13.
23. te Pas AB, Siew M, Wallace MJ, et al. Effect of sustained inflation length on establishing functional residual capacity at birth in ventilated premature rabbits. Pediatr Res 2009;66:295–300.
24. Sobotka KS, Hooper SB, Allison BJ, et al. An initial sustained inflation improves the respiratory and cardiovascular transition at birth in preterm lambs. Pediatr Res 2011;70(1):56–60.
25. te Pas AB, Siew M, Wallace MJ, et al. Establishing functional residual capacity at birth: the effect of sustained inflation and positive end-expiratory pressure in a preterm rabbit model. Pediatr Res 2009;65:537–41.
26. te Pas AB, Walther FJ. A randomized, controlled trial of delivery-room respiratory management in very preterm infants. Pediatrics 2007;120:322–9.
27. Lista G, Boni L, Scopesi F, et al. Sustained lung inflation at birth for preterm infants: a randomized clinical trial. Pediatrics 2015;135:e457–64.
28. Lindner W, Hogel J, Pohlandt F. Sustained pressure-controlled inflation or intermittent mandatory ventilation in preterm infants in the delivery room? A

randomized, controlled trial on initial respiratory support via nasopharyngeal tube. Acta Paediatr 2005;94:303–9.

29. Vyas H, Milner AD, Hopkin IE, et al. Physiologic responses to prolonged and slow-rise inflation in the resuscitation of the asphyxiated newborn infant. J Pediatr 1981;99:635–9.

30. Klingenberg C, Sobotka KS, Ong T, et al. Effect of sustained inflation duration; resuscitation of near-term asphyxiated lambs. Arch Dis Child Fetal Neonatal Ed 2013;98:F222–7.

31. Sobotka KS, Ong T, Polglase GR, et al. The effect of oxygen content during an initial sustained inflation on heart rate in asphyxiated near-term lambs. Arch Dis Child Fetal Neonatal Ed 2015;100:F337–43.

32. Pillow JJ, Hillman NH, Polglase GR, et al. Oxygen, temperature and humidity of inspired gases and their influences on airway and lung tissue in near-term lambs. Intensive Care Med 2009;35(12):2157–63.

33. Vento M, Asensi M, Sastre J, et al. Resuscitation with room air instead of 100% oxygen prevents oxidative stress in moderately asphyxiated term neonates. Pediatrics 2001;107:642–7.

34. Lakshminrusimha S, Russell JA, Steinhorn RH, et al. Pulmonary arterial contractility in neonatal lambs increases with 100% oxygen resuscitation. Pediatr Res 2006;59:137–41.

35. Munkeby BH, Borke WB, Bjornland K, et al. Resuscitation of hypoxic piglets with 100% O2 increases pulmonary metalloproteinases and IL-8. Pediatr Res 2005;58: 542–8.

36. Del TJ, Louis PT, Goddard-Finegold J. Cerebrovascular regulation and neonatal brain injury. Pediatr Neurol 1991;7:3–12.

37. Fellman V, Raivio KO. Reperfusion injury as the mechanism of brain damage after perinatal asphyxia. Pediatr Res 1997;41:599–606.

38. Saugstad OD, Ramji S, Soll RF, et al. Resuscitation of newborn infants with 21% or 100% oxygen: an updated systematic review and meta-analysis. Neonatology 2008;94:176–82.

39. Saugstad OD, Vento M, Ramji S, et al. Neurodevelopmental outcome of infants resuscitated with air or 100% oxygen: a systematic review and meta-analysis. Neonatology 2012;102:98–103.

40. Gluckman PD, Johnston BM. Lesions in the upper lateral pons abolish the hypoxic depression of breathing in unanaesthetized fetal lambs in utero. J Physiol 1987; 382:373–83.

41. Davey MG, Moss TJ, McCrabb GJ, et al. Prematurity alters hypoxic and hypercapnic ventilatory responses in developing lambs. Respir Physiol 1996;105: 57–67.

42. Bookatz GB, Mayer CA, Wilson CG, et al. Effect of supplemental oxygen on reinitiation of breathing after neonatal resuscitation in rat pups. Pediatr Res 2007;61: 698–702.

43. Saugstad OD, Rootwelt T, Aalen O. Resuscitation of asphyxiated newborn infants with room air or oxygen: an international controlled trial: the Resair 2 study. Pediatrics 1998;102:e1.

44. Barber CA, Wyckoff MH. Use and efficacy of endotracheal versus intravenous epinephrine during neonatal cardiopulmonary resuscitation in the delivery room. Pediatrics 2006;118:1028–34.

45. Wyckoff MH, Berg RA. Optimizing chest compressions during delivery-room resuscitation. Semin Fetal Neonatal Med 2008;13:410–5.

46. Harrington DJ, Redman CW, Moulden M, et al. The long-term outcome in surviving infants with Apgar zero at 10 minutes: a systematic review of the literature and hospital-based cohort. Am J Obstet Gynecol 2007;196:463–5.
47. Solevag AL, Cheung PY, Lie H, et al. Chest compressions in newborn animal models: a review. Resuscitation 2015;96:151–5.
48. Hemway RJ, Christman C, Perlman J. The 3:1 is superior to a 15:2 ratio in a newborn manikin model in terms of quality of chest compressions and number of ventilations. Arch Dis Child Fetal Neonatal Ed 2013;98:F42–5.
49. Schmolzer GM, O'Reilly M, LaBossiere J, et al. 3:1 compression to ventilation ratio versus continuous chest compression with asynchronous ventilation in a porcine model of neonatal resuscitation. Resuscitation 2014;85:270–5.
50. Foglia E, Patel J, Niles D, et al. Provider adherence to neonatal resuscitation program recommendations for coordinated neonatal chest compressions and ventilations. Analg Resusc 2013;(Suppl 1):2324-903X.S1-010.
51. Schmolzer GM, O'Reilly M, LaBossiere J, et al. Cardiopulmonary resuscitation with chest compressions during sustained inflations: a new technique of neonatal resuscitation that improves recovery and survival in a neonatal porcine model. Circulation 2013;128:2495–503.

Cardiovascular Alterations and Multiorgan Dysfunction After Birth Asphyxia

Graeme R. Polglase, PhD[a],*, Tracey Ong, PhD[a],
Noah H. Hillman, MD[b]

KEYWORDS

- Asphyxia • Cardiovascular • Multiorgan failure • Kidneys • Liver

KEY POINTS

- The cardiovascular consequences of asphyxia likely underlie downstream multiorgan injury.
- The major mechanism is redistribution of blood flow and oxygen delivery to vital organs, resulting in poor perfusion and hypoxia in other organs.
- Current clinical management needs to consider the cardiovascular effects of therapeutic hypothermia on the asphyxia-mediated organ dysfunction and recovery.

INTRODUCTION

Birth asphyxia causes hypoxic-ischemic encephalopathy and multiorgan failure. The most studied organ affected by hypoxia is the cardiovascular system, and the resulting hemodynamic instability that occurs because of hypoxia, either in utero or during resuscitation and newborn transition, causes downstream effects on other organs. The clinical focus during the resuscitation of asphyxiated infants is largely on the immediate changes in heart rate and systemic blood pressure that occur at delivery, based on the seminal findings of Dawes,[1] Cross,[2] and Dawes and colleagues.[3] The acute cardiorespiratory consequences of asphyxia require rapid intervention in the form of stimulation, ventilation, and in extreme cases cardiac resuscitation.[4]

However, other cardiovascular consequences of asphyxia can also have long-term consequences to asphyxic newborns. One of the profound cardiovascular responses to asphyxia is the redistribution of cardiac output. Hypoxia diverts blood, partially through a primitive diving reflex, from less vital organs, such as the liver, kidney,

Disclosure: The authors have nothing to disclose.
[a] The Ritchie Centre, Hudson Institute of Medical Research, 27-31 Wright Street, Clayton, Victoria 3168, Australia; [b] Department of Pediatrics, Saint Louis University, 1100 South Grand Boulevard, St Louis, MO 63124, USA
* Corresponding author.
E-mail address: graeme.polglase@monash.edu

and gut, to maintain oxygen delivery to critical organs such as the adrenal gland, heart, and brain, at the expense of other organs.[5–7] Within these organs now deprived of blood flow, local vasoconstriction and redistribution of blood flow results in a decrease in oxygen delivery.[7] If prolonged, this can cause cellular injury and inadequate tissue function and can result in multiorgan dysfunction after birth. Further, the fetal cardiovascular response to asphyxia can also lead to redistribution of blood volume toward the placenta, leaving the asphyxic newborn volume depleted and prone to circulatory shock.

All the clinical manifestations of organ failure must be managed in the setting of therapeutic hypothermia. Although much of perinatology has been focused on the downstream consequences of asphyxia on the brain, and the serious consequences of hypoxic-ischemic encephalopathy (HIE), a growing appreciation of the consequences of asphyxia on other organs is emerging (**Table 1**),[8–11] which further complicates the care of asphyxiated infants.

This article describes the circulatory responses to asphyxia and how they can lead to multiorgan dysfunction. It focuses on the physiologic derangements that occur in response to hypoxia, and the end-organ damage caused by both the hypoxia and the hypoperfusion caused by responsive shunting of blood. It also briefly outlines the current clinical strategies for minimizing multiorgan injury to attempt to reduce lifelong morbidity.

CARDIOVASCULAR RESPONSE TO ASPHYXIA

Irrespective of the cause of impaired gas exchange, there is a sequence of cardiovascular and respiratory changes that ensue in asphyxiated infants at birth. Shortly after the onset of asphyxia, the newborn undergoes a period of primary apnea that is also associated with a profound bradycardia.[1,2,12,13] Blood pressure is usually maintained during primary apnea because of peripheral vasoconstriction and the redirection of blood from nonvital organs toward the heart, central nervous system, and adrenal glands.[5,6,14–18]

If asphyxia continues, after a period of gasping the fetus enters secondary apnea or terminal apnea.[15,19] Secondary apnea is associated with a large decrease in blood pressure[12,19] and, without intervention, the newborn eventually has cardiac arrest.[12,19]

Table 1
Multiorgan failure after birth asphyxia in randomized therapeutic hypothermia trials

Study	Selective Head CoolCap[8]		Whole-body NICHD[9]		Whole-body TOBY Trial[10]		Selective Head Chinese Trial[11]	
	Cooled	Control	Cooled	Control	Cooled	Control	Cooled	Control
Increased Liver Enzyme Levels (%)	38[a]	53	20	15	NR	NR	35	28
Thrombocytopenia (%)	33	22	NR	NR	58	50	6	2
Prolonged Coagulation (%)	50	42	18	11	41	43	NR	NR
Hemorrhage/ Bleeding (%)	NR	NR	3	2	NR	NR	3	2
Renal Failure (%)	65	70	22	26	ND	ND	23	22

Abbreviations: ND, none requiring dialysis; NICHD, National Institute of Child Health and Human Development; NR, not reported.
[a] *P*<.05 verses control infants.

The downstream consequences of asphyxia are detrimental to multiple organ systems. The underlying cause of multiorgan dysfunction is likely the cardiovascular sequelae of asphyxia.

HEART RATE

The heart rate response to asphyxia has been well described in studies in fetal sheep. An immediate bradycardia is initiated with acute hypoxia and this is augmented by acidosis when the induced asphyxia is acute and severe.[20] The bradycardia associated with fetal asphyxia is mediated by the vagus nerve, supplying parasympathetic efferent innervation to the heart. Vagotomy inhibits the bradycardic response to asphyxia and similar results are obtained using a pharmacologic approach with atropine (a competitive acetylcholine muscarinic receptor antagonist).[21–24]

Debate has arisen previously over the afferent stimulus for the bradycardic response to asphyxia. Arterial chemoreceptors and/or baroreceptors likely provide the afferent input into the cardiovascular control center, resulting in increased parasympathetic drive that mediates the heart rate response. Although peripheral chemoreceptors and baroreceptors are active and functional in the fetal sheep from 90 days gestational age, it is likely that the bradycardic response is primarily initiated by a chemoreflex for several reasons.[25,26] First, the increases in arterial blood pressure are gradual and occur after the more rapid decrease in heart rate.[24] The bradycardic response occurs during brief episodes of fetal hypoxia without changes in blood pressure.[27] In addition, there is an absence of fetal heart rate decrease or arterial pressure increase to acute hypoxia in carotid body and aortic body denervated fetal lambs, suggesting that the fetal bradycardic response is chemoreflex mediated.[28]

Similar bradycardic responses to asphyxia have been shown in newborn animal model studies.[3,21,29,30] These studies were conducted in animals of varying postnatal ages (from birth to 10 days) and the asphyxia was induced by placing the animal's head in a liquid-filled environment (water or normal saline) to prevent gaseous exchange. Recent studies have shown that the heart rate response to asphyxia is altered if the asphyxia occurs with the fetus in utero compared with ex utero.[31]

ARTERIAL BLOOD PRESSURE AND PERIPHERAL VASOCONSTRICTION

The knowledge of the distribution of fetal cardiac output comes largely from the seminal work of Rudolph and colleagues.[16,32,33] The normal organ distribution of fetal cardiac output is shown in **Fig. 1**. Blood is oxygenated within the placenta and returns to the heart through the umbilical veins, bypasses the kidneys through the ductus venosus, and enters the inferior vena cava. Inferior vena caval blood flow represents about two-thirds of total venous return and is highly oxygenated; ~65% saturation. The oxygenated blood preferentially is directed through the foreman ovale to the left atrium. Left ventricular output in the fetus is only 33% of combined ventricular output and is distributed to the heart and upper body, including the brain, with only a quarter of left ventricular output flowing into the descending aorta. Right ventricular output makes up 66% of combined ventricular output in the fetus. Most of the right ventricular output bypasses the lungs via the ductus arteriosus, whereupon it is distributed to the placenta, abdomen, and lower body.

In response to severe hypoxemia fetal cardiac output decreases but umbilical flow remains constant.[34] In order to maintain arterial blood pressure and adequate oxygen supply to vital organs there is a redirection of cardiac output to preferentially direct blood away from nonvital organs (the gut, kidney, lungs, and skin) toward the heart, central nervous system, and adrenal glands (**Fig. 2**).[5,33,34] This redistribution of cardiac

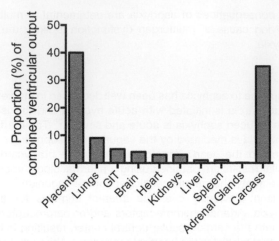

Fig. 1. Distribution of cardiac output in the fetus. GIT, gastrointestinal tract. (*Data from* Refs.[5,33,34])

output is the direct result of vasoconstriction in nonvital organs and vasodilation in vital organs such as the brain and heart. Increases in catecholamine levels and increased sympathetic activity via hypoxia-induced activation of the sympathetic-adrenergic system likely mediate these changes in peripheral vascular resistance.[24,35]

The carotid arterial chemoreceptor role in mediating peripheral vasoconstriction has been confirmed in studies in which carotid denervation abolished femoral vasoconstriction during hypoxia.[24] In addition, femoral vasoconstriction is inhibited using phentolamine (an α-adrenergic antagonist), confirming an adrenergic efferent mechanism mediating this pathway.[24] Pulmonary blood flow decreases via pulmonary vasoconstriction in asphyxiated fetal and newborn studies.[36,37] The increase in pulmonary

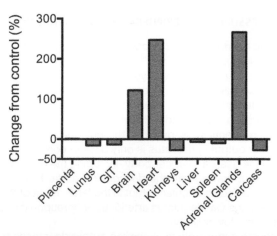

Fig. 2. Change in cardiac output from control values during reduction in uterine blood flow resulting in hypoxemia in fetal sheep, showing the redistribution of cardiac output to the brain, adrenals, and heart at the expense of other organs. (*Data from* Jensen A, Roman C, Rudolph AM. Effects of reducing uterine blood flow on fetal blood flow distribution and oxygen delivery. J Dev Physiol 1991;15(6):309-23.)

vascular resistance was negated in sinoaortic denervated fetuses, suggesting similar chemoreflexive mechanisms.[38]

The high peripheral vasoconstriction also can result in the preferential redistribution of blood from the high-resistance fetus, toward the low-resistance placenta, resulting in a reduction in the blood volume to the newborn.[39] As asphyxia progresses, arterial blood pressure cannot be maintained in spite of peripheral vasoconstriction, because ventricular function begins to decline. As a result, during secondary apnea, blood pressure begins to decrease, and this eventually leads to myocardial dysfunction and cardiac arrest.

VENTRICULAR OUTPUT AND MYOCARDIAL DYSFUNCTION

The relative roles of heart rate and the Frank-Starling mechanism in effectively altering cardiac output in newborns remain controversial. In adults, the Frank-Starling mechanism refers to the direct influence of end-diastolic volume on stroke volume; the intrinsic length-tension relationship of increasing cardiac muscle length by increasing end-diastolic volume increases contractile force and therefore increases stroke volume. Some fetal studies have shown that heart rate is the major determinant of fetal cardiac output rather than stroke volume.[40–42] These studies found that increasing preload as a means of increasing stroke volume via blood or saline infusion had little effect on cardiac output.[41] Rudolph and Heyman[42] further showed that altering heart rate (from 160–180 beats/min [bpm] to 240–270 bpm) via left atrial pacing increased right ventricular output by just 12%. It has been suggested that the inability of the fetal heart to increase stroke volume is caused by immaturity of the fetal myocardium.[43] However, structural immaturity cannot solely be responsible for limiting the cardiac response because left ventricular output is able to double immediately after birth.[44] Further, increasing heart rate via left atrial pacing in the fetus decreased right to left shunting through the foramen ovale.[45] As a result, increases in right ventricular output associated with left atrial pacing in the studies by Rudolph and Heyman[42] were likely to be exaggerated.

Kirkpatrick and colleagues[46] showed that spontaneous changes in fetal heart rate (114–180 bpm) were not associated with significant changes in fetal left ventricular output. Further, Anderson and colleagues[47] found that changes in end-diastolic ventricular volume influenced ventricular stroke volume and left ventricular output in chronically instrumental fetal lambs. These studies suggest that the Frank-Starling mechanism is a major determinant of fetal cardiac output.[46,47]

Irrespective of the precise mechanisms effecting newborn cardiac output, ongoing severe asphyxia is associated with significantly reduced ventricular output and stroke volume.[39,48] It is likely that the causes of eventual myocardial dysfunction and subsequent reduced cardiac output in asphyxiated neonates are multifactorial; these include the low heart rate associated with asphyxia, acidosis,[49] and reduced myocardial contractility caused by poor perfusion and ischemic cardiac injury. Asphyxiated newborns are at increased risk of ischemic cardiac injury caused by decreased cardiac output and decreased coronary perfusion.[50] Asphyxiated newborns have increased troponin levels (a protein located on the actin filament of myocardium and that is an indicator of myocardial cell death and myocardial damage).[51–53] Increased serum troponin levels (taken within 24 hours of delivery) in asphyxiated human infants have been associated with increased myocardial damage and consequently lower left ventricular output and stroke volume.[52]

Therefore, progressive asphyxia in newborns without intervention results in ongoing circulatory deterioration, eventually leading to myocardial dysfunction, circulatory shock, right and left ventricular failure, tricuspid regurgitation, and hypotension and eventual cardiac arrest. Clinical management of cardiac dysfunction relies on maintaining adequate perfusion to organs, maintaining blood pressure, and assisting in cardiac contractility. Review of cardiac management and blood pressure control in newborns is beyond the scope of this article but has been nicely summarized in a recent review article by Giesinger and McNamara.[54]

LIVER INJURY, COAGULOPATHY, AND BLEEDING

Liver injury is likely caused by hypoperfusion rather than hypoxia.[55] Transaminase levels (aspartate transaminase and alanine transaminase) often increase from initial measurements, but typically significantly improve by the end of 72 hours of therapeutic hypothermia.[56,57] Some correlation between the severity of the perinatal asphyxia and the increase of liver transaminase levels has been seen.[58] In contrast, in a piglet model of HIE, there was a poor correlation between the serum transaminase levels and the degree of tissue damage on pathologic specimens, suggesting that significant liver dysfunction can occur in the setting of normal transaminase levels.[59] In a selective head-cooling trial, 53% of noncooled asphyxiated infants had increased liver enzyme levels versus 38% in the cooled group ($P = .02$).[8] There were no differences in coagulopathies (17%) and prolonged coagulation times (46%) between infants who received therapeutic cooling and those who did not.[31] The overall rate of death or disability was higher in both groups of the CoolCap study than in other HIE cooling trials, suggesting that the infants were overall sicker than in the other studies, which may explain the higher percentage of hepatic dysfunction[9–11](see **Table 1**). A head-cooling trial from China also showed no difference between groups, with 30% showing increased liver enzyme levels.[11]

Coagulation dysfunction in hypoxic infants was reported as early as 1971 in a subset of infants with birth asphyxia, with the cause associated with a consumptive coagulopathy (increased fibrin degradation products) followed by disseminated intravascular coagulation.[60,61] The effect on coagulation was of short duration and may only play a minor role in the overall morbidity of birth asphyxia. Levels of factor XIII are lower in infants with birth asphyxia. Plasma levels of thrombin-antithrombin complexes, D-dimer, fibrinogen, and fibrin degradation products are higher in infants with birth asphyxia.[62] Note that levels of coagulation factors II, VII, IX, and X; protein C; protein S; and antithrombin are also reduced in preterm compared with term plasma.[63] Prothrombin time and activated partial thromboplastin time are higher in preterm infants, but there is no correlation with increased risk of intraventricular hemorrhage (IVH) with higher coagulation times.[63] Coagulopathy requiring fresh frozen plasma occurred in up to 50% of infants with HIE (see **Table 1**).[8–11,56] In the National Institute of Child Health and Human Development (NICHD) whole-body cooling trial, 17% of infants had hepatic dysfunction and 14% had disseminated intravascular coagulation.[9] Although it is difficult to determine the cause of coagulation abnormalities in the setting of perinatal asphyxia, therapeutic cooling does not seem to increase coagulopathy. This finding is reassuring because hypothermia impairs coagulation in whole-blood samples and accelerates microvascular coagulation in mice.[64,65] In a retrospective analysis of bleeding in 76 infants with birth asphyxia undergoing therapeutic cooling, 54% had some form of active bleeding, with an even distribution of intracranial, pulmonary, and gastrointestinal bleeding and hematuria.[66] Infants with bleeding had a lower platelet count, fibrinogen level, and higher maximum International Normalized Ratio (INR), and investigators suggest that the levels associated with increased bleeding were minimum fibrinogen level of 1.54 g/L, minimum platelet count of

130,000 $\times$ 10^6/L, and INR of 1.98.[66] The bleeding was not severe enough to require surgery or neurosurgical intervention, and the rate of major bleeding was consistent with the lower rates in the randomized trials.[66] There is a wide range of clinical practice with regard to maintaining coagulation laboratory values in the normal range in asphyxiated children and no clinical guidelines have been determined. Fresh frozen plasma is often transfused in these infants to correct INR values or as part of fluid resuscitation for blood pressure control.

THROMBOCYTOPENIA

Thrombocytopenia, as defined by a platelet count of less than 100,000 $\times$ 10^6/L, is common in ill infants and infants with birth asphyxia (see **Table 1**). It is difficult to gain consensus among neonatologists about the level of thrombocytopenia that is dangerous for ill neonates or infants with birth asphyxia. In a prospective, observational study of thrombocytopenia in all infants admitted to 7 neonatal intensive care units (NICUs), 5% of all admissions had platelet count less than 60,000 $\times$ 10^6/L and 78% of these infants were less than 28 weeks' gestational age.[67] Although a large percentage of infants born weighing less than 1500 g had severe thrombocytopenia, only 9% developed a major hemorrhage.[67] In late preterm and term asphyxiated infants, a large retrospective study found that 31% had thrombocytopenia.[68] The nadir for the platelet count in these asphyxiated infants was on day 3, but normalization of thrombocytopenia took an average of 19 days.[68] There is a large variation in the rate of thrombocytopenia in the clinical trials of therapeutic hypothermia, with rates ranging from 6% to 55% of asphyxiated infants.[8–11,56]

Hypoxia is thought to have a direct effect on platelet formation for a clinical presentation termed thrombocytopenia of perinatal asphyxia.[68] Hypoxia in adult mice causes a decrease in the size and production of the megakaryocytes in the bone marrow.[69] Although the megakaryocytes seem to not be injured by hypoxia, the cells in the bone marrow surrounding them are affected and decrease the release of platelet promoting factors.[70] Increased destruction of platelets contributes importantly to thrombocytopenia of birth asphyxia, as is evident by the rapid decrease in platelet numbers after platelet transfusions in infants with birth asphyxia.[71] Thrombocytopenia was more common in infants with more chronic hypoxia (>24 hours), as classified by increased nucleated red blood cell count.[66] Infants with thrombocytopenia after asphyxia were more likely to die in one study, but the cause of death was not active bleeding or hemorrhagic consequences.[66]

There are large variations in indications for platelet transfusion between NICUs in the United States and Canada, with many units transfusing platelets in nonbleeding infants with platelet counts greater than 50,000 $\times$ 10^6/L.[72] The average response to a platelet transfusion is an increase of 52,000 $\times$ 10^6/L.[67] When preterm infants were randomized at a platelet count of 50,000 $\times$ 10^6/L to ether platelet transfusion to 150,000 $\times$ 10^6/L or left alone, there were no differences in bleeding or IVH. Because bleeding is often not severe in infants with thrombocytopenia (3% of infants in the NICHD whole-body cooling study[9]), the National Institutes of Health conducted an expert conference to determine whether platelet transfusions were necessary for many of these infants. No consensus could be given because no clear randomized trial on platelet use has been performed.[73] British guidelines suggest keeping platelet counts greater than 20,000 $\times$ 10^6/L to 30,000 $\times$ 10^6/L in stable newborns, and transfusing platelets if less than 50,000 $\times$ 10^6/L in sick infants with active bleeding or coagulation defects.[74,75] The Platelets for Neonatal Transfusion – Study 2 (PlaNeT-2) is a randomized study of high and low platelet transfusion thresholds in newborns and is currently being conducted in Europe.[76] Until further studies are performed, individual clinicians must decide whether treating thrombocytopenia in stable, nonbleeding asphyxiated infants is necessary.

RENAL DYSFUNCTION AND ELECTROLYTE DISTURBANCES AFTER BIRTH ASPHYXIA

There are poor definitions for acute kidney injury (AKI) in neonates because of the variation in serum creatinine levels at birth, which often reflect the maternal levels for the first 48 hours, and the large changes in glomerular filtration rates (GFRs) that occur at birth and cause variations in urine production.[77,78] However, AKI after neonatal asphyxia occurs in as many as 56% of asphyxiated infants, with a combination of oliguric and nonoliguric renal failure complicating the clinical management. All nephrons are formed by 34 weeks' gestational age but the GFR increases 6-fold from birth until 1 year of life.[79] The renal blood flow rate is low at 4% of cardiac output in infants at birth and increases slowly over the first 6 weeks to about 15% of cardiac output (adult levels are 20%–25%).[78] Some studies define AKI as creatinine level greater than 1.5 mg/dL and decreasing urine output (<1 mL/kg/h), but oliguria only occurs in 50% of infants with AKI.[80] Infants can often maintain urine output greater than 1 mL/kg/h and still have renal dysfunction.[77] Oliguric renal failure is associated with higher mortality than nonoliguric failure,[81] but there is no evidence that converting oliguric renal failure to nonoliguric renal failure improves prognosis.[77]

Kidney injury is common in infants with birth asphyxia (see **Table 1**). In hypothermia trials, 50% of asphyxiated infants had increased creatinine levels and 18% to 39% had urine output less than 0.5 mL/kg/h for greater than 24 hours.[56] In selective head cooling (CoolCap), 67% of the infants had abnormal renal function, whereas in the whole-body cooling study only 19% had oliguria and 5% were anuric.[9] The percentage of infants with oliguria is similar to the 20% of infants in a head-cooling trial from China, which had increased blood urea nitrogen and creatinine levels.[11] The differences in the incidence of AKI between studies may have been caused by the severity of HIE in the CoolCap study. In a small study of 36 infants, AKI persisted in 17% of infants at 96 hours after birth asphyxia.[82] The degree of kidney injury is correlated with the clinical severity of the birth asphyxia and infants with AKI were more likely to have abnormal findings on the brain MRI.[83,84] Asphyxiated infants with AKI are also ventilated on average for 4 days longer than infants without kidney disease.[82] Electrolyte abnormalities were seen in more than 50% of infants, with hyponatremia, hypokalemia, and hypocalcemia the most prominent.[8,56]

Because the definition of AKI is not refined in the newborn period, the assessments of biomarkers of kidney injury are often suboptimal. Serum creatinine level does not begin to increase until 25% to 50% of renal function is lost, thus significant injury can occur without changes in creatinine level.[85] The change in serum creatinine levels over the first few days is predictive of renal injury, with normal values of greater than 50% decline or serum creatinine level less than 0.6 mg/dl found in 70% of infants after HIE.[86] A fractional excretion of sodium of greater than 3% is moderately specific for AKI after 48 hours.[77] Although cystatin C and neutrophil gelatinase-associated lipocalin (NGAL) are both specific markers of other pediatric kidney injury, their levels can be increased by birth asphyxia, making it impossible to determine whether an infant will develop AKI.[86,87] A recent study showed that an NGAL level greater than 250 ng/mL was significantly associated with severe HIE and mortality.[88] Researchers are continuing to develop new assays for determining AKI in the hope that earlier detection might alter the high rate of persistent renal failure in survivors of pediatric acute kidney disease.

The response to asphyxia-associated kidney disease depends on the clinical scenario because some infants have initial oliguria followed by high-output renal failure from acute tubular necrosis. Close monitoring of fluid balance, serum electrolyte levels, and body weight can prevent situations of hypovolemia or fluid overload.[78] Fluid overload at the time of renal replacement therapy is associated with increased mortality in multiple pediatric critical care settings.[89] Because renal dysfunction can occur with normal urine output, it is important to monitor drug levels and avoid nephrotoxic medications. Although prophylactic theophylline was shown in multiple randomized studies to improve AKI after birth asphyxia, it is not heavily used for this purpose in NICUs in the United States because long-term follow-up is not available and studies were done before the introduction of therapeutic hypothermia.[90] The use of diuretics in AKI was not shown to be beneficial and could be harmful.[78] Rapid fluid and electrolyte shifts can occur after birth asphyxia, so care needs to be given to correction of the hyponatremia, hypokalemia, and hypocalcemia that are often seen in HIE.

LUNG AND GASTROINTESTINAL COMPLICATIONS

Most infants with significant birth asphyxia have injury to the lungs and many require mechanical ventilation. Because mechanical ventilation may be necessary because of injury to the lung parenchyma, alterations in the blood vessels in the lung, or alterations in the respiratory drive in the brainstem, respiratory management varies significantly from one patient to the next. As with any critically ill infants, infants after birth asphyxia should have oxygenation maximized to decrease shunting away from vital organs. If allowed to recover using minimal mechanical ventilation, the lungs often respond well and many infants with severe brain injury remain on room air. Pulmonary hypertension is also common in birth asphyxia and may be caused by the underlying cause of the birth asphyxia (in utero hypoxia with vascular hypertrophy) or may be a response to the concurrent hypoxia.[8,9,56] Whether pulmonary hypertension occurs during therapeutic hypothermia or during the rewarming process, it can be treated with nitric oxide, muscle relaxation, and medications for pain and anxiety. Occasionally infants with birth asphyxia require extracorporeal membrane oxygenation (ECMO) for pulmonary reasons, but many centers use severe birth asphyxia as a contraindication for ECMO. Pulmonary hemorrhage has been reported in severe asphyxia and with significant coagulopathy.[66] Overall, the lung can repair itself quickly. Prolonged ventilation is often necessary for neurologic reasons instead of intrinsic issues with the lungs.

The gut has multiple watershed regions that are prone to hypoxic injury from birth asphyxia. Necrotizing enterocolitis has been reported in these infants, but is a rare complication.[91] Current guidelines for therapeutic hypothermia have infants receiving nothing by mouth until completion of the hypothermia and this delay in feeding may allow the gut mucosa to repair. Hypothermia might improve gut morbidities after HIE and has been considered as therapy in older infants with necrotizing enterocolitis.[92] The ability to use total parenteral nutrition in these infants has allowed clinicians to rest the gut mucosa for multiple days and allow for reconstituting the gut barrier lost in hypoxic events.[93]

THERAPEUTIC HYPOTHERMIA AND MULTIORGAN FAILURE

In most of the clinical trials of therapeutic hypothermia to prevent death or poor neurologic outcome, there were no differences in markers of organ failure between the asphyxiated infants who received cooling and those who did not (see **Table 1**).[8–11] A slight improvement in liver function tests was measured in selective head cooling, but not in other trials that included slightly less ill infants.[8–11] Proponents of selective head cooling argue that selective head cooling has fewer systemic effects, whereas clinicians at whole-body cooling centers may think that the overall lower metabolic rate from hypothermia should be beneficial to all organs. In a single-center comparative study, there were no differences in end-organ damage over the first 72 hours of cooling between whole-body and selective head cooling[56] The rates of multiorgan system failure also did not differ between infants with HIE who had good or poor neurologic outcomes, suggesting that multiorgan failure is not a good predictor of overall outcome.[57]

SUMMARY

Multiorgan failure is common in infants born after acute or prolonged asphyxia, and likely results from downstream consequences of cardiovascular redistribution. The redistribution of blood flow and oxygen delivery results in regionalized hypoxia and consequently cellular death. Current clinical therapies of multiorgan dysfunction are now conducted on a background of therapeutic hypothermia. The efficacy of many of these therapies is yet to be shown in this environment. Understanding the circulatory consequences of asphyxia may lead to improved cardiovascular stability after birth with potential benefit on multiple organ systems.

Best practices box

What is the current practice?

Current newborn resuscitation guidelines recommend therapeutic hypothermia for severe birth asphyxia. Although neonatologists have focused on decreasing neurologic injury, the cardiovascular derangements from birth asphyxia lead to multiorgan failure. Therapeutic hypothermia has not changed the rate of multiorgan failure, and coagulopathy and kidney injury can lead to increased morbidity and mortalities.

What changes in current practice are likely to improve outcomes?

Improvements in management of blood pressure and perfusion will improve multiorgan failure

Although many clinicians have expanded the criteria for the use of therapeutic hypothermia, clinical studies are warranted to study whether later use (>6 hours) or use on infants with lower gestational age is beneficial.

Major recommendations
   Maintaining adequate circulatory support after birth asphyxia, based on blood pressure and echocardiographic data, helps to decrease multiorgan failure.
   Supportive measures to maintain adequate platelet counts and correction of coagulopathy should decrease bleeding events, but this has not been shown in clinical studies.
   Renal dysfunction should be closely monitored in infants with birth asphyxia and medication doses adjusted
   Rating for the strength of the evidence: moderate

Summary statement: birth asphyxia leads to cardiovascular changes in heart rate, cardiac output, and vasoconstriction that lead to multiorgan failure. In the setting of therapeutic hypothermia, clinicians need to provide symptomatic support to other affected organ systems as the organs recover from the hypoperfusion event.

REFERENCES

1. Dawes GS. Foetal and neonatal physiology: a comparative study of the changes at birth. Chicago: Year Book Medical Publishers; 1968.

2. Cross KW. Resuscitation of the asphyxiated infant. Br Med Bull 1966;22(1):73–8.
3. Dawes GS, Jacobson HN, Mott JC, et al. Some observations on foetal and new-born rhesus monkeys. J Physiol 1960;152:271–98.
4. Wyllie J, Perlman JM, Kattwinkel J, et al. Part 7: neonatal resuscitation: 2015 International Consensus on Cardiopulmonary Resuscitation and Emergency Cardiovascular Care Science with Treatment Recommendations. Resuscitation 2015;95:e169–201.
5. Peeters LL, Sheldon RE, Jones MD Jr, et al. Blood flow to fetal organs as a function of arterial oxygen content. Am J Obstet Gynecol 1979;135(5):637–46.
6. Sheldon RE, Peeters LL, Jones MD Jr, et al. Redistribution of cardiac output and oxygen delivery in the hypoxemic fetal lamb. Am J Obstet Gynecol 1979;135(8): 1071–8.
7. Jensen A, Garnier Y, Berger R. Dynamics of fetal circulatory responses to hypoxia and asphyxia. Eur J Obstet Gynecol Reprod Biol 1999;84(2):155–72.
8. Gluckman PD, Wyatt JS, Azzopardi D, et al. Selective head cooling with mild systemic hypothermia after neonatal encephalopathy: multicentre randomised trial. Lancet 2005;365(9460):663–70.
9. Shankaran S, Laptook AR, Ehrenkranz RA, et al. Whole-body hypothermia for neonates with hypoxic-ischemic encephalopathy. N Engl J Med 2005;353(15): 1574–84.
10. Azzopardi DV, Strohm B, Edwards AD, et al. Moderate hypothermia to treat perinatal asphyxial encephalopathy. N Engl J Med 2009;361(14):1349–58.
11. Zhou WH, Cheng GQ, Shao XM, et al. Selective head cooling with mild systemic hypothermia after neonatal hypoxic-ischemic encephalopathy: a multicenter randomized controlled trial in China. J Pediatr 2010;157(3):367–72, 372.e1–3.
12. Wyllie J. Applied physiology of newborn resuscitation. Curr Paediatr 2006;16(6): 379–85.
13. Gupta JM, Tizard JP. The sequence of events in neonatal apnoea. Lancet 1967; 2(7506):55–9.
14. Low JA. Intrapartum fetal asphyxia: definition, diagnosis, and classification. Am J Obstet Gynecol 1997;176(5):957–9.
15. Wall SN, Lee AC, Carlo W, et al. Reducing intrapartum-related neonatal deaths in low- and middle-income countries–what works? Semin Perinatol 2010;34(6): 395–407.
16. Jensen A, Roman C, Rudolph AM. Effects of reducing uterine blood flow on fetal blood flow distribution and oxygen delivery. J Dev Physiol 1991;15(6):309–23.
17. Itskovitz J, LaGamma EF, Rudolph AM. Effects of cord compression on fetal blood flow distribution and O_2 delivery. Am J Physiol 1987;252(1 Pt 2):H100–9.
18. Zaichkin J, Weiner GM. Neonatal Resuscitation Program (NRP) 2011: new science, new strategies. Adv Neonatal Care 2011;11(1):43–51.
19. Lakshminrusimha S, Carrion V. Perinatal physiology and principles of neonatal resuscitation. Clin Pediatr Emerg Med 2008;9(3):131–9.
20. Bennet L, Rossenrode S, Gunning MI, et al. The cardiovascular and cerebrovascular responses of the immature fetal sheep to acute umbilical cord occlusion. J Physiol 1999;517(1):247–57.
21. Adamsons K, Behrman R, Dawes GS, et al. The treatment of acidosis with alkali and glucose during asphyxia in foetal rhesus monkeys. J Physiol 1963;169(3): 679–89.
22. Thakor AS, Giussani DA. Effects of acute acidemia on the fetal cardiovascular defense to acute hypoxemia. Am J Physiol Regul Integr Comp Physiol 2009;296(1): R90–9.

23. Reeves JT, Daoud FS, Eastin C. Effects of vagotomy on arterial pressure and blood gases in the fetal calf. Am J Physiol 1971;221:349–55.
24. Giussani DA, Spencer JA, Moore PJ, et al. Afferent and efferent components of the cardiovascular reflex responses to acute hypoxia in term fetal sheep. J Physiol 1993;461:431–49.
25. Blanco C, Dawes GS, Hanson MA, et al. Carotid baroreceptors in fetal and newborn sheep. Pediatr Res 1988;24(3):342–6.
26. Blanco C, Dawes GS, Hanson MA, et al. The response to hypoxia of arterial chemoreceptors in fetal sheep and new-born lambs. J Physiol 1984;351(1):25–37.
27. Parer J, Dijkstra HR, Vredebregt PP, et al. Increased fetal heart rate variability with acute hypoxia in chronically instrumented sheep. Eur J Obstet Gynecol Reprod Biol 1980;10(6):393–9.
28. Itskovitz J, LaGamma EF, Bristow J, et al. Cardiovascular responses to hypoxemia in sinoaortic-denervated fetal sheep. Pediatr Res 1991;30(4):381–7.
29. Born G, Dawes G, Mott JC. Oxygen lack and autonomic nervous control of the foetal circulation in the lamb. J Physiol 1956;134(1):149–66.
30. Dawes G, Jacobson HN, Mott JC, et al. The treatment of asphyxiated, mature foetal lambs and rhesus monkeys with intravenous glucose and sodium carbonate. J Physiol 1963;169(1):167–84.
31. Sobotka KS, Morley C, Ong T, et al. Circulatory responses to asphyxia differ if the asphyxia occurs in utero or ex utero in near-term lambs. PLoS One 2014;9(11): e112264.
32. Rudolph AM, Heymann MA. The circulation of the fetus in utero. Methods for studying distribution of blood flow, cardiac output and organ blood flow. Circ Res 1967;21(2):163–84.
33. Rudolph AM. Distribution and regulation of blood flow in the fetal and neonatal lamb. Circ Res 1985;57(6):811–21.
34. Cohn HE, Sacks EJ, Heymann MA, et al. Cardiovascular responses to hypoxemia and acidemia in fetal lambs. Am J Obstet Gynecol 1974;120(6):817–24.
35. Mulder AL, van Goor CA, Giussani DA, et al. Alpha-adrenergic contribution to the cardiovascular response to acute hypoxemia in the chick embryo. Am J Physiol Regul Integr Comp Physiol 2001;281(6):R2004–10.
36. Campbell A, Dawes GS, Fishman AP, et al. Pulmonary vasoconstriction and changes in heart rate during asphyxia in immature foetal lambs. J Physiol 1967;192(1):93.
37. Cassin S, Dawes G, Ross B. Pulmonary blood flow and vascular resistance in immature foetal lambs. J Physiol 1964;171(1):80–9.
38. Moore P, Hanson M. The role of peripheral chemoreceptors in the rapid response of the pulmonary vasculature of the late gestation sheep fetus to changes in PaO_2. J Dev Physiol 1991;16(3):133–8.
39. Van Bel F, Walther FJ. Myocardial dysfunction and cerebral blood flow velocity following birth asphyxia. Acta Paediatr Scand 1990;79(8–9):756–62.
40. Kenny J, Plappert T, Doubilet P, et al. Effects of heart rate on ventricular size, stroke volume, and output in the normal human fetus: a prospective Doppler echocardiographic study. Circulation 1987;76(1):52–8.
41. Gilbert RD. Control of fetal cardiac output during changes in blood volume. Am J Physiol 1980;238(1):H80–6.
42. Rudolph AM, Heyman M. Fetal and neonatal circulation and respiration. Annu Rev Physiol 1974;36(1):187–207.
43. Friedman WF. The intrinsic physiologic properties of the developing heart. Prog Cardiovasc Dis 1972;15(1):87–111.

44. Teitel D, Rudolph A. Perinatal oxygen delivery and cardiac function. Adv Pediatr 1984;32:321–47.
45. Pitlick PT, Kirkpatrick SE, Friedman WF. Distribution of fetal cardiac output: importance of pacemaker location. Am J Physiol 1976;231(1):204–8.
46. Kirkpatrick SE, Pitlick PT, Naliboff J, et al. Frank-Starling relationship as an important determinant of fetal cardiac output. Am J Physiol 1976;231(2):495–500.
47. Anderson P, Glick KL, Killam AP, et al. The effect of heart rate on in utero left ventricular output in the fetal sheep. J Physiol 1986;372(1):557–73.
48. Walther FJ, Siassi B, Ramadan NA, et al. Cardiac output in newborn infants with transient myocardial dysfunction. J Pediatr 1985;107(5):781–5.
49. Fisher DJ. Left ventricular oxygen consumption and function in hypoxemia in conscious lambs. Am J Physiol 1983;244(5):H664–71.
50. Sehgal A, Wong F, Mehta S. Reduced cardiac output and its correlation with coronary blood flow and troponin in asphyxiated infants treated with therapeutic hypothermia. Eur J Pediatr 2012;171(10):1511–7.
51. Costa S, Zecca E, De Rosa G, et al. Is serum troponin T a useful marker of myocardial damage in newborn infants with perinatal asphyxia? Acta Paediatr 2007;96(2):181–4.
52. Wei Y, Xu J, Xu T, et al. Left ventricular systolic function of newborns with asphyxia evaluated by tissue Doppler imaging. Pediatr Cardiol 2009;30(6):741–6.
53. Clark S, Newland P, Yoxall CW, et al. Cardiac troponin T in cord blood. Arch Dis Child Fetal Neonatal Ed 2001;84(1):F34–7.
54. Giesinger RE, McNamara PJ. Hemodynamic instability in the critically ill neonate: an approach to cardiovascular support based on disease pathophysiology. Semin Perinatol 2016;40(3):174–88.
55. Beath SV. Hepatic function and physiology in the newborn. Semin Neonatol 2003; 8(5):337–46.
56. Sarkar S, Barks JD, Bhagat I, et al. Effects of therapeutic hypothermia on multiorgan dysfunction in asphyxiated newborns: whole-body cooling versus selective head cooling. J Perinatol 2009;29(8):558–63.
57. Shah P, Riphagen S, Beyene J, et al. Multiorgan dysfunction in infants with post-asphyxial hypoxic-ischaemic encephalopathy. Arch Dis Child Fetal Neonatal Ed 2004;89(2):F152–5.
58. Islam MT, Islam MN, Mollah AH, et al. Status of liver enzymes in babies with perinatal asphyxia. Mymensingh Med J 2011;20(3):446–9.
59. Karlsson M, Satas S, Stone J, et al. Liver enzymes cannot be used to predict liver damage after global hypoxia-ischemia in a neonatal pig model. Neonatology 2009;96(4):211–8.
60. Chessells JM, Wigglesworth JS. Coagulation studies in severe birth asphyxia. Arch Dis Child 1971;46(247):253–6.
61. Chadd MA, Elwood PC, Gray OP, et al. Coagulation defects in hypoxic full-term newborn infants. Br Med J 1971;4(5786):516–8.
62. Suzuki S, Morishita S. Hypercoagulability and DIC in high-risk infants. Semin Thromb Hemost 1998;24(5):463–6.
63. Neary E, McCallion N, Kevane B, et al. Coagulation indices in very preterm infants from cord blood and postnatal samples. J Thromb Haemost 2015;13(11): 2021–30.
64. Dirkmann D, Hanke AA, Görlinger K, et al. Hypothermia and acidosis synergistically impair coagulation in human whole blood. Anesth Analg 2008;106(6): 1627–32.

65. Lindenblatt N, Menger MD, Klar E, et al. Sustained hypothermia accelerates microvascular thrombus formation in mice. Am J Physiol Heart Circ Physiol 2005;289(6):H2680–7.

66. Forman KR, Diab Y, Wong EC, et al. Coagulopathy in newborns with hypoxic ischemic encephalopathy (HIE) treated with therapeutic hypothermia: a retrospective case-control study. BMC Pediatr 2014;14:277.

67. Stanworth SJ, Clarke P, Watts T, et al. Prospective, observational study of outcomes in neonates with severe thrombocytopenia. Pediatrics 2009;124(5): e826–34.

68. Christensen RD, Baer VL, Yaish HM. Thrombocytopenia in late preterm and term neonates after perinatal asphyxia. Transfusion 2015;55(1):187–96.

69. McDonald TP, Cottrell MB, Clift RE, et al. Effects of hypoxia on megakaryocyte size and number of C3H and BALB/c mice. Proc Soc Exp Biol Med 1992; 199(3):287–90.

70. Saxonhouse MA, Rimsza LM, Stevens G, et al. Effects of hypoxia on megakaryocyte progenitors obtained from the umbilical cord blood of term and preterm neonates. Biol Neonate 2006;89(2):104–8.

71. Bauman ME, Cheung PY, Massicotte MP. Hemostasis and platelet dysfunction in asphyxiated neonates. J Pediatr 2011;158(2 Suppl):e35–9.

72. Josephson CD, Su LL, Christensen RD, et al. Platelet transfusion practices among neonatologists in the United States and Canada: results of a survey. Pediatrics 2009;123(1):278–85.

73. Josephson CD, Glynn SA, Kleinman SH, et al. A multidisciplinary "think tank": the top 10 clinical trial opportunities in transfusion medicine from the National Heart, Lung, and Blood Institute-sponsored 2009 state-of-the-science symposium. Transfusion 2011;51(4):828–41.

74. Carr R, Kelly AM, Williamson LM. Neonatal thrombocytopenia and platelet transfusion - a UK perspective. Neonatology 2015;107(1):1–7.

75. Gibson BE, Todd A, Roberts I, et al. Transfusion guidelines for neonates and older children. Br J Haematol 2004;124(4):433–53.

76. Curley A, Venkatesh V, Stanworth S, et al. Platelets for neonatal transfusion - study 2: a randomised controlled trial to compare two different platelet count thresholds for prophylactic platelet transfusion to preterm neonates. Neonatology 2014; 106(2):102–6.

77. Durkan AM, Alexander RT. Acute kidney injury post neonatal asphyxia. J Pediatr 2011;158(2 Suppl):e29–33.

78. Selewski DT, Charlton JR, Jetton JG, et al. Neonatal acute kidney injury. Pediatrics 2015;136(2):e463–73.

79. Vanpee M, Blennow M, Linné T, et al. Renal function in very low birth weight infants: normal maturity reached during early childhood. J Pediatr 1992;121(5 Pt 1):784–8.

80. Karlowicz MG, Adelman RD. Nonoliguric and oliguric acute renal failure in asphyxiated term neonates. Pediatr Nephrol 1995;9(6):718–22.

81. Agras PI, Tarcan A, Baskin E, et al. Acute renal failure in the neonatal period. Ren Fail 2004;26(3):305–9.

82. Kaur S, Jain S, Saha A, et al. Evaluation of glomerular and tubular renal function in neonates with birth asphyxia. Ann Trop Paediatr 2011;31(2):129–34.

83. Aggarwal A, Kumar P, Chowdhary G, et al. Evaluation of renal functions in asphyxiated newborns. J Trop Pediatr 2005;51(5):295–9.

84. Sarkar S, Askenazi DJ, Jordan BK, et al. Relationship between acute kidney injury and brain MRI findings in asphyxiated newborns after therapeutic hypothermia. Pediatr Res 2014;75(3):431–5.
85. Askenazi DJ, Ambalavanan N, Goldstein SL. Acute kidney injury in critically ill newborns: what do we know? what do we need to learn? Pediatr Nephrol 2009;24(2):265–74.
86. Gupta C, Massaro AN, Ray PE. A new approach to define acute kidney injury in term newborns with hypoxic ischemic encephalopathy. Pediatr Nephrol 2016; 31(7):1167–78.
87. Sweetman DU, Molloy EJ. Biomarkers of acute kidney injury in neonatal encephalopathy. Eur J Pediatr 2013;172(3):305–16.
88. Essajee F, Were F, Admani B. Urine neutrophil gelatinase-associated lipocalin in asphyxiated neonates: a prospective cohort study. Pediatr Nephrol 2015;30(7): 1189–96.
89. Sutherland SM, Zappitelli M, Alexander SR, et al. Fluid overload and mortality in children receiving continuous renal replacement therapy: the prospective pediatric continuous renal replacement therapy registry. Am J Kidney Dis 2010;55(2): 316–25.
90. Al-Wassia H, Alshaikh B, Sauve R. Prophylactic theophylline for the prevention of severe renal dysfunction in term and post-term neonates with perinatal asphyxia: a systematic review and meta-analysis of randomized controlled trials. J Perinatol 2013;33(4):271–7.
91. Goldberg RN, Thomas DW, Sinatra FR. Necrotizing enterocolitis in the asphyxiated full-term infant. Am J Perinatol 1983;1(1):40–2.
92. Thornton KM, Dai H, Septer S, et al. Effects of whole body therapeutic hypothermia on gastrointestinal morbidity and feeding tolerance in infants with hypoxic ischemic encephalopathy. Int J Pediatr 2014;2014:643689.
93. Grenz A, Clambey E, Eltzschig HK. Hypoxia signaling during intestinal ischemia and inflammation. Curr Opin Crit Care 2012;18(2):178–85.

Neonatal Encephalopathy

Update on Therapeutic Hypothermia and Other Novel Therapeutics

Ryan M. McAdams, MD*, Sandra E. Juul, MD, PhD

KEYWORDS

- Dexmedetomidine • Erythropoietin • Melatonin • N-acetylcysteine
- Neurodevelopment • Stem cells • Umbilical cord milking • Xenon

KEY POINTS

- Although limited in number, the available long-term follow-up studies of neonates with neonatal encephalopathy (NE) treated with therapeutic hypothermia (TH) demonstrate sustained benefits through middle childhood.
- Neonates with severe NE remain at high risk for death and disability despite treatment with TH, emphasizing the need for adjunctive neuroprotective treatments.
- Clinical trials of erythropoietin neuroprotection have raised no safety concerns, and suggest that erythropoietin treatment plus TH may improve neurologic outcomes in neonates with NE.
- Although preclinical trials seemed promising, the benefits of xenon, melatonin, and stem cell therapies in neonates with NE treated with TH need to be clarified.
- Studies investigating clinical management strategies in neonates with NE, such as umbilical cord milking and sedative, antiepileptics, and pressor medications are needed to optimize outcomes.

INTRODUCTION

Intrapartum hypoxic events are a major cause of neonatal mortality responsible for approximately 1 in 5 of all neonatal deaths worldwide, causing an estimated 717,000 deaths in 2010.[1] Intrapartum-related hypoxic events ("birth asphyxia") may result in neonatal encephalopathy (NE), defined as a disturbance of neurologic function evident in the first days after birth in a newborn, characterized by a subnormal level of consciousness and depressed tone and reflexes, with or without seizures and

The authors have no conflict of interest, financial support, or other potential conflicts of interest to declare.
Division of Neonatology, Department of Pediatrics, University of Washington, Box 356320, Seattle, WA 98195-6320, USA
* Corresponding author.
E-mail address: mcadams@uw.edu

often with impaired respiration and feeding abilities (both of presumed central origin).[2] NE is characterized as mild, moderate, or severe based on the Sarnat scoring system.[3] Neonates with moderate to severe NE who survive are at risk for motor disabilities and long-term neurodevelopmental impairments, including cognitive, neuropsychological, educational, and behavioral problems.[4,5] Although preterm infants are at even higher risk of NE than term infants, this review is restricted to discussion of term and near term infants.

Throughout this article, we use the terms NE and hypoxic ischemic encephalopathy (HIE) interchangeably to describe the published studies discussed in this review. Although debate continues over which of these terms to use,[6,7] HIE specifically refers to encephalopathy associated with intrapartum injury from hypoxia and ischemia, mechanisms that can be difficult to prove, whereas NE is a broader term denoting a syndrome of neurologic disturbance owing to an intrapartum hypoxic insult or other causes.[2]

Considerable research has been conducted in the past decade on NE as demonstrated by the co-word analysis study by Huang and colleagues,[8] which identified 1892 scientific studies (1568 articles and 324 reviews) that included the cooccurrence of keywords related to HIE published between January 2005 to December 2014 in the Web of Science database. Multiple randomized controlled trials (RCTs) have investigated induced hypothermia for newborns with NE, which has led to therapeutic hypothermia (TH) becoming a standard treatment for newborns 36 weeks of gestation or greater with NE related to intrapartum hypoxic events.[9,10] Although TH seems to be effective at improving outcomes, neonates with severe NE remain at significant risk of death or severe neurodevelopmental impairment despite being cooled, emphasizing the urgent need for additional adjunctive treatment strategies.

This review discusses the evidence supporting TH for term or near term neonates with NE, including findings of recent long-term outcome studies. Clinical strategies and novel adjunctive therapies to augment neurodevelopmental outcomes for neonates with NE who receive TH are also discussed.

CLINICAL TRIALS OF THE BENEFITS OF THERAPEUTIC HYPOTHERMIA FOR NEONATAL ENCEPHALOPATHY

Numerous RCTs have investigated the benefit of TH for improving outcomes of newborns with NE.[11–21] TH methods for NE include whole body and selective head cooling, with both methods demonstrating similar effects regarding long-term neurologic outcomes based on metaanalysis.[22]

A recent Cochrane systematic metaanalysis review by Jacobs and colleagues[23] included 11 RCTs, comprising 1505 term and late preterm infants with moderate to severe encephalopathy and evidence of intrapartum asphyxia. This Cochrane review demonstrated that TH resulted in improvement of the primary outcome measure of less death and better neurodevelopmental outcomes for survivors. Findings from 8 of the 11 studies (1344 infants) demonstrated that TH decreased the combined outcome of mortality or major neurodevelopmental disability to 18 months of age (46% [312/678] vs 61% [409/666] in controls; typical risk ratio (RR), 0.75; 95% CI, 0.68–0.83; typical risk difference (RD) −0.15; 95% CI, −0.20 to −0.10).[11–18] The number needed to treat (NNT) to benefit 1 newborn is 7 (95% CI, 5–10).

Secondary outcomes of the Cochrane review included mortality, major neurodevelopmental disability, adverse effects of cooling, and additional indicators of neurodevelopmental outcome (eg, severity of electroencephalographic abnormality, seizures, MRI findings).

Eleven studies (1468 infants) supported a decreased mortality with TH (25% [186/736] vs 34% [250/732] in controls; typical RR, 0.75; 95% CI, 0.64–0.88; typical RD, −0.09; 95% CI, −0.13 to −0.04), for an NNT of 11 (95% CI, 8–25).[11–21] Findings from 8 studies (917 infants) demonstrated that TH decreases neurodevelopmental disability in infants who survived (26% [130/495] vs 39% [166/422] in controls; typical RR, 0.77; 95% CI, 0.63–0.94; typical RD −0.13; 95% CI, −0.19 to −0.07), for an NNT of 8 (95% CI, 5–14).[11–18] Based on the available RCT studies, TH seems to increase survival without increasing major disability in survivors.

Metaanalysis of Adverse Effects of Cooling

Significant adverse effects that can occur as a result of TH include sinus bradycardia (heart rate <80 bpm), which occurred in 5% of infants (62/1292; RR, 11.59; 95% CI, 4.94–27.17; RD, 0.09; 95% CI, 0.07–0.11), for an NNT of 11,[11–16,18,21] and thrombocytopenia (platelet counts <150 × 10^9/L), which occurred in 31% of infants (438/1392; RR, 1.21; 95% CI, 1.05–1.40; RD, 0.06; 95% CI, 0.02–0.10), for an NNT of 17 (95% CI, 10–50).[11–18] Based on the Cochrane metaanalysis review, TH was not associated with a significant increase in major cardiac arrhythmia, hypotension (mean arterial pressure <40 mm Hg), or need for blood pressure support with inotropic agents.

One challenge for neonatal care providers assessing newborns with suspected intrapartum hypoxic events is that not all babies with brain injury are symptomatic after birth. Some newborns who may be depressed at birth seem to recover adequately, but then become symptomatic, manifesting seizure activity after the 6-hour postbirth window when TH is typically offered. Recognizing and treating these at-risk neonates remains a challenge and requires further research to establish reliable biomarkers to accurately identify these neonates in a timely manner.

Long-term Outcomes

There are a limited number of long-term follow-up studies assessing the sustained benefits of TH on reducing death and cognitive or motor disabilities later in childhood.

At the time of this review, long-term outcome data were available on 379 of the 1505 infants (25.2%) included in the Cochrane metaanalysis review.[23–26] Shankaran and colleagues[13] reported long-term outcome data on 190 of 208 child participants (91.3%) in the US National Institute of Child Health and Human Development study who were assessed subsequently at the ages of 6 to 7 years.[24] The primary outcome of death or an IQ of less than 70, which had been significant at 18 to 22 months of age, was lower in the TH group (46 of 97 children; 47%) compared with the control group (58 of 93 children; 62%), but no longer significant (RR in TH group, 0.78; 95% CI, 0.61–1.01). Death remained significantly lower in the TH group (28% vs 44% of controls; $P = .04$) as did death or severe disability (41% vs 60% of controls; $P = .03$). There was no difference in moderate or severe disability (35% of TH group vs 38% of controls; $P = .87$) or rates of cerebral palsy (CP; 17% of TH group vs 29% of controls; $P = .14$). Based on this study, it seems that TH increases survival without increasing major disability, rates of an IQ score of less than 70, or CP in surviving children.

Another follow-up study that assessed children at the ages of 6 to 7 years was published by Azzopardi and colleagues,[25] who reported data from 127 of 325 newborn infants (39%) originally enrolled in the European Total Body Hypothermia for Neonatal Encephalopathy (TOBY) RCT. At 18 months, children in the TOBY trial who had received TH had reduced risks of CP and better Mental Developmental Index and Psychomotor Developmental Index scores based on Bayley Scales of Infant

Development II.[14] At 6 to 7 years of age, children who had received TH (75 of 145; 52%) had a significantly higher frequency of survival with an IQ score of 85 or higher, compared with children not treated with TH (52 of 132; 39%), which was the primary study outcome (RR, 1.31; $P = .04$).[25] The percent of children who died in the TH group (29%) and the control group (30%) were similar. However, among the children who survived, normal neurologic outcomes were more common in the TH group (65 of 145; 45%) compared with the control group (37 of 132 [28%]; RR, 1.60; 95% confidence interval, 1.15–2.22). The risk for CP was significantly lower in surviving children from the TH group (21%) compared with the control group (36%). Children from the TH groups also had less moderate or severe disability (22%) than the control group (37%).

Similar to the TOBY trial, follow-up of children from the Cool Cap trial demonstrated that 18-month neurodevelopmental assessments are predictive of long-term functional outcomes. Guillet and colleagues[26] reported outcomes on 62 (32 cooled; 30 controls) of 135 surviving children (46%) enrolled in the Cool Cap trial who were reassessed at 7 to 8 years of age. Using the Functional Independence Measure for Children (WeeFIM) to measure self-care, mobility, and cognitive function qualitatively, this follow-up analysis demonstrated that disability status at 18 months was strongly associated with WeeFIM ratings at 7 to 8 years of age ($P<.001$), supporting a sustained treatment effect of TH for NE. However, this follow-up study had insufficient power to determine whether treatment with TH affected long-term outcome.

Cooling Duration and Depth

The standard of care for full-term neonates with moderate or severe NE is to initiate TH within 6 hours of birth for a 72-hour duration to a depth of 33.0°C to 34.0°C.[27] However, not all neonates with moderate, and most with severe, NE do not benefit from TH. Because animal studies suggest that extending TH beyond 72 hours and below 33.5°C may provide increased neuroprotection,[28] a trial was conducted in human neonates to determine whether TH for a longer duration and at a greater depth might show further benefit.

The National Institute of Child Health and Human Development trial by Shankaran and colleagues[29] studied the effects of longer and deeper cooling in full-term neonates with moderate or severe HIE. The trial was stopped early, owing to safety and futility concerns, with 364 neonates enrolled (of 726 planned). Analysis of the predefined secondary outcomes, safety, and deaths in the neonatal intensive care unit, was done by marginal comparisons of 72 hours versus 120 hours duration and 33.5°C depth versus 32.0°C depth (predefined secondary outcomes). Both longer and deeper cooling were associated with increased mortality. Death rates increased from 7% (7 of 95 neonates) to 16% (15 of 96 neonates) when cooling at 33.5°C was extended from 72 to 120 hours. Similarly, death rates increased from 14% (13 of 90 neonates) to 17% (14 of 83 neonates) when cooling at 32.0°C was extended from 72 hours to 120 hours. The adjusted RR for deaths in the neonatal intensive care unit for the 120-hour group versus the 72-hour group was 1.37 (95% CI, 0.92–2.04) and for the 32.0°C group versus 33.5°C group was 1.24 (95% CI, 0.69–2.25). Future analyses will determine the primary outcome of death or disability at 18 to 22 months. Although this trial was stopped early, available results suggest that more is not necessarily better regarding the effect of duration and depth of TH on survival.

Cooling Newborns Who Do Not Meet Standard Cooling Criteria

Current clinical standards for TH were derived from RCTs that used strict study entry criteria. To practice evidence-based medicine, most centers offering TH for neonates with NE adhere to treatment protocols based on similar criteria developed by published RCTs.[9] However, like many practices in medicine, therapeutic drift has occurred such that patients not quite meeting entry criteria for cooling are still treated, or cooling protocols are not strictly followed. For example, in the TOBY trial, in 2.2% of infants (29/1331), cooling was initiated at greater than 12 postnatal hours, and 65% of subjects (887/1368) were cooled to less than 33°C with 4% (61/1368) reaching temperatures less than 31°C at some point. Allowing initiation of TH up to 12 hours after birth for neonates with suspected NE has been advocated given the potential for benefit, the low risk of TH, and limited alternative treatment options.[30]

An observational study by Smit and colleagues[31] analyzed prospective data on 165 infants collected over a 6-year period in a regional cooling center (St Michael's Hospital, Bristol, UK) to compare complications and outcomes between infants who were cooled despite not fulfilling the standard inclusion and exclusion criteria as set out in the CoolCap/TOBY protocol (n = 36; 21%) and infants who fulfilled the standard entry criteria (n = 129).

Cooled infants not meeting standard entry criteria included infants cooled greater than 6 postnatal hours (n = 11), late preterm infants (n = 6), and infants with postnatal collapse (n = 10), major cranial hemorrhage (n = 5), congenital cardiac disease (n = 2), and surgical conditions (n = 2). In the 11 infants cooled at greater than 6 postnatal hours, cooling was started at a median age of 7.8 hours (interquartile range, 6.8–8.5), and target temperature was reached at a median time of 10.5 hours (interquartile range, 10–15). The mean gestational age of the 6 late preterm that received TH was 34^{+6} weeks (range, 34^{+0} to 35^{+4}). In the infants not fulfilling compared with those fulfilling the cooling entry criteria, 11% (4 of 36) versus 16% (20 of 129) died and 33% (9 of 27 assessed) versus 29% (22 of 76 assessed) had a Mental Developmental Index and/or Psychomotor Developmental Index score of less than 70. A combined poor outcome of death or disability at 18 months occurred in 44% of infants cooled not fulfilling the entry criteria compared with 45% who did meet entry criteria. All 5 infants with major cranial hemorrhage had coagulation abnormalities and 80% (4 of 5) died or had disability.

Although the study by Smit and colleagues provides insight into patients not fulfilling the standard TH treatment criteria, this small study was observational, which precludes the ability to make any strong conclusions about patients that deviate from current evidence-based practices. Based on the multiple available RCTs, TH (33.5°C to 34.5°C) for 72 hours seems to be effective and safe when used to treat newborns 36 weeks of gestational age or greater with moderate to severe NE. It is not advisable to deviate from this proven protocol because such deviations may result in increased adverse outcomes, as shown by Shankaran and colleagues[29] investigating longer duration and deeper TH.

When caring for critically ill infants with suspected brain injury, the practitioner is often placed in a time-sensitive conundrum of trying to decide who to offer TH to and who not to treat. In these scenarios, the desire to do good may lead to harm, emphasizing the importance of understanding the infrequent but serious risks that may exist by treating newborns outside of standard TH guidelines, risks that typically require well-designed, properly powered studies to be revealed.

ADJUNCTIVE NEUROPROTECTIVE TREATMENTS PLUS THERAPEUTIC HYPOTHERMIA
Erythropoietin

Erythropoietin (Epo), a glycoprotein originally identified for its role in erythropoiesis, has remarkable neuroprotective and reparative effects in the central nervous system.[32–37] Epo functions by binding to its homodimeric cell surface receptor. Epo receptors are expressed by multiple cell types in the central nervous system,[38,39] including neuronal progenitor cells,[35] subsets of mature neurons,[40] astrocytes,[41] oligodendrocytes,[41–43] microglia,[44] and endothelial cells.[35] Epo is expressed in brain, primarily by astrocytes. In the setting of hypoxia–ischemia, Epo receptor expression is upregulated rapidly, with Epo production increasing only if significant hypoxia is prolonged. If Epo is available to bind to the upregulated receptor, cell survival is promoted; however, in the absence of Epo, the pathway of programmed cell death predominates.[45,46] This creates an important rationale for exogenous Epo administration, given that upregulation of Epo may take several hours, whereas brain injury can occur after brief but catastrophic insults that are insufficient to stimulate an increase in endogenous Epo synthesis.[47]

Preclinical studies of Epo neuroprotection after hypoxic–ischemic brain injury show robust histologic and functional evidence for benefit.[43,48–57] Epo has both early and late beneficial effects. Early benefits include antiapoptotic and antiinflammatory effects,[58–62] whereas later effects include increased neurogenesis, oligodendrogenesis, and angiogenesis, all of which contribute to tissue remodeling after hypoxia–ischemia.[63–67] In nonhuman primates, Epo reduces the combined outcome of death or CP, and improves neurologic function in animals undergoing TH for HIE.[68] Although insufficiently powered to prove efficacy, phase I and II clinical trials of Epo neuroprotection raise no safety concerns, and suggest that infants with HIE treated with multiple doses of Epo during the first week of life have better neurologic outcomes.[69,70] The High-Dose Erythropoietin for Neuroprotection in Neonatal Encephalopathy (NEAT) and Neonatal Erythropoietin And Therapeutic Outcomes in Newborn Brain Injury (NEATO) trials (https://clinicaltrials.gov, NCT00719407 and NCT01913340) have demonstrated safety, feasibility,[71] and beneficial outcomes as measured by early MRI, biomarkers, 6 month, and 1- and 2-year outcomes (even among infants with significant brain injury seen on MRI).[72,73] Epo is available commercially and safe in infants. Several phase III trials are now in the planning or early stages of execution internationally (PAEAN [Preventing Adverse Outcomes of Neonatal Hypoxic Ischaemic Encephalopathy with Erythropoietin], HEAL [High-dose Epo for Asphyxia and Encephalopathy]).

Xenon

Xenon, a noble gas that crosses the placenta and the blood–brain barrier, binds to N-methyl-D-aspartate glutamate receptors to inhibit function, thus decreasing neuronal apoptosis.[74,75] Significant benefit was demonstrated in preclinical studies of HIE,[76] so a multicenter Total Body hypothermia plus Xenon (TOBY-Xe) trial was conducted in the UK. Ninety-two infants (36–43 weeks) were enrolled, 46 of whom were randomly assigned to cooling only and 46 to xenon plus cooling.[77] The primary outcomes were assessment of reduced thalamic lactate to N-acetyl aspartate (NAA) ratios measured with magnetic resonance (MR) spectroscopy and preserved fractional anisotropy in the posterior limb of the internal capsule determined by MRI within 15 days of birth. Lactate to NAA ratios have been demonstrated to be good predictive imaging biomarker of neurodevelopmental outcomes.[78] Changes in fractional anisotropy, a measure of brain connectivity derived from the diffusion tensor imaging that assesses the degree of regional anisotropic diffusion, correlate well with subsequent outcomes in neonates with HIE.[79] The TOBY-Xe trial was underpowered to detect changes in the lactate to NAA ratios, but well-powered to detect changes in fractional anisotropy. Although no serious adverse events were recorded, no MR differences were detected between groups. Based on the MR results of 37 infants in the cooling only group and 41 in the cooling plus xenon group, early TH plus treatment with 30% xenon for 24 hours begun greater than 6 hours after birth combined are not likely to improve clinical outcomes compared with TH alone for newborns with NE. Multiple factors that may impact inhaled xenon treatment outcomes, including the timing, dose, and duration of treatment, need further study. Study results of the CoolXenon3 Study (https://clinicaltrials.gov, NCT02071394) combining TH with 18 hours of xenon inhalation in cooled infants with HIE are pending.

Melatonin

Melatonin (N-acetyl-5-methoxytryptamine), a neurohormone derived from the amino acid tryptophan and secreted by the pineal gland, is a strong antioxidant capable of scavenging free radicals and stimulating several antioxidative enzymes, including glutathione, glutathione reductase, peroxidase, and superoxide dismutase.[80] Melatonin can directly stimulate cellular membrane G protein-coupled high-affinity melatonin receptors (melatonin receptors 1 and 2) that activate numerous second messenger cascades, which vary in cell-, tissue-, and species-specific ways, and also induce receptor-independent intracellular activities by targeting calcium-binding proteins, cytoskeletal and scaffold proteins, and components of mitochondrial signaling.[81] Melatonin's safety profile and antioxidant, antiinflammatory, and antiapoptotic properties have made it an attractive neuroprotective candidate for treating neonates with NE.[82,83]

The postnatal neuroprotective benefits of melatonin have been demonstrated in an HIE piglet model, in which intravenous melatonin plus TH significantly improved cerebral energy metabolism based on proton MR spectroscopy studies, reduced apoptosis in deep brain structures, and decreased microglial activation in the cortex at 48 hours after injury.[45] In uncooled full term human newborns with NE (n = 10), oral melatonin (8 doses of 10 mg each separated by 2-hour intervals) administration within the first 6 hours after delivery reduced serum malondialdehyde, a lipid peroxidation product, and nitrite/nitrate levels at 12 and 24 hours compared with untreated, uncooled controls (n = 10), suggesting a role for melatonin in reducing oxidative damage.[84] In a recent prospective trial by Aly and colleagues,[85] involving 45 term newborns, 30 with HIE and 15 healthy controls, compared with TH alone (n = 15), melatonin (10 mg/kg daily × 5 enteral doses) plus TH (n = 15) was associated with decreased seizures per electroencephalographic monitoring and decreased white matter abnormalities on MRI after 2 weeks of age and improved survival without neurologic or developmental abnormalities at 6 months of age ($P<.001$).[85]

Melatonin remains an attractive potential antenatal neuroprotectant that could be administered to pregnant mothers because it seems to be safe, crosses the placenta,[86] and crosses the blood–brain barrier (based on adult rat studies).[87] Further research is needed to clarify the mechanisms by which the pleiotropic neurohormone melatonin may regulate neuronal cell survival, brain tissue homeostasis, and neuroprotection in neonates with NE.

2-Iminobiotin

The biotin (vitamin B_7) analog 2-iminobiotin (2-IB) is a combined neuronal and inducible (but not endothelial) nitric oxide synthase inhibitor that has been demonstrated to improve neuroprotection in animal models of HIE.[46,88,89] Although the exact mechanism of action has yet to be defined, 2-IB potentially protects against hypoxic–ischemic brain damage by preventing nitric oxide or peroxynitrite-induced mitochondrial damage.[89] Interestingly, after cerebral hypoxia–ischemia, the 2-IB treatment response seems to be gender dependent, with neuroprotection demonstrated in female, but not male immature P3 rats.[47,90]

A small phase II pilot trial (n = 6) of neonates at least 36 and less than 44 weeks' gestation with moderate to severe HIE has been completed in Turkey (https://clinicaltrials.gov, NCT01626924). Study subjects were enrolled within 6 hours after birth and received 6 pulse doses of 2-IB within 20 hours. The primary study outcomes include the basal ganglia lactate/NAA ratio as measured by single or multiple voxel MR spectroscopy and the composite endpoint of survival at 48 hours with a normal ambulatory electroencephalogram. To explore the short-term safety and tolerability of 2-IB and the pharmacokinetic profile of 2-IB when given on top of TH, a related phase II trial, the 2-STEP study, will be performed in the Netherlands (www.trialregister.nl/trialreg/admin/rctview.asp?TC=5221).

Physiologic Placental Transfusion

Delayed cord clamping (DCC) and umbilical cord milking (UCM) are 2 methods of augmenting redistribution of blood from the placenta back to the newborn after fetal delivery. In preterm infants, both DCC (delaying cord clamping for 30–60 seconds) and UCM (stripping the unclamped umbilical cord toward the infant) have been associated with decreased hypotension requiring volume expanders and a decreased need for inotrope support after delivery, as well as decreased intraventricular hemorrhage of all grades.[91,92] DCC and UCM have not been studied in the context of newborns 36 weeks' gestation or greater with NE. The current practice in depressed newborns suspected of having an intrapartum hypoxic event is to immediately clamp the umbilical cord, making DCC, which is typically performed over 1 to 3 minutes after delivery in term infants, an unlikely option for health care providers eager to initiate neonatal resuscitation.

However, in depressed newborns with NE, it is not clear if immediate cord clamping has a beneficial or adverse effect on an already compromised cardiovascular system. Immediate cord clamping may not be ideal in newborns with NE who have inadequate pulmonary ventilation, are severely bradycardic, and who are at risk for hypovolemic shock. UCM, which can be performed in less than 10 seconds, may provide a beneficial strategy to augment cardiac preload by promoting placental to fetal transfusion. Although clinical trials studying the potential benefits of placental transfusion strategies may be challenging to conduct in newborns with NE, UCM techniques with unclamped or immediately clamped and milked cords may provide a strategy to increase placental transfusion and allow for prompt neonatal resuscitation.[93,94] Studies looking at the role of placental transfusion as the first therapeutic intervention after delivery of a newborn (eg, https://clinicaltrials.gov, NCT02287077) with NE are warranted.

Stem Cells

Stem cell therapies seem to hold significant potential for newborns with NE based on animal data demonstrating neuroprotection from hypoxic ischemic brain injury.[95] Umbilical cord blood (UCB) and tissue derived (Wharton jelly) cells, which contain endothelial progenitor cells,[96] mesenchymal stem cells,[97,98] and UCB-mononuclear cells,[99] are an attractive therapy given their ease of acquisition from cord blood at birth.

Neural stemlike cells have been derived from human UCBs[100]; however, whether these UCB-derived progenitors may be effectively differentiated into functional neuronlike cells in human newborns with brain injury remains unknown.

In a recent study, Cotten and colleagues[101] reported on 23 infants 35 weeks' gestation or greater with NE who received TH fresh autologous UCB cells. This study demonstrated safety and feasibility of UCB cell administration in cooled newborns with NE, but was not able to provide definitive conclusions regarding long-term neurodevelopmental outcomes or mortality. Current ongoing clinical trials (https://clinicaltrials.gov, NCT01962233, NCT00593242, and NCT01506258) will further inform us of potential clinical outcomes. Future research will hopefully improve our understanding of stem cell-associated cellular mechanisms that may be involved in neuronal protection, rescue, or repair in the contest of TH. Although stem cell therapies for NE hold promise, numerous preclinical questions need to be addressed regarding the optimal stem cell type, delivery route, therapeutic window, safety profile, and short- and long-term outcomes before stem cell therapy is used in routine clinical practice.

N-Acetylcysteine

N-Acetylcysteine (NAC), a membrane-permeable cysteine precursor, is a free radical scavenger and major contributor to cellular maintenance of glutathione that has shown promise as an emerging treatment of adult vascular and nonvascular neurologic disorders.[102] In a neonatal rodent model (P7 rats) of hypoxic ischemic brain injury, NAC plus TH reduced brain volume loss with increased myelin expression and improved reflexes.[103] Further research in a rabbit model of CP has shown that conjugating NAC to a polyamidoamine dendrimer, a synthetic biomimic of globular proteins that can function as a drug delivery vehicle, is more effective than systemically administered free NAC.[104] Information on the NAC-associated neuroprotection for neonates with NE is lacking.

Clinical Management Strategies

Along with seizures, neonates with NE frequently demonstrate cardiovascular instability evidenced by hypotension, metabolic acidosis, and pulmonary hypertension. Unlike the more standardized TH guidelines, clinical approaches regarding antiepileptic use, fluid resuscitation, pressor support (including hydrocortisone treatment), the use of base replacement (eg, sodium bicarbonate), ventilation strategies, oxygen saturation targets, inhaled nitric oxide use, and blood transfusion parameters may all influence outcomes in the setting of TH.

Additionally, the use of medications to provide sedation and prevent shivering in cooled newborns with NE needs to be studied. The current use of morphine during TH is not evidence based and may not be ideal owing to its side effect profile (eg, respiratory depression, urinary retention, constipation) and because it does not specifically prevent shivering. Dexmedetomidine (DEX) and clonidine, both α2-adrenergic receptor agonists, are promising alternative sedatives because they specifically prevent shivering without suppressing respirations. DEX reduces inflammation,[105,106] does not produce abnormal brain histology (neonatal rats),[107] and produces neuroprotection in animal models of HIE.[108–110] Currently, trials to assess the pharmacokinetics and safety of DEX (Cool DEX study, NCT02529202) and clonidine (NCT02252848) in newborns with NE during TH are underway.

SUMMARY

Preventing NE related brain injury remains a monumental problem, because there is currently no way to predict whom NE will affect or when they will be affected. Although animal models often demonstrate effective prenatal pharmacologic treatments, this approach is often not feasible because NE is a postinjury event diagnosis. Whether safe and effective treatments (eg, melatonin) could be adminis-tered prophylactically to all pregnant mothers requires further investigation. Deciding which infants need cooling, how long to cool, and the method of cooling remain important unanswered questions. In addition to further analysis of existing data (eg, metaanalyses), to better understand the pathophysiology and how to treat NE, ongoing research is needed to assess biomarkers and different therapeutic interventions.

A tremendous amount of effort and sound research led to the establishment of TH as the standard of care for neonates with NE, yet many questions remain unan-swered regarding this treatment. Although neonates with NE typically present with a common phenotype, which can be classified by Sarnat scoring, a myriad of acute and chronic in utero events may contribute to this phenotype. Our inability to identify the diverse and complex events that precede the manifestation of NE in human new-borns is a contributing factor that may explain why effective neuroprotective treat-ments in animal models may not translate into clinical practice. Countless newborns had died or been devastated by NE and millions worldwide remain at risk for death and disability from NE despite the capabilities of modern-day medicine. The concerted efforts of researchers and funding agencies to develop effective ther-apeutic strategies that can be combined with TH is needed to mitigate this perpetual tragedy.

Best practices

What is the current practice?

Therapeutic hypothermia is the standard treatment for newborns 36 weeks of gestation or greater with moderate to severe neonatal encephalopathy related to intrapartum hypoxic events.

What changes in current practice are likely to improve outcomes?

Therapeutic hypothermia plus adjunctive neuroprotective treatments, (eg, erythropoietin, melatonin, stem cell therapies) and optimal clinical practice strategies are needed to improve survival and outcomes of newborns with moderate and severe.

Is there a Clinical Algorithm?

Major Recommendations
Newborns 36 weeks of gestation or greater with moderate to severe neonatal encephalopathy should receive therapeutic hypothermia (33°C to 34°C) for 72 hours duration based on results from multiple randomized, controlled trials.

Summary Statement

Surviving neonates with severe neonatal encephalopathy remain at significant risk of death or severe neurodevelopmental impairment despite being cooled, emphasizing the need for well-studied additional adjunctive treatment strategies.

REFERENCES

1. Liu L, Johnson HL, Cousens S, et al. Global, regional, and national causes of child mortality: an updated systematic analysis for 2010 with time trends since 2000. Lancet 2012;379(9832):2151–61.

2. Executive summary: neonatal encephalopathy and neurologic outcome. American College of Obstetricians and Gynecologists. Obstet Gynecol 2014;123:896–901.

3. Sarnat HB, Sarnat MS. Neonatal encephalopathy following fetal distress. A clinical and electroencephalographic study. Arch Neurol 1976;33(10):696–705.

4. Marlow N, Rose AS, Rands CE, et al. Neuropsychological and educational problems at school age associated with neonatal encephalopathy. Arch Dis Child Fetal Neonatal Ed 2005;90(5):F380–7.

5. van Handel M, Swaab H, de Vries LS, et al. Long-term cognitive and behavioral consequences of neonatal encephalopathy following perinatal asphyxia: a review. Eur J Pediatr 2007;166(7):645–54.

6. Dammann O, Ferriero D, Gressens P. Neonatal encephalopathy or hypoxic-ischemic encephalopathy? Appropriate terminology matters. Pediatr Res 2011;70(1):1–2.

7. Volpe JJ. Neonatal encephalopathy: an inadequate term for hypoxic-ischemic encephalopathy. Ann Neurol 2012;72(2):156–66.

8. Huang J, Tang J, Qu Y, et al. Mapping the knowledge structure of neonatal hypoxic-ischemic encephalopathy over the past decade: a co-word analysis based on keywords. J Child Neurol 2015;31(6):797–803.

9. Kattwinkel J, Perlman JM, Aziz K, et al. Neonatal resuscitation: 2010 American Heart Association Guidelines for Cardiopulmonary Resuscitation and Emergency Cardiovascular Care. Pediatrics 2010;126(5):e1400–13.

10. Perlman JM, Wyllie J, Kattwinkel J, et al. Neonatal resuscitation: 2010 International Consensus on Cardiopulmonary Resuscitation and Emergency Cardiovascular Care Science with Treatment Recommendations. Pediatrics 2010; 126(5):e1319–44.

11. Gunn AJ, Gluckman PD, Gunn TR. Selective head cooling in newborn infants after perinatal asphyxia: a safety study. Pediatrics 1998;102(4 Pt 1):885–92.

12. Eicher DJ, Wagner CL, Katikaneni LP, et al. Moderate hypothermia in neonatal encephalopathy: safety outcomes. Pediatr Neurol 2005;32(1):18–24.

13. Shankaran S, Laptook AR, Ehrenkranz RA, et al. Whole-body hypothermia for neonates with hypoxic-ischemic encephalopathy. N Engl J Med 2005;353(15): 1574–84.

14. Azzopardi DV, Strohm B, Edwards AD, et al. Moderate hypothermia to treat perinatal asphyxial encephalopathy. N Engl J Med 2009;361(14):1349–58.

15. Simbruner G, Mittal RA, Rohlmann F, et al, neo.nEURO.network Trial Participants. Systemic hypothermia after neonatal encephalopathy: outcomes of neo.nEURO.network RCT. Pediatrics 2010;126(4):e771–8.

16. Jacobs SE, Morley CJ, Inder TE, et al. Whole-body hypothermia for term and near-term newborns with hypoxic-ischemic encephalopathy: a randomized controlled trial. Arch Pediatr Adolesc Med 2011;165(8):692–700.

17. Zhou WH, Cheng GQ, Shao XM, et al. Selective head cooling with mild systemic hypothermia after neonatal hypoxic-ischemic encephalopathy: a multicenter randomized controlled trial in China. J Pediatr 2010;157(3):367–72, 372.e1–3.

18. Gluckman PD, Wyatt JS, Azzopardi D, et al. Selective head cooling with mild systemic hypothermia after neonatal encephalopathy: multicentre randomised trial. Lancet 2005;365(9460):663–70.

19. Shankaran S, Laptook A, Wright LL, et al. Whole-body hypothermia for neonatal encephalopathy: animal observations as a basis for a randomized, controlled pilot study in term infants. Pediatrics 2002;110(2 Pt 1):377–85.

20. Lin ZL, Yu HM, Lin J, et al. Mild hypothermia via selective head cooling as neuro-protective therapy in term neonates with perinatal asphyxia: an experience from a single neonatal intensive care unit. J Perinatol 2006;26(3):180–4.
21. Akisu M, Huseyinov A, Yalaz M, et al. Selective head cooling with hypothermia suppresses the generation of platelet-activating factor in cerebrospinal fluid of newborn infants with perinatal asphyxia. Prostaglandins Leukot Essent Fatty Acids 2003;69(1):45–50.
22. Tagin MA, Woolcott CG, Vincer MJ, et al. Hypothermia for neonatal hypoxic ischemic encephalopathy: an updated systematic review and meta-analysis. Arch Pediatr Adolesc Med 2012;166(6):558–66.
23. Jacobs SE, Berg M, Hunt R, et al. Cooling for newborns with hypoxic ischaemic encephalopathy. Cochrane Database Syst Rev 2013;(1):CD003311.
24. Shankaran S, Pappas A, McDonald SA, et al. Childhood outcomes after hypo-thermia for neonatal encephalopathy. N Engl J Med 2012;366(22):2085–92.
25. Azzopardi D, Strohm B, Marlow N, et al. Effects of hypothermia for perinatal asphyxia on childhood outcomes. N Engl J Med 2014;371(2):140–9.
26. Guillet R, Edwards AD, Thoresen M, et al. Seven- to eight-year follow-up of the CoolCap trial of head cooling for neonatal encephalopathy. Pediatr Res 2012; 71(2):205–9.
27. Committee on Fetus and Newborn, Papile LA, Baley JE, et al. Hypothermia and neonatal encephalopathy. Pediatrics 2014;133(6):1146–50.
28. Iwata O, Thornton JS, Sellwood MW, et al. Depth of delayed cooling alters neu-roprotection pattern after hypoxia-ischemia. Ann Neurol 2005;58(1):75–87.
29. Shankaran S, Laptook AR, Pappas A, et al. Effect of depth and duration of cool-ing on deaths in the NICU among neonates with hypoxic ischemic encephalop-athy: a randomized clinical trial. JAMA 2014;312(24):2629–39.
30. Saliba E. Should we extend the indications for therapeutic hypothermia? Acta Paediatr 2015;104(2):114–5.
31. Smit E, Liu X, Jary S, et al. Cooling neonates who do not fulfil the standard cool-ing criteria - short- and long-term outcomes. Acta Paediatr 2015;104(2):138–45.
32. Villa P, Bigini P, Mennini T, et al. Erythropoietin selectively attenuates cytokine production and inflammation in cerebral ischemia by targeting neuronal apoptosis. J Exp Med 2003;198(6):971–5.
33. Agnello D, Bigini P, Villa P, et al. Erythropoietin exerts an anti-inflammatory effect on the CNS in a model of experimental autoimmune encephalomyelitis. Brain Res 2002;952(1):128–34.
34. Arvin B, Neville LF, Barone FC, et al. The role of inflammation and cytokines in brain injury. Neurosci Biobehav Rev 1996;20(3):445–52.
35. Wang L, Zhang Z, Wang Y, et al. Treatment of stroke with erythropoietin en-hances neurogenesis and angiogenesis and improves neurological function in rats. Stroke 2004;35(7):1732–7.
36. Yamaji R, Okada T, Moriya M, et al. Brain capillary endothelial cells express two forms of erythropoietin receptor mRNA. Eur J Biochem 1996;239(2):494–500.
37. Chong ZZ, Kang JQ, Maiese K. Angiogenesis and plasticity: role of erythropoi-etin in vascular systems. J Hematother Stem Cell Res 2002;11(6):863–71.
38. Bernaudin M, Marti HH, Roussel S, et al. A potential role for erythropoietin in focal permanent cerebral ischemia in mice. J Cereb Blood Flow Metab 1999; 19(6):643–51.
39. Mu D, Chang YS, Vexler ZS, et al. Hypoxia-inducible factor 1alpha and erythro-poietin upregulation with deferoxamine salvage after neonatal stroke. Exp Neu-rol 2005;195(2):407–15.

40. Wallach I, Zhang J, Hartmann A, et al. Erythropoietin-receptor gene regulation in neuronal cells. Pediatr Res 2009;65(6):619–24.
41. Sugawa M, Sakurai Y, Ishikawa-Ieda Y, et al. Effects of erythropoietin on glial cell development; oligodendrocyte maturation and astrocyte proliferation. Neurosci Res 2002;44(4):391–403.
42. Genc K, Genc S, Baskin H, et al. Erythropoietin decreases cytotoxicity and nitric oxide formation induced by inflammatory stimuli in rat oligodendrocytes. Physiol Res 2006;55(1):33–8.
43. Iwai M, Stetler RA, Xing J, et al. Enhanced oligodendrogenesis and recovery of neurological function by erythropoietin after neonatal hypoxic/ischemic brain injury. Stroke 2010;41(5):1032–7.
44. Chong ZZ, Kang JQ, Maiese K. Erythropoietin fosters both intrinsic and extrinsic neuronal protection through modulation of microglia, Akt1, Bad, and caspase-mediated pathways. Br J Pharmacol 2003;138(6):1107–18.
45. Robertson NJ, Faulkner S, Fleiss B, et al. Melatonin augments hypothermic neuroprotection in a perinatal asphyxia model. Brain 2013;136(Pt 1):90–105.
46. Bjorkman ST, Ireland Z, Fan X, et al. Short-term dose-response characteristics of 2-iminobiotin immediately postinsult in the neonatal piglet after hypoxia-ischemia. Stroke 2013;44(3):809–11.
47. Nijboer CH, Kavelaars A, van Bel F, et al. Gender-dependent pathways of hypoxia-ischemia-induced cell death and neuroprotection in the immature P3 rat. Dev Neurosci 2007;29(4–5):385–92.
48. McPherson RJ, Demers EJ, Juul SE. Safety of high-dose recombinant erythropoietin in a neonatal rat model. Neonatology 2007;91(1):36–43.
49. Sola A, Rogido M, Lee BH, et al. Erythropoietin after focal cerebral ischemia activates the Janus kinase-signal transducer and activator of transcription signaling pathway and improves brain injury in postnatal day 7 rats. Pediatr Res 2005;57(4):481–7.
50. Chang YS, Mu D, Wendland M, et al. Erythropoietin improves functional and histological outcome in neonatal stroke. Pediatr Res 2005;58(1):106–11.
51. Gonzalez FF, McQuillen P, Mu D, et al. Erythropoietin enhances long-term neuroprotection and neurogenesis in neonatal stroke. Dev Neurosci 2007;29(4–5): 321–30.
52. Demers EJ, McPherson RJ, Juul SE. Erythropoietin protects dopaminergic neurons and improves neurobehavioral outcomes in juvenile rats after neonatal hypoxia-ischemia. Pediatr Res 2005;58(2):297–301.
53. Kumral A, Uysal N, Tugyan K, et al. Erythropoietin improves long-term spatial memory deficits and brain injury following neonatal hypoxia-ischemia in rats. Behav Brain Res 2004;153(1):77–86.
54. Sargin D, Friedrichs H, El-Kordi A, et al. Erythropoietin as neuroprotective and neuroregenerative treatment strategy: Comprehensive overview of 12 years of preclinical and clinical research. Best Pract Res Clin Anaesthesiol 2010;24(4): 573–94.
55. Pett GC, Juul SE. The potential of erythropoietin to treat asphyxia in newborns. Res Rep Neonatol 2014;4:195–207.
56. Rangarajan V, Juul SE. Erythropoietin: emerging role of erythropoietin in neonatal neuroprotection. Pediatr Neurol 2014;51(4):481–8.
57. Juul SE, Pet GC. Erythropoietin and neonatal neuroprotection. Clin Perinatol 2015;42(3):469–81.

58. Digicaylioglu M, Lipton SA. Erythropoietin-mediated neuroprotection involves cross-talk between Jak2 and NF-kappaB signalling cascades. Nature 2001; 412(6847):641–7.

59. Xiong T, Qu Y, Mu D, et al. Erythropoietin for neonatal brain injury: opportunity and challenge. Int J Dev Neurosci 2011;29(6):583–91.

60. Kellert BA, McPherson RJ, Juul SE. A comparison of high-dose recombinant erythropoietin treatment regimens in brain-injured neonatal rats. Pediatr Res 2007;61(4):451–5.

61. Sun Y, Calvert JW, Zhang JH. Neonatal hypoxia/ischemia is associated with decreased inflammatory mediators after erythropoietin administration. Stroke 2005;36(8):1672–8.

62. Juul SE, Beyer RP, Bammler TK, et al. Microarray analysis of high-dose recombinant erythropoietin treatment of unilateral brain injury in neonatal mouse hippocampus. Pediatr Res 2009;65(5):485–92.

63. Reitmeir R, Kilic E, Kilic U, et al. Post-acute delivery of erythropoietin induces stroke recovery by promoting perilesional tissue remodelling and contralesional pyramidal tract plasticity. Brain 2011;134(Pt 1):84–99.

64. Iwai M, Cao G, Yin W, et al. Erythropoietin promotes neuronal replacement through revascularization and neurogenesis after neonatal hypoxia/ischemia in rats. Stroke 2007;38(10):2795–803.

65. Ransome MI, Turnley AM. Systemically delivered Erythropoietin transiently enhances adult hippocampal neurogenesis. J Neurochem 2007;102(6):1953–65.

66. Wang L, Chopp M, Gregg SR, et al. Neural progenitor cells treated with EPO induce angiogenesis through the production of VEGF. J Cereb Blood Flow Metab 2008;28(7):1361–8.

67. Yang Z, Covey MV, Bitel CL, et al. Sustained neocortical neurogenesis after neonatal hypoxic/ischemic injury. Ann Neurol 2007;61(3):199–208.

68. Traudt CM, McPherson RJ, Bauer LA, et al. Concurrent erythropoietin and hypothermia treatment improve outcomes in a term nonhuman primate model of perinatal asphyxia. Dev Neurosci 2013;35(6):491–503.

69. Zhu C, Kang W, Xu F, et al. Erythropoietin improved neurologic outcomes in newborns with hypoxic-ischemic encephalopathy. Pediatrics 2009;124(2): e218–26.

70. Elmahdy H, El-Mashad AR, El-Bahrawy H, et al. Human recombinant erythropoietin in asphyxia neonatorum: pilot trial. Pediatrics 2010;125(5):e1135–42.

71. Wu YW, Bauer LA, Ballard RA, et al. Erythropoietin for neuroprotection in neonatal encephalopathy: safety and pharmacokinetics. Pediatrics 2012; 130(4):683–91.

72. Rogers EE, Bonifacio SL, Glass HC, et al. Erythropoietin and hypothermia for hypoxic-ischemic encephalopathy. Pediatr Neurol 2014;51(5):657–62.

73. Wu YW, Mathur AM, Chang T, et al. High-dose erythropoietin and hypothermia for hypoxic-ischemic encephalopathy: A Phase II Trial. Pediatrics 2016;137(6): e20160191.

74. Franks NP, Dickinson R, de Sousa SL, et al. How does xenon produce anaesthesia? Nature 1998;396(6709):324.

75. Ma D, Williamson P, Januszewski A, et al. Xenon mitigates isoflurane-induced neuronal apoptosis in the developing rodent brain. Anesthesiology 2007; 106(4):746–53.

76. Lobo N, Yang B, Rizvi M, et al. Hypothermia and xenon: novel noble guardians in hypoxic-ischemic encephalopathy? J Neurosci Res 2013;91(4):473–8.

77. Azzopardi D, Robertson NJ, Bainbridge A, et al. Moderate hypothermia within 6 h of birth plus inhaled xenon versus moderate hypothermia alone after birth asphyxia (TOBY-Xe): a proof-of-concept, open-label, randomised controlled trial. Lancet Neurol 2015;15(2):145–53.

78. Thayyil S, Chandrasekaran M, Taylor A, et al. Cerebral magnetic resonance biomarkers in neonatal encephalopathy: a meta-analysis. Pediatrics 2010;125(2): e382–95.

79. Tusor N, Wusthoff C, Smee N, et al. Prediction of neurodevelopmental outcome after hypoxic-ischemic encephalopathy treated with hypothermia by diffusion tensor imaging analyzed using tract-based spatial statistics. Pediatr Res 2012;72(1):63–9.

80. Reiter RJ, Tan DX, Osuna C, et al. Actions of melatonin in the reduction of oxidative stress. A review. J Biomed Sci 2000;7(6):444–58.

81. Luchetti F, Canonico B, Betti M, et al. Melatonin signaling and cell protection function. FASEB J 2010;24(10):3603–24.

82. Alonso-Alconada D, Alvarez A, Arteaga O, et al. Neuroprotective effect of melatonin: a novel therapy against perinatal hypoxia-ischemia. Int J Mol Sci 2013; 14(5):9379–95.

83. Biran V, Phan Duy A, Decobert F, et al. Is melatonin ready to be used in preterm infants as a neuroprotectant? Dev Med Child Neurol 2014;56(8):717–23.

84. Fulia F, Gitto E, Cuzzocrea S, et al. Increased levels of malondialdehyde and nitrite/nitrate in the blood of asphyxiated newborns: reduction by melatonin. J Pineal Res 2001;31(4):343–9.

85. Aly H, Elmahdy H, El-Dib M, et al. Melatonin use for neuroprotection in perinatal asphyxia: a randomized controlled pilot study. J Perinatol 2015;35(3):186–91.

86. Okatani Y, Okamoto K, Hayashi K, et al. Maternal-fetal transfer of melatonin in pregnant women near term. J Pineal Res 1998;25(3):129–34.

87. Vitte PA, Harthe C, Lestage P, et al. Plasma, cerebrospinal fluid, and brain distribution of 14C-melatonin in rat: a biochemical and autoradiographic study. J Pineal Res 1988;5(5):437–53.

88. Peeters-Scholte C, Koster J, Veldhuis W, et al. Neuroprotection by selective nitric oxide synthase inhibition at 24 hours after perinatal hypoxia-ischemia. Stroke 2002;33(9):2304–10.

89. van den Tweel ER, van Bel F, Kavelaars A, et al. Long-term neuroprotection with 2-iminobiotin, an inhibitor of neuronal and inducible nitric oxide synthase, after cerebral hypoxia-ischemia in neonatal rats. J Cereb Blood Flow Metab 2005; 25(1):67–74.

90. Nijboer CH, Groenendaal F, Kavelaars A, et al. Gender-specific neuroprotection by 2-iminobiotin after hypoxia-ischemia in the neonatal rat via a nitric oxide independent pathway. J Cereb Blood Flow Metab 2007;27(2):282–92.

91. Raju TN. Timing of umbilical cord clamping after birth for optimizing placental transfusion. Curr Opin Pediatr 2013;25(2):180–7.

92. Al-Wassia H, Shah PS. Efficacy and safety of umbilical cord milking at birth: a systematic review and meta-analysis. JAMA Pediatr 2015;169(1):18–25.

93. Bora R, Akhtar SS, Venkatasubramaniam A, et al. Effect of 40-cm segment umbilical cord milking on hemoglobin and serum ferritin at 6 months of age in full-term infants of anemic and non-anemic mothers. J Perinatol 2015;35(10): 832–6.

94. Yadav AK, Upadhyay A, Gothwal S, et al. Comparison of three types of intervention to enhance placental redistribution in term newborns: randomized control trial. J Perinatol 2015;35(9):720–4.

95. Fleiss B, Guillot PV, Titomanlio L, et al. Stem cell therapy for neonatal brain injury. Clin Perinatol 2014;41(1):133–48.
96. Ingram DA, Mead LE, Tanaka H, et al. Identification of a novel hierarchy of endothelial progenitor cells using human peripheral and umbilical cord blood. Blood 2004;104(9):2752–60.
97. Lee MW, Yang MS, Park JS, et al. Isolation of mesenchymal stem cells from cryopreserved human umbilical cord blood. Int J Hematol 2005;81(2):126–30.
98. Van Pham P, Truong NC, Le PT, et al. Isolation and proliferation of umbilical cord tissue derived mesenchymal stem cells for clinical applications. Cell Tissue Bank 2016;17(2):289–302.
99. Pereira-Cunha FG, Duarte AS, Reis-Alves SC, et al. Umbilical cord blood CD34(+) stem cells and other mononuclear cell subtypes processed up to 96 h from collection and stored at room temperature maintain a satisfactory functionality for cell therapy. Vox Sang 2015;108(1):72–81.
100. Buzanska L, Jurga M, Domanska-Janik K. Neuronal differentiation of human umbilical cord blood neural stem-like cell line. Neurodegener Dis 2006;3(1–2): 19–26.
101. Cotten CM, Murtha AP, Goldberg RN, et al. Feasibility of autologous cord blood cells for infants with hypoxic-ischemic encephalopathy. J Pediatr 2014;164(5): 973–9.e1.
102. Bavarsad Shahripour R, Harrigan MR, Alexandrov AV. N-acetylcysteine (NAC) in neurological disorders: mechanisms of action and therapeutic opportunities. Brain Behav 2014;4(2):108–22.
103. Jatana M, Singh I, Singh AK, et al. Combination of systemic hypothermia and N-acetylcysteine attenuates hypoxic-ischemic brain injury in neonatal rats. Pediatr Res 2006;59(5):684–9.
104. Kannan S, Dai H, Navath RS, et al. Dendrimer-based postnatal therapy for neuroinflammation and cerebral palsy in a rabbit model. Sci Transl Med 2012; 4(130):130ra146.
105. Taniguchi T, Kurita A, Kobayashi K, et al. Dose- and time-related effects of dexmedetomidine on mortality and inflammatory responses to endotoxin-induced shock in rats. J Anesth 2008;22(3):221–8.
106. Yang CL, Tsai PS, Huang CJ. Effects of dexmedetomidine on regulating pulmonary inflammation in a rat model of ventilator-induced lung injury. Acta Anaesthesiol Taiwan 2008;46(4):151–9.
107. McAdams RM, McPherson RJ, Kapur R, et al. Dexmedetomidine reduces cranial temperature in hypothermic neonatal rats. Pediatr Res 2015;77(6):772–8.
108. Laudenbach V, Mantz J, Lagercrantz H, et al. Effects of alpha(2)-adrenoceptor agonists on perinatal excitotoxic brain injury: comparison of clonidine and dexmedetomidine. Anesthesiology 2002;96(1):134–41.
109. Paris A, Mantz J, Tonner PH, et al. The effects of dexmedetomidine on perinatal excitotoxic brain injury are mediated by the alpha2A-adrenoceptor subtype. Anesth Analg 2006;102(2):456–61.
110. Sato K, Kimura T, Nishikawa T, et al. Neuroprotective effects of a combination of dexmedetomidine and hypothermia after incomplete cerebral ischemia in rats. Acta Anaesthesiol Scand 2010;54(3):377–82.

Inflammatory Biomarkers of Birth Asphyxia

Lina F. Chalak, MD, MSCS

KEYWORDS

- Asphyxia • Placenta • Cytokines • GFAP • Ubiquitin

KEY POINTS

- Hypothermia is a recognized standard-of-care neuroprotective therapy for newborns with hypoxic-ischemic encephalopathy, but about 45% of infants have abnormal outcomes despite treatment.
- Biomarkers could help the bedside clinician identify responders and nonresponders to hypothermia who could benefit from added neuroprotective strategies.
- The author's observations suggest an important role of the placenta through inflammatory mechanisms to the severity of the hypoxic-asphyxial insult and therapeutic responses following hypothermia therapy.
- Using a serum panel of inflammatory and neuronal biomarkers, rather than a single biomarker, seems the most promising once validated in large cohorts.

INTRODUCTION

Perinatal asphyxia remains a frequent cause of cerebral palsy, mental retardation, learning disability, epilepsy, and death.[1] The worldwide burden is 4 million newborns every year, of which one million die and an additional million have significant disabilities.[2,3] Neonatal brain injury is recognized by a distinctive clinical encephalopathy that evolves from hyperexcitability to lethargy and stupor during the first 3 days of life.[4,5] Large trials have shown that hypothermia therapy results in a significant reduction in death or disability with a relative risk of 0.76 (confidence interval [CI] 0.65–0.89).[6–12] Hypothermia is the current standard of care for hypoxic neonatal encephalopathy (NE). However, 45% of cooled newborns have significant disabilities at 12 to 18 months of age,[13] when tested by the Bayley Scales of Infant and Toddler Development gold standard neurodevelopmental tools.

Because hypothermia does not protect all affected neonates from neurocognitive delay and mental retardation, adjuvant therapies are being sought; but the real

Disclosure Statement: The author has nothing to disclose.
Department of Pediatrics, University of Texas Southwestern Medical Center, 5323 Harry Hines Boulevard, Room F3.312B, Dallas, TX 75390-9063, USA
E-mail address: Lina.chalak@utsouthwestern.edu

Clin Perinatol 43 (2016) 501–510
http://dx.doi.org/10.1016/j.clp.2016.04.008   perinatology.theclinics.com
0095-5108/16/$ – see front matter © 2016 Elsevier Inc. All rights reserved.

challenge is to define which neonates will need these therapies shortly after birth. Despite the complex pathophysiology related to the uncertain timing, severity, and patterns of the fetal insult,[14] neonates with NE are currently viewed dichotomously[15]: those who do, or do not, qualify for cooling. Hypothermia is offered uniformly in a one-size-fits-all strategy based on the early neurologic examination, which has a limited predictive value, and the striking heterogeneity between the moderate and severe groups.[6-12] Infants with mild NE are not currently cooled, yet 20% to 30% may have abnormal outcomes.[16] Amplitude electroencephalogram[17] is a good physiologic marker of neuronal integrity, but its predictive values are attenuated during hypothermia.[18,19] Although brain MRI is considered the best short-term marker of early childhood outcome,[20-23] the sensitivity improves beyond the first week of life. An ideal biomarker would be measured in real time and directly reflect the neurovascular unit function[23] linking it to outcomes.[24-26] Such a biomarker would enhance the ability to stratify the insult severity by identifying neonates with mild NE who might benefit from hypothermia and those with moderate-severe NE who need added interventions to improve outcomes. The quest for such biomarkers is still mostly research based. This review covers promising biomarkers of injury to the neurovascular unit during hypothermia therapy including (1) biomarkers of placental inflammation, (2) neuronal biomarkers, as well as (3) general inflammatory cytokines in the serum.

PLACENTAL INFLAMMATORY BIOMARKERS

The placenta mediates interactions between mother and fetus throughout gestation and provides a historical record of maternal and fetal interactions. Its fetal composition makes it an ideal storyteller of perinatal distress. In 1955, Eastman and De Leon first described the association of intrapartum infection and cerebral palsy (CP). Over the years, there has been growing evidence to support an association between placental inflammation, elevated cytokines and CP.[27-29] A multitude of elegant animal studies have shown a variable response of the developing brain to inflammation, depending on the critical timing of exposure.[30,31] When administered either 72 hours before or 6 hours after the insult, lipopolysaccharide (LPS) resulted in increased hypoxic-ischemic (HI) injury, in contrast to a reduced injury when administered 24 hours before the insult.[30] Therapeutic hypothermia was not neuroprotective in another LPS-sensitized unilateral strokelike HI brain injury model in newborn rats.[31] In a recent clinical study, postnatal sepsis was associated with increased watershed evidence of brain injury, whereas reports of isolated prenatal maternal chorioamnionitis were associated with lower incidence of MRI abnormalities in newborns with encephalopathy.[32]

The placental milieu can have various influences on outcomes, as well as the extent of responses to therapies, depending on the severity and timing of the inflammatory sensitization. The author and colleagues recently reported findings of a large cohort that included all 120 neonates born with a gestational age of 36 weeks or greater and a birth weight greater than 1800 g who were admitted to the neonatal intensive care unit at Parkland Hospital from January 2006 through November 2011 with evidence of perinatal acidosis and NE.[33] As it was routine practice for all placentas associated with specific maternal-fetal complications of pregnancy and need for presence of the neonatal resuscitation team to be sent to pathology, placentas from all the infants during the study time period were examined. Gross and histologic examinations were reported according to the 2005 Redline classification.[34] Major pathology was identified to include (1) intervillous fibrin deposition/retroplacental hemorrhage/infarction involving 20% of placental volume; (2) fetal vascular thrombo-occlusive disease with greater than 1 focus of avascular villi/thrombotic vasculopathy; (3)

chorioamnionitis including a fetal response; and (4) patchy/diffuse chronic villitis. Chronic villitis was divided into low-grade (focal/multifocal villitis) and high-grade villitis (patchy/diffuse villitis). Low-grade lesions included focal villitis, a small cluster of 10 or less affected villi and multifocal villitis, and 2 or more small clusters of 10 or less affected villi. High-grade lesions included patchy villitis defined as a large cluster of more than 10 affected villi but less than 25% of the terminal villi plus diffuse villitis and the presence of extensive inflammation with multiple large clusters detected on all slides. In this high-risk inborn patient population with metabolic acidosis and encephalopathy, most (95%) had placental abnormalities and 65% met criteria for a diagnosis of a major placental pathology. There was a high incidence of inflammatory pathology observed with chorioamnionitis in 61 of 114 (54%) and chronic patchy/ diffuse villitis in 13 of 114 (11%).

The frequency of occurrence increased with severity of NE. Following univariate regression analysis, which included clinical and placental variables, chronic active/ patchy villitis was the only predictive variable that was significantly associated with abnormal 2-year neurodevelopmental outcomes after hypothermia (odds ratio 9.29; 95% CI 1.11–77.73). These findings suggest an important contribution by placental inflammatory mechanisms to the severity of the asphyxia and therapeutic responses following hypothermia.

SERUM BIOMARKERS OF THE NEUROVASCULAR UNIT

The neurovascular unit includes the blood-brain barrier (BBB), a key interface of molecular and cellular exchange between blood and neural tissues.[19] The BBB is dynamic and can be modified by circulating factors secreted by microglia or transferred from distant organs.[35] Microglia are activated in the setting of HI encephalopathy (HIE) and develop macrophagelike capabilities, including phagocytosis, cytokine and chemokine production, antigen presentation, and the release of matrix metalloproteinases that weaken the BBB. As a result, peripheral leukocytes infiltrate into the brain, leading to increased inflammation and neuronal injury. Commonly known factors upregulated after hypoxia can impair BBB permeability, such as interleukins (IL-1α, IL-1β, IL-6), tumor necrosis factor α (TNFα), free radicals, and nitric oxide, to list a few.[19] Multiple organ dysfunction is an integral part of HIE; therefore, multiple organs, in addition to the leaky BBB, can contribute to the inflammatory response.[36]

Brain-Specific Biomarkers

The microglia and astrocytes from the neurovascular unit can further produce glial fibrillary acidic protein (GFAP), ubiquitin carboxyl-terminal hydrolase L1 (UCH-L1), S100B, neuron-specific enolase (NSE), as well as cytokines, chemokines, and other factors.[19,37] **Table 1** summarizes reports of neuronal biomarkers detected in the serum of neonates with HIE. All of the studies,[38–45] although novel, represent small pilot studies and are not powered to detect long-term outcome predictions. GFAP is an intermediate filament protein released from astrocytes into the blood on astrocyte death and has been correlated with poor outcomes in adult patients after stroke, cardiac arrest, extracorporeal membrane oxygenation, or traumatic brain injury.[43] Serum GFAP has been recently reported by Ennen and colleagues[45] to be significantly elevated in newborns with NE undergoing hypothermia therapy when compared with controls. A GFAP threshold level greater than 0.15 ng/mL following hypothermia therapy was associated with an abnormal brain MRI. UCH-L1 is a neuron-specific cytoplasmic enzyme and marker of neuronal apoptosis that is concentrated in dendrites. Serum UCH-L1 reflects the extent of neuronal injury because it is expressed

Table 1
Biomarkers of the neurovascular unit: sources, functions, and conditions detected focusing on hypoxic-ischemic encephalopathy

Neurovascular Unit Biomarkers	Sources and Functions	Conditions Where Detected	Neonatal HIE Studies
GFAP			
Ennen et al,[45] 2011 Massaro et al,[41] 2013 Chalak et al,[13,38] 2014	Intermediate filament protein from astrocyte • Role in astrocyte growth • CSF, serum	In stroke, cardiac arrest, ECMO, TBI, HIE	• 23 HIE high with cutoff >0.15 ng/mL with abnormal MRI • 20 HIE optimal ROC at 72 h for death and abn MRI • 30 HIE (cooled vs mild noncooled) cord art bld and during 72 h associated with abn Bayley 2 y
UCH-L1			
Douglas-escobar et al,[39] 2010 Massaro et al,[41] 2013 Chalak et al,[13,38] 2014	Neuronal protein • Released with neuronal death • CSF, serum	In subarachnoid hemorrhage, TBI, HIE	• 14 HIE highest in 2 who died • 20 HIE optimal ROC at 24 h for death and abn MRI • 30 HIE highest with severe HIE only in cord art bld, decreases afterbirth
SB100			
Gazzalo 2004 and 2009; Risso 2011 Massaro et al,[40,42] 2012, 2014	Protein binding calcium • Released in astrocytes • In urine, serum, CSF, saliva, milk, and multiple other cells	In newborns higher, decrease with age, increased with HIE	• Levels in 40 HIE>CTL • 132 w HIE cutoff value 0.41 mcg/L for abn outcomes • 75 cooled w HIE cutoff 1.6 ng/mL on day 1 predicted death/MRI but sensitivity <40% and no controls • 2.5 odds of Bayley <85 outcomes
NSE			
Celtik et al,[46] 2004 Massaro et al,[40,42] 2012, 2014	Glycolytic enzyme in neurons • Released from neurons and platelets	Cardiac arrest, TBI, stroke, cardiac surgery, HIE	• Cutoff >45 mcg/L associated with abn outcomes in HIE and > no or mild HIE • 75 cooled w HIE cutoff 110 ng/mL on day 1 predicted death/MRI but sensitivity <40% and no controls • ×2 Odds of Bayley <85 outcomes

Abbreviations: abn, abnormal; art, arterial; CSF, cerebrospinal fluid; CTL, control; ECMO, extracorporeal membrane oxygenation; ROC, receiver operator curve-blood; TBI, traumatic brain injury.

in neurons and then released into the circulation after breakdown of the BBB and is easily measured.[44] In another study, UCH-L1 serum values were greater than 100 ng/mL in neonates with NE who subsequently died.[39] Additionally, serum NSE cutoff point concentrations of 45.4 mcg/L have also been associated with severity of NE and could help distinguish infants with poor outcomes.[46]

Brain-specific biomarkers in the serum and neurodevelopmental outcomes after hypothermia

Particular emphasis is placed on the review of relatively more brain-specific GFAP and UCH-L1, whereby limited long-term outcomes were initially reported beyond death and/or MRI abnormalities. The author and colleagues recently conducted a prospective pilot cohort study to assess GFAP, along with UCH-L1, and cytokines in the serum from the cord arterial blood as well as an indwelling umbilical artery at 6 to 24, 48, 72, and 78 hours of age. Neurodevelopmental outcomes (Bayley Scales of Infant and Toddler Development III) were performed at 18 to 24 months. The umbilical arterial cord serum GFAP and ubiquitin levels correlated with severity of NE, with higher levels in moderate to severe NE, as compared with those not cooled with mild NE.[38] At birth, serum GFAP and UCH-L1 were increased with the severity of NE as seen in **Fig. 1** (P<.001). UCH-L1 decreased after the first 6 to 24 hours of hypothermia compared with the cord blood values at birth, possibly reflecting the effect of hypothermia on this specific neuronal marker of apoptosis. In contrast, serial GFAP values remained elevated in neonates with moderate to severe NE who were undergoing hypothermia. In addition, GFAP levels of greater than 0.05 ng/mL beyond 72 hours of age were associated with abnormal Bayley III neurodevelopmental outcomes at 24 months of age.[38] Another recent study reported UCH-L1 to also be acutely elevated in the umbilical arterial cord plasma, whereas GFAP was significantly elevated later at 72 hours in cooled infants who developed adverse outcomes.[41] The sustained increase in GFAP over the

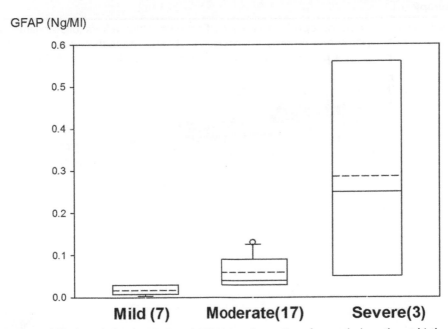

GFAP (Ng/Ml)

Mild (7)   Moderate(17)   Severe(3)

Fig. 1. Umbilical cord plasma GFAP and UCH-L1 and severity of encephalopathy at birth. A box and whisker plot gives median as solid line, mean as dotted line, and 25th and 75th quartiles as lower and upper borders. Analyses include neonates with mild, moderate, and severe encephalopathy. P = .001 (GFAP) and P = .03 (UCH-L1) by Jonckheere-Terpstra test. (*From* Chalak LF, Sanchez PJ, Adams-Huet B, et al. Biomarkers for severity of neonatal hypoxic-ischemic encephalopathy and outcomes in newborns receiving hypothermia therapy. J Pediatrics 2014;164 (3):468; with permission.)

duration of hypothermia could result from its multiple functions, which also involve repair and growth beyond the acute injury phase.

GENERAL INFLAMMATORY BIOMARKERS

The term cytokine encompasses a variety of proteins including interleukins, colony-stimulating factors, interferons (IFNs), TNF, and chemokines[47] which link the neural, endocrine, and immune systems.[48] Cytokines are mediators in the common pathways associated with perinatal brain injury induced by a variety of insults.[49-53] Cytokines are chemotactic for blood-borne neutrophils and monocytes/macrophages, potentially increasing leukocyte recruitment as well as directly amplifying inflammatory cascades in the injured central nervous system.[27] Hypoxia-asphyxia and infection seem to potentiate the systemic inflammatory response associated with elevated cytokines.[28,54,55] Serum cytokines from the neonatal screening were reported to be elevated in infants who later developed CP.[27] Elevated concentrations of IL-6 and IL-8 have been demonstrated in the CSF and serum of asphyxiated full-term infants.[56] Higher concentrations of IL-1β, IL-6, TNF-α, and IL-8 in the blood of neonates with HIE have also been associated with abnormal neurodevelopmental outcomes.[57,58] Before the hypothermia era, meta-analysis highlighted both serum IL-1β and serum IL-6, when measured before 96 hours in infants with encephalopathy,[59] as biomarkers predictive of abnormal outcomes.

Inflammatory Cytokines and Neurodevelopmental Outcomes After Hypothermia Therapy

The focus of this current report is to review inflammatory biomarkers following implementation of hypothermia therapy for newborns of HIE. The author and colleagues recently reported in a cohort of 30 newborns with encephalopathy that IL-1, IL-6,

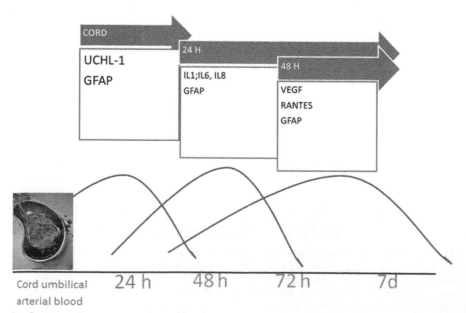

Fig. 2. Biomarkers temporal profile changes during hypothermia therapy in the first 72 hours of life. RANTES, Regulated on Activation, Normal T Cell Expressed and Secreted.

IL-8, TNF, and INF were elevated at 6 to 24 hours after birth in the infants with later abnormal neurologic outcomes at 18 to 24 months.[38] The author and colleagues and others[60] have further investigated the temporal relationships of biomarkers in injury and recovery and the variability of those phases during hypothermia. Some biomarkers, such as IL-1, IL-6, IL-8, and MCP1 (monocyte chemotactic protein 1), were found to have early peaks within the first 24 to 48 hours of life, as compared with others, such as vascular endothelial growth factor (VEGF) and MIP1α (macrophage inflammatory protein 1 alpha), which peaked later, around 72 hours. The recent study by Celtik and colleagues[46] found no differences between the effect of total and selective head cooling on inflammatory biomarkers after HIE.

SUMMARY

Understanding of the modulation of serum cytokines and neuronal and placental biomarkers is needed to better delineate the injury-repair pathways and responses to neuroprotective therapies. Given the complexity of the presentation and spectrum of NE/HIE, it is unlikely that a single biomarker at birth will be able to predict clinical outcomes following therapy (**Fig. 2**). Future neuroprotective strategies targeting inflammation will likely benefit from development of such biomarkers, as proxy to long-term outcomes, to help evaluate therapeutic efficacy and responses in real time.

Best practices

What is the current practice?

- Hypothermia is the standard of care for neuroprotective therapy for newborns with HIE, but about 45% of infants have abnormal outcomes despite treatment.

- Biomarkers are being evaluated in research studies to help the bedside clinician identify responders and nonresponders to hypothermia who could benefit from added neuroprotective strategies.

What changes in current practice are likely to improve outcomes?

- Placental examination for neonates with NE, if results were available in a timely manner, could identify a subgroup of patients who might benefit from strategies targeting antiinflammatory therapies in addition to hypothermia.

- Although GFAP and UCH-L1 seem to be promising as brain-specific biomarkers, there is no currently available biomarker to be recommended for clinical use.

- Future serum biomarker studies will need to be conducted in multiple centers to have sufficient patient numbers for large dataset validation for clinical practice.

REFERENCES

1. Levene ML, Kornberg J, Williams TH. The incidence and severity of post-asphyxial encephalopathy in full-term infants. Early Hum Dev 1985;11(1):21–6.
2. Bryce J, Boschi-Pinto C, Shibuya K, et al. WHO estimates of the causes of death in children. Lancet 2005;365(9465):1147–52.
3. Pryds O, Greisen G, Lou H, et al. Vasoparalysis associated with brain damage in asphyxiated term infants. J Pediatr 1990;117(1 Pt 1):119–25.
4. Sarnat HB, Sarnat MS. Neonatal encephalopathy following fetal distress. A clinical and electroencephalographic study. Arch Neurol 1976;33(10):696–705.

5. Miller SP, Latal B, Clark H, et al. Clinical signs predict 30-month neurodevelopmental outcome after neonatal encephalopathy. Am J Obstet Gynecol 2004; 190(1):93–9.

6. Jacobs SE, Morley CJ, Inder TE, et al. Whole-body hypothermia for term and near-term newborns with hypoxic-ischemic encephalopathy: a randomized controlled trial. Arch Pediatr Adolesc Med 2011;165(8):692–700.

7. Zhou WH, Cheng GQ, Shao XM, et al. Selective head cooling with mild systemic hypothermia after neonatal hypoxic-ischemic encephalopathy: a multicenter randomized controlled trial in China. J Pediatr 2010;157(3): 367–72, 372.e1–3.

8. Simbruner G, Mittal RA, Rohlmann F, et al. Systemic hypothermia after neonatal encephalopathy: outcomes of neo.nEURO.network RCT. Pediatrics 2010; 126(4):e771–8.

9. Azzopardi DV, Strohm B, Edwards AD, et al. Moderate hypothermia to treat perinatal asphyxial encephalopathy. N Engl J Med 2009;361(14):1349–58.

10. Gluckman PD, Wyatt JS, Azzopardi D, et al. Selective head cooling with mild systemic hypothermia after neonatal encephalopathy: multicentre randomised trial. Lancet 2005;365(9460):663–70.

11. Spitzmiller RE, Phillips T, Meinzen-Derr J, et al. Amplitude-integrated EEG is useful in predicting neurodevelopmental outcome in full-term infants with hypoxic-ischemic encephalopathy: a meta-analysis. J Child Neurol 2007;22(9): 1069–78.

12. Shankaran S, Laptook AR, Ehrenkranz RA, et al. Whole-body hypothermia for neonates with hypoxic-ischemic encephalopathy. N Engl J Med 2005;353(15): 1574–84.

13. Chalak LF, DuPont TL, Sanchez PJ, et al. Neurodevelopmental outcomes after hypothermia therapy in the era of Bayley-III. J Perinatol 2014;34(8):629–33.

14. Ferriero DM. Neonatal brain injury. N Engl J Med 2004;351(19):1985–95.

15. Ferriero DM, Bonifacio SL. The search continues for the elusive biomarkers of neonatal brain injury. J Pediatr 2014;164(3):438–40.

16. Dupont TL, Chalak LF, Morriss MC, et al. Short-term outcomes of newborns with perinatal acidemia who are not eligible for systemic hypothermia therapy. J Pediatr 2012;162(1):35–41.

17. Shalak LF, Laptook AR, Velaphi SC, et al. Amplitude-integrated electroencephalography coupled with an early neurologic examination enhances prediction of term infants at risk for persistent encephalopathy. Pediatrics 2003;111(2):351–7.

18. Thoresen M, Hellstrom-Westas L, Liu X, et al. Effect of hypothermia on amplitude-integrated electroencephalogram in infants with asphyxia. Pediatrics 2010; 126(1):e131–9.

19. McAdams RM, Juul SE. The role of cytokines and inflammatory cells in perinatal brain injury. Neurol Res Int 2012;2012:561494.

20. Barkovich AJ, Hajnal BL, Vigneron D, et al. Prediction of neuromotor outcome in perinatal asphyxia: evaluation of MR scoring systems. AJNR Am J Neuroradiol 1998;19(1):143–9.

21. Thayyil S, Chandrasekaran M, Taylor A, et al. Cerebral magnetic resonance biomarkers in neonatal encephalopathy: a meta-analysis. Pediatrics 2010;125(2): e382–95.

22. Rutherford M, Srinivasan L, Dyet L, et al. Magnetic resonance imaging in perinatal brain injury: clinical presentation, lesions and outcome. Pediatr Radiol 2006;36(7):582–92.

23. Rutherford M, Ramenghi LA, Edwards AD, et al. Assessment of brain tissue injury after moderate hypothermia in neonates with hypoxic-ischaemic encephalopathy: a nested substudy of a randomised controlled trial. Lancet Neurol 2010; 9(1):39–45.

24. Higgins RD, Raju T, Edwards AD, et al. Hypothermia and other treatment options for neonatal encephalopathy: an executive summary of the Eunice Kennedy Shriver NICHD workshop. J Pediatr 2011;159(5):851–8.e1.

25. Kratzer I, Chip S, Vexler ZS. Barrier mechanisms in neonatal stroke. Front Neurosci 2014;8:359.

26. Juul SE, Ferriero DM. Pharmacologic neuroprotective strategies in neonatal brain injury. Clin Perinatol 2014;41(1):119–31.

27. Nelson KB, Dambrosia JM, Grether JK, et al. Neonatal cytokines and coagulation factors in children with cerebral palsy. Ann Neurol 1998;44(4):665–75.

28. Shalak LF, Laptook AR, Jafri HS, et al. Clinical chorioamnionitis, elevated cytokines, and brain injury in term infants. Pediatrics 2002;110(4):673–80.

29. Wu YW, Colford JM Jr. Chorioamnionitis as a risk factor for cerebral palsy: a meta-analysis. JAMA 2000;284(11):1417–24.

30. Eklind S, Mallard C, Arvidsson P, et al. Lipopolysaccharide induces both a primary and a secondary phase of sensitization in the developing rat brain. Pediatr Res 2005;58(1):112–6.

31. Osredkar D, Thoresen M, Maes E, et al. Hypothermia is not neuroprotective after infection-sensitized neonatal hypoxic-ischemic brain injury. Resuscitation 2014; 85(4):567–72.

32. Jenster M, Bonifacio SL, Ruel T, et al. Maternal or neonatal infection: association with neonatal encephalopathy outcomes. Pediatr Res 2014;76(1):93–9.

33. Mir IN, Johnson-Welch SF, Nelson DB, et al. Placental pathology is associated with severity of neonatal encephalopathy and adverse developmental outcomes following hypothermia. Am J Obstet Gynecol 2015;213(6):849.e1-8.

34. Redline RW, Heller D, Keating S, et al. Placental diagnostic criteria and clinical correlation - a workshop report. Placenta 2005;26:S114–7.

35. Abbott NJ, Ronnback L, Hansson E. Astrocyte-endothelial interactions at the blood-brain barrier. Nat Rev Neurosci 2006;7(1):41–53.

36. Vela JM, Molina-Holgado E, Arevalo-Martin A, et al. Interleukin-1 regulates proliferation and differentiation of oligodendrocyte progenitor cells. Mol Cell Neurosci 2002;20(3):489–502.

37. Mir IN, Chalak LF. Serum biomarkers to evaluate the integrity of the neurovascular unit. Early Hum Dev 2014;90(10):707–11.

38. Chalak LF, Sanchez PJ, Adams-Huet B, et al. Biomarkers for severity of neonatal hypoxic-ischemic encephalopathy and outcomes in newborns receiving hypothermia therapy. J Pediatr 2014;164(3):468–74.e1.

39. Douglas-Escobar M, Yang C, Bennett J, et al. A pilot study of novel biomarkers in neonates with hypoxic-ischemic encephalopathy. Pediatr Res 2010;68(6):531–6.

40. Massaro AN, Chang T, Kadom N, et al. Biomarkers of brain injury in neonatal encephalopathy treated with hypothermia. J Pediatr 2012;161(3):434–40.

41. Massaro AN, Jeromin A, Kadom N, et al. Serum biomarkers of MRI brain injury in neonatal hypoxic ischemic encephalopathy treated with whole-body hypothermia: a pilot study. Pediatr Crit Care Med 2013;14(3):310–7.

42. Massaro AN, Chang T, Baumgart S, et al. Biomarkers S100B and neuron-specific enolase predict outcome in hypothermia-treated encephalopathic newborns*. Pediatr Crit Care Med 2014;15(7):615–22.

43. Pelinka LE, Kroepfl A, Leixnering M, et al. GFAP versus S100B in serum after traumatic brain injury: relationship to brain damage and outcome. J Neurotrauma 2004;21(11):1553–61.

44. Papa L, Akinyi L, Liu MC, et al. Ubiquitin C-terminal hydrolase is a novel biomarker in humans for severe traumatic brain injury. Crit Care Med 2010; 38(1):138–44.

45. Ennen CS, Huisman TA, Savage WJ, et al. Glial fibrillary acidic protein as a biomarker for neonatal hypoxic-ischemic encephalopathy treated with whole-body cooling. Am J Obstet Gynecol 2011;205(3):251.e1-7.

46. Celtik C, Acunas B, Oner N, et al. Neuron-specific enolase as a marker of the severity and outcome of hypoxic ischemic encephalopathy. Brain Dev 2004; 26(6):398–402.

47. Tayal V, Kalra BS. Cytokines and anti-cytokines as therapeutics–an update. Eur J Pharmacol 2008;579(1–3):1–12.

48. Rostene W, Dansereau MA, Godefroy D, et al. Neurochemokines: a menage a trois providing new insights on the functions of chemokines in the central nervous system. J Neurochem 2011;118(5):680–94.

49. Dammann O, O'Shea TM. Cytokines and perinatal brain damage. Clin Perinatol 2008;35(4):643–63.

50. Foster-Barber A, Dickens B, Ferriero DM. Human perinatal asphyxia: correlation of neonatal cytokines with MRI and outcome. Dev Neurosci 2001;23(3):213–8.

51. Elovitz MA, Brown AG, Breen K, et al. Intrauterine inflammation, insufficient to induce parturition, still evokes fetal and neonatal brain injury. Int J Dev Neurosci 2011;29(6):663–71.

52. Malaeb S, Dammann O. Fetal inflammatory response and brain injury in the preterm newborn. J Child Neurol 2009;24(9):1119–26.

53. Shalak LF, Perlman JM. Infection markers and early signs of neonatal encephalopathy in the term infant. Ment Retard Dev Disabil Res Rev 2002;8(1):14–9.

54. Ellison VJ, Mocatta TJ, Winterbourn CC, et al. The relationship of CSF and plasma cytokine levels to cerebral white matter injury in the premature newborn. Pediatr Res 2005;57(2):282–6.

55. Volpe JJ. Cerebral white matter injury of the premature infant-more common than you think. Pediatrics 2003;112(1 Pt 1):176–80.

56. Savman K, Blennow M, Gustafson K, et al. Cytokine response in cerebrospinal fluid after birth asphyxia. Pediatr Res 1998;43(6):746–51.

57. Chiesa C, Pellegrini G, Panero A, et al. Umbilical cord interleukin-6 levels are elevated in term neonates with perinatal asphyxia. Eur J Clin Invest 2003;33(4): 352–8.

58. Bartha AI, Foster-Barber A, Miller SP, et al. Neonatal encephalopathy: association of cytokines with MR spectroscopy and outcome. Pediatr Res 2004;56(6):960–6.

59. Ramaswamy V, Horton J, Vandermeer B, et al. Systematic review of biomarkers of brain injury in term neonatal encephalopathy. Pediatr Neurol 2009;40(3):215–26.

60. Jenkins DD, Rollins LG, Perkel JK, et al. Serum cytokines in a clinical trial of hypothermia for neonatal hypoxic-ischemic encephalopathy. J Cereb Blood Flow Metab 2012;32(10):1888–96.

Neuroimaging and Other Neurodiagnostic Tests in Neonatal Encephalopathy

Stephanie L. Merhar, MD, MS[a],*, Vann Chau, MD[b]

KEYWORDS

- Hypoxic-ischemic encephalopathy • Birth asphyxia • MRI • MR spectroscopy
- Amplitude integrated EEG • Near-infrared spectroscopy

KEY POINTS

- Neonatal hypoxic-ischemic brain injury is associated with a high rate of death and disability despite the introduction of therapeutic hypothermia to clinical practice.
- Hypoxic-ischemic brain injury evolves over days and weeks, and interpreting magnetic resonance (MR) scans of infants with suspected birth asphyxia should take this concept of progression into account in order to avoid underestimating the extent of brain injury.
- Therapeutic hypothermia affects MRI, amplitude-integrated electroencephalogram, and near-infrared spectroscopy findings but should not impact the overall predictive values of these tests.
- Amplitude-integrated electroencephalogram and near-infrared spectroscopy are noninvasive tools that can help monitor brain functions at the bedside and predict long-term outcomes.
- Advanced MR techniques are promising in that they can help us better understand the pathophysiology of brain injury and assess its progression, in addition to fine-tuning clinicians' ability to predict outcomes.

NEUROIMAGING

The prediction of long-term outcomes in infants with neonatal encephalopathy is of great importance to families and clinicians, whether this information is used to pursue comfort care or to justify more invasive interventions. In addition, stratification of these infants may allow for identification of infants who will benefit from further

Disclosure Statement: The authors have nothing to disclose.
[a] Division of Neonatology, Cincinnati Children's Hospital Medical Center, Perinatal Institute, ML 7009, Cincinnati, OH 45229, USA; [b] Division of Neurology (Pediatrics), The Hospital for Sick Children, University of Toronto and Neuroscience & Mental Health Research Institute, 555 University Avenue, Room 6536B, Hill Wing, Toronto, Ontario M5G 1X8, Canada
* Corresponding author.
E-mail address: stephanie.merhar@cchmc.org

Clin Perinatol 43 (2016) 511–527
http://dx.doi.org/10.1016/j.clp.2016.04.009
0095-5108/16/$ – see front matter © 2016 Elsevier Inc. All rights reserved.
perinatology.theclinics.com

neuroprotective therapies, some of which are currently being tested (eg, erythropoietin and stem cells). This review addresses the role of neuroimaging, amplitude-integrated electroencephalography (aEEG), and near-infrared spectroscopy (NIRS) for neurodevelopmental prognostication in term newborns with encephalopathy. This review also discusses the effect of therapeutic hypothermia on the predictive values of these tests.

Sensitivity means the ability of a test to correctly classify an individual as having a disease, in this case the ability of an abnormal MRI/aEEG/NIRS to classify an infant as having later disability. Specificity refers to the ability of a test to correctly classify a person as disease free, in this case the ability of normal MRI, aEEG, or NIRS to predict that an infant will *not* die or have severe disability. Unlike sensitivity and specificity, predictive values depend on the prevalence of the disease (in this case, abnormal neurologic outcome) in the population. Positive predictive value (PPV) is the percentage of patients with a positive test who actually have the disease, in this case the percentage of all infants with death or disability who had an abnormal MRI/aEEG/NIRS in the neonatal period. Negative predictive value (NPV) is the percentage of patients with a negative test who do not have the disease or the percentage of all infants with a good/normal outcome who had a normal MRI/aEEG/NIRS in the neonatal period.

MRI

With technology advances, the capacity to safely repeat brain imaging in critically ill infants has enabled studies confirming the clinical and experimental observations that neonatal brain injury evolves over days and weeks.[1] With the development of magnetic resonance (MR)-compatible incubators and monitoring equipment, MRI is now the modality of choice, although head ultrasound and computed tomography (CT) still have a role to play in specific circumstances. Despite its ability to detect the predominant patterns of brain injury after birth asphyxia, sensitivity and specificity of CT for injury are significantly lower than MRI[2]; there are important concerns of radiation exposure with its routine use.[3] Head ultrasound is often normal even in cases of severe birth asphyxia but can be used to rule out antenatal injury and intracranial hemorrhage. Imaging infants with birth asphyxia is important to confirm the diagnosis and exclude other causes of neonatal encephalopathy, such as metabolic disorders or neonatal stroke. Of note, MRI with diffusion-weighted imaging (DWI) seems to be the most sensitive imaging method to detect abnormalities associated with other causes of neonatal encephalopathy, such as cerebral dysgenesis, infections, stroke, and metabolic disorders. Imaging can also guide clinical decision-making and counsel families. The standard neonatal brain MRI protocol includes conventional anatomic sequences (T1- and T2-weighted imaging) and DWI. Brain imaging has revealed patterns of brain injury following a hypoxic-ischemic insult that are unique to the immature brain and that depend on the age at which it occurs and the severity and duration of the insult (**Fig. 1**).[4,5] These clinical investigations have confirmed the prolonged temporal evolution of brain injury that was initially revealed by neonatal animal models. This time course suggests a therapeutic window for interventions that could be instituted hours or days after the hypoxic-ischemic insult.[1]

In order to confirm the diagnosis of hypoxic-ischemic brain injury and determine the extent of injury, MRI and DWI are optimally acquired between 3 and 5 days of life in term newborns with encephalopathy.[6–8] In newborns treated with hypothermia, the *optimal* timing of MRI is unclear and will require further investigation.[9] In a neonatal primate model of brain injury, the distribution of injury is associated with the duration and severity of ischemia. Although acute and profound asphyxia produces injury in the basal ganglia and thalamus, prolonged and partial asphyxia causes diffuse injury in

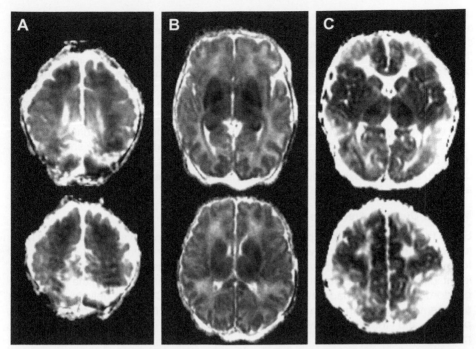

Fig. 1. Predominant patterns of brain injury in term hypoxic-ischemic encephalopathy. In (*A*), watershed-predominant pattern of injury in a newborn with perinatal asphyxia imaged on the third day of life. Cortical and subcortical brain injury is demonstrated (hypointense, *dark areas*) on these apparent diffusion coefficient (ADC) maps in the watershed regions, affecting both the cortex and the white matter. In (*B*), basal ganglia–predominant pattern of injury in a newborn with perinatal asphyxia imaged on the third day of life. Brain injury is demonstrated on the ADC maps as areas of restricted diffusion (hypointense, *dark areas*) in the thalami, basal ganglia, and optic radiations. Both the basal nuclei and watershed-predominant patterns can lead to the total predominant pattern (*C*), if severe enough, as shown by diffuse areas of restricted diffusion (hypointense, *dark areas*) on these ADC maps.

the white matter.[10] Similar patterns of injury are found in term newborns following hypoxia-ischemia (see **Fig. 1**). The *basal ganglia*–predominant pattern involves the basal ganglia and thalamus and perirolandic cortex.[5,6,11] The *watershed* pattern predominantly involves the vascular watershed, from the white matter and extending to the cerebral cortex.[5,11] Maximal injury in both the watershed region and basal ganglia leads to the total pattern of brain injury.[5,11]

Determining the Onset and Progression of Injury

Determining the onset and progression of brain injury has been facilitated with the use of diffusion MR techniques. DWI detects alterations in free water diffusion. With acute injury, intracellular water increases and water movement is restricted by the cell membrane. Diffusion imaging will show an area of restricted diffusion as increased signal intensity. Recent studies have shown that the reduction in diffusion due to brain injury in term newborns evolves over the initial days of life, reaching its peak by 2 to 4 days after injury.[8,12] On days 1 and 2 after injury, T1/T2 changes are very subtle, whereas diffusion changes are more apparent.[8] By day of life 3, T1/T2 changes are more apparent and diffusion changes are even more apparent. Scans on day of life 7 continue to show more obvious T1/T2 changes, but diffusion values begin to normalize (known as pseudonormalization). In line with this concept, diffusion images acquired before 2 to 4 days may underestimate the full extent of injury. As diffusion abnormalities persist only for 7 to 8 days before pseudonormalization, imaging around this time period may also underestimate the extent of injury.[12,13] Exceptionally, brain injury may progressively worsen over the first 2 weeks of life to involve new brain areas, particularly the white matter tracts. Quantitative MR techniques now offer a dynamic measure of brain injury in the newborn that can be safely used to determine the short-term effects of novel intervention strategies. It is critical that MR interpretation takes into account this dynamic association between the onset of brain injury and time of imaging acquisition.

MRI and Outcome Prediction

Since the first description of predominant patterns of injury, several investigators have looked at their association with the long-term outcomes of asphyxiated infants. At follow-up, 56% of 173 surviving infants with basal ganglia/thalamus (BG/T)–predominant injury had spastic quadriplegia, whereas only 11% of infants with the watershed-predominant pattern had severe cerebral palsy (CP).[5] Cognitive deficits were more apparent at 30 months than 12 months in infants with the watershed-predominant pattern, and these cognitive deficits often occurred in the absence of motor problems.[5]

Other investigators have found that abnormal signal intensity in the posterior limb of the internal capsule (PLIC) on T1/T2 imaging seems to be an accurate predictor of motor outcome after birth asphyxia.[14] Rutherford and colleagues[14] studied 73 term infants with birth asphyxia and reported that all with abnormal signal intensity in the PLIC on T1/T2-weighted images had neurodevelopmental impairment (defined as any Griffith score <85 or any neurologic abnormality on examination) at 12 months of age. The absence of normal signal in the PLIC predicted abnormal outcomes with a sensitivity of 0.90, specificity of 1.0, PPV of 1.0, and NPV of 0.89.

A large meta-analysis evaluated 32 studies of MRI in 860 noncooled infants with neonatal encephalopathy.[15] Conventional MRI, mostly using scoring systems based on T1- and T2-weighted imaging, had a pooled sensitivity of 0.91 and specificity of 0.51 to predict adverse outcome (death and/or moderate/severe disability, depending on the individual study) at 12 or more months of age. Late MRI (defined as MRI between day of life 8 and 30) had higher sensitivity but lower specificity than early MRI (performed between day of life 1 and 7). However, there was significant statistical heterogeneity between studies.

More recently, Hayes and colleagues[16] studied 73 infants who were not cooled with neonatal MRI and follow-up. Almost one-third of the infants with a normal MRI of the brain in the neonatal period were at risk of developmental problems at 2 to 4 years of age. Death/CP occurred only in the children with more extensive damage in the BG/T or severe watershed injury. Seventy-seven percent of infants with isolated BG/T injury died or developed CP. Involvement of the PLIC was a poor prognostic sign usually associated with neurologic sequelae, as all 23 children with PLIC injury had some developmental problems.

Hypothermia does not seem to alter the prognostic value of MRI, although 2 studies showed that it may alter the timing of changes seen on MRI. In a small series of 23 infants with hypoxic-ischemic encephalopathy (HIE), pseudonormalization of

DWI seems to occur later in infants undergoing hypothermia.[17] The return of mean diffusivity to normal values occurred after the 10th day in infants treated with hypothermia versus 6 to 8 days in infants with HIE not treated with hypothermia. Another prospective study using serial MRI found that the T1/T2 changes appeared later (by day of life 3 in noncooled infants but not until the MRI on day of life 10 in 2 of the cooled infants).[9] Despite these limitations, recent analyses showed that predictive values of MRI do not seem to be affected by therapeutic hypothermia. Rutherford and colleagues[18] studied 131 infants from the TOBY cooling trial (TOtal Body hYpothermia). They found that in the infants treated with therapeutic hypothermia, less BG/T lesions and fewer abnormalities in the PLIC were identified. Infants who were cooled were more likely to have normal scans. They calculated the ability of major MRI abnormalities to predict death or major disability at 18 months in both groups. In the cooled infants, sensitivity was 0.88, specificity was 0.82, PPV was 0.76, and NPV was 0.91, whereas in the noncooled group the sensitivity was 0.94, specificity was 0.68, PPV was 0.74, and NPV 0.92.[18] In the Infant Cooling Evaluation (ICE) trial, fewer newborns in the hypothermia group had moderate/severe white matter or gray matter abnormalities on T1/T2-weighted scans as compared with infants in the normothermia group; but abnormal MRI findings were still predictive of outcome in both the normothermia and the hypothermia groups.[19] The sensitivity of T1/T2 and diffusion abnormalities to predict adverse outcome was low (0.27–0.60) but specificity was high (0.92–0.95).[19] Even in the longer term, MRI seems to demonstrate good predictive values. In the National Institute of Child Health and Human Development cooling trial, the sensitivity, specificity, PPV, and NPV of moderate/severe brain injury on neonatal MRI to predict death or IQ less than 70 at 6 to 7 years of age were similar between the hypothermia group (0.77, 0.85, 0.71, and 0.89, respectively) and the control group (0.85, 0.66, 0.69, and 0.83, respectively).[20] Death or IQ less than 70 occurred in 4 of 50 children with normal MRI in the neonatal period. A recent systematic review has analyzed these studies in detail and determined the pooled sensitivity, specificity, PPV, and NPV of these different studies (**Table 1**).[21]

Advanced Magnetic Resonance Techniques

Advanced MR techniques, such as diffusion and spectroscopic imaging, allow clinicians to observe the progression of brain injury more objectively than visual inspection.[22] Additionally, diffusion tensor imaging (DTI) and MR spectroscopy can be used to measure brain maturation. In newborns with brain injury, DTI may detect abnormalities of microstructural brain development remote from the primary injuries, in areas of the brain that appear normal on T_1- and T_2-weighted images.[23]

Quantitative Diffusion-Weighted Imaging and Diffusion Tensor Imaging

DTI measures the amount (apparent diffusion coefficient [ADC], or average diffusivity) and the directionality (fractional anisotropy [FA]) of water motion. With brain maturation, ADC decreases in gray and white matter with the development of cell membranes that restrict water diffusion.[24,25] Over this period, FA increases in white matter, even before myelin is evident on T_1- and T_2-weighted images.[23,26] FA values in the white matter and basal ganglia are decreased with significant injury during the first week of life in term newborns with encephalopathy.[27]

ADC can be measured by drawing regions of interest on the ADC map outputted by most commercial radiology software. Using this region-of-interest–based technique, reduced ADC values in the PLIC were found to be associated with a greater risk of adverse neurodevelopmental outcome in term newborns with encephalopathy.[28] In another study, mean diffusivity in various areas of the brain, including the corpus

Table 1
Predictive values of different ancillary tests in newborns at 36 or more weeks' gestation with hypoxic-ischemic encephalopathy with follow-up to greater than 18 months of age

Study (Design)	Abnormal Findings	Outcome Studied	Pooled Sensitivity and Specificity[21]
MRI			
Alderliesten et al,[43] 2011 (R)	MRI: basal ganglia ADC ≤1031 × 10^{-6} mm²/s; MRS: basal ganglia lactate/NAA >0.08	Griffiths and neurological examination (18–46-mo follow-up)	
Ferrari et al,[67] 2011 (P)	MRI: abnormal T1/T2 in basal ganglia, white matter, cortex or PLIC	Griffiths and neurological examination (2-y follow-up)	
Twomey et al,[68] 2010 (P)	MRI: abnormalities T1/T2 or DWI: diffuse, watershed, central, atypical	Bayley II and WPPSI (2-y follow-up)	
Rutherford et al,[18] 2010 (P)	MRI: abnormalities T1/T2 in basal ganglia, PLIC, white matter, cortex	Bayley and GMFCS (18-mo follow-up)	
Ancora et al,[69] 2010 (P)	MRS: ratio lactate/creatine >0.3, ratio NAA/creatine <0.5	Griffiths Mental Developmental Scale (2-y follow-up)	*DWI:* ≤1 wk: sensitivity 0.58 and specificity 0.89
Liauw et al,[70] 2009 (R)	MRI: ADC basal ganglia <1018.5 × 10^{-6} mm²/s	van Wiechen examination (2-y follow-up)	*ADC:* ≤1 wk: sensitivity 0.79 and specificity 0.85
Vermeulen et al,[71] 2008 (P)	MRI: T1/T2 or DWI abnormal cortex, basal ganglia, brainstem, PLIC or cerebellum	Bayley II (2-y follow-up)	*T1/T2:* ≤1 wk: sensitivity 0.84 and specificity 0.90, ≤2 wk: sensitivity 0.98 and specificity 0.76, ≤6 wk: sensitivity 0.83 and specificity 0.53
L'Abee et al,[72] 2005 (P)	MRI: abnormalities T1/T2 or DWI in cortex, basal ganglia, or white matter; Abnormal ADC in basal ganglia or white matter; MRS: elevated lactate/NAA in basal ganglia	Griffiths and neurological examination (2-y follow-up)	
Belet et al,[73] 2004 (P)	MRI: abnormalities T1/T2 white matter, deep gray matter, encephalomalacia/atrophy	Bayley II and Denver developmental test (3.5–4.0-y follow-up)	
Khong et al,[74] 2004 (P)	MRI: abnormal T1/T2 or DWI in white matter, deep gray nuclei, brainstem; abnormal ADC in basal ganglia	Griffiths and neurological examination (18–24-mo follow-up)	
Biagioni et al,[75] 2001 (P)	MRI: abnormal T1/T2 in BG/T, PLIC, white matter	Griffiths and neurological examination (2-y follow-up)	
Roelants-van Rijn et al,[39] 2001 (P)	MRI: abnormal T1/T2 in BG/T, PLIC, cortex	Griffiths and neurological examination (2-y follow-up)	
Groenendaal et al,[76] 1996 (P)	MRS: lactate in basal ganglia or periventricular white matter	Griffiths and neurological examination (18-mo follow-up)	

EEG and aEEG

Study	Abnormal finding	Outcome measure	Sensitivity/specificity
Murray et al,[77] 2009 (P)	Moderate, major abnormalities EEG background; seizures or inactive EEG	Griffiths and neurological examination (2-y follow-up)	
Toet et al,[78] 2006 (P) (232)	Abnormal EEG pattern: flat trace, continuous low-voltage, burst suppression, seizures	Griffiths and Movement ABC (2-y follow-up)	
van Rooij et al,[57] 2005 (R)	Abnormal EEG pattern: flat trace, continuous low voltage, burst suppression	Griffiths and neurological examination (2-y follow-up)	
ter Horst et al,[58] 2004 (R)	Abnormal EEG pattern: flat trace, continuous low voltage, burst suppression	Touwen test (2-y follow-up)	
Toet et al,[79] 1999 (P)	Abnormal EEG pattern: flat trace, continuous low voltage, burst suppression	Griffiths and neurological examination (5-y follow-up)	aEEG: ≤6 h: sensitivity 0.95 and specificity 0.92, ≤72 h: sensitivity 0.93 and specificity 0.90
Eken et al,[80] 1995 (P)	Abnormal EEG pattern: flat trace, continuous low voltage, burst suppression; seizures on aEEG	Griffiths and neurological examination (2-y follow-up)	EEG: ≤72 h: sensitivity 0.92 and specificity 0.83
van Lieshout et al,[81] 1995 (R)	Abnormal EEG: isoelectric, low-voltage pattern, burst suppression, diffuse delta pattern, interhemispheric asynchrony	WHO disability staging (7-y follow-up)	
Thornberg & Ekstrom-Jodal,[82] 1994 (P)	Abnormal aEEG background (burst suppression) or seizures	Denver developmental test (18-mo follow-up)	
Prechtl et al,[83] 1993 (P)	EEG: electrical discharges, severely depressed and/or severely discontinuous interictal EEG	Griffiths and neurological examination (17–24-mo follow-up)	

Adverse outcome defined by 1 or more of the following: (1) CP; (2) ≥2 standard deviations less than the mean on Bayley Mental and Developmental Scales or Griffiths Mental Developmental Index; (3) death during the specified follow-up period.

Abbreviations: ABC, Movement Assessment Battery for Children; ADC, apparent diffusion coefficient; GMFCS, Gross Motor Function Classification Scale; MRS, MR spectroscopy; NAA, N-acetylaspartate; P, prospective; R, retrospective; WHO, World Health Organization; WPPSI, Wechsler Preschool and Primary Scale of Intelligence.

Data from van Laerhoven H, de Haan TR, Offringa M, et al. Prognostic tests in term neonate with hypoxic-ischemic encephalopathy: a systematic review. Pediatrics 2013;131(1):88–98.

callosum and thalamus, in 20 infants with HIE had a PPV of 1.0 and a NPV of 0.83 to predict death or severe CP or death at 2 years of age.[29] In Thayyil and colleagues'[15] meta-analysis evaluating 4 studies using ADC, measurement of ADC had a sensitivity of 0.66 and specificity of 0.64 to predict neurologic outcome after 12 months of age. It should be noted, however, that therapeutic hypothermia is associated with preserved brain microstructure, particularly in the BG/T.[30] For example, although restricted diffusion in the posterior corpus callosum predicts an adverse outcome following HIE, therapeutic hypothermia modifies this association, such that greater restriction is needed for an adverse outcome.[31]

Tract-based spatial statistics (TBSS) is an automated whole-brain approach to evaluating DTI images, which aligns white matter tract skeletons from multiple subjects. In a small cohort of 43 term newborns with HIE studied with TBSS, infants with unfavorable outcomes at 12 to 28 months of age had significantly lower FA values in multiple areas of the brain than infants with favorable outcomes.[32]

Diffusion tensor tractography, another technique derived from DTI, also provides new insights into recovery and resilience by measuring microstructural development of specific functional pathways.[33] In encephalopathic newborns, impaired microstructural organization of the corpus callosum and corticospinal tract predicts poorer cognitive and motor performance, respectively, at 15 and 21 months.[34]

Magnetic Resonance Spectroscopy

MR spectroscopy (MRS) acquires signals from metabolites in predefined regions of the brain. The strongest signals in normal brain tissue are from choline (Cho), creatine (Cr), and N-acetylaspartate (NAA). NAA levels decrease with cerebral injury or impaired cerebral metabolism.[35] Lactate (Lac) levels are elevated with disturbed brain energy substrate delivery and oxidative metabolism as seen with hypoxia-ischemia. In the first 24 hours following brain injury in the term newborn, Lac increases followed by a decrease in NAA in the 3 days following injury.[13] Results can be reported as absolute concentrations of metabolites or ratios of metabolites. Elevated Lac and reduced NAA levels are highly predictive of neurodevelopmental outcome following neonatal brain injury.[35] Given this, Lac/NAA ratios are especially discriminatory of newborns with adverse outcomes.[35,36]

Several small studies have evaluated MRS in infants with HIE and found that, compared with infants with normal outcomes or mild delays, infants with severe neurologic abnormalities or death have significantly decreased NAA and increased Lac.[37,38] One study found that the NAA/Cho at an echo time of 136 milliseconds had the best predictive value, with an area under the receiver operating characteristic (ROC) curve of 0.90, PPV of 0.85, and an NPV of 1.0 using a NAA/Cho cutoff value of 0.62.[39] However, in many MRS studies there is a significant overlap between the good and poor outcome groups. In their meta-analysis of biomarkers in HIE, Thayyil and colleagues[15] pooled 10 studies that evaluated the Lac/NAA ratio in the basal ganglia, with a median cutoff value between normal and abnormal of 0.29. The pooled sensitivity was 0.82 and specificity was 0.95 for a value greater than 0.29 to predict a poor outcome (death or disability measured at $\geq$12 months). To these investigators, the Lac/NAA ratio in the deep gray matter seemed to be the most accurate MR biomarker for outcome prediction.

The earliest MRS study evaluated 28 infants with presumed HIE (not cooled) within 48 hours of birth. Infants were followed to 1 year of age.[40] The maximum Lac/NAA ratio (cutoff value of 0.34) predicted adverse outcomes at 1 year with a specificity of 0.90 and PPV of 0.92. Similar results were found by Shanmugalingam and colleagues[36] a few years later in 21 noncooled term infants with HIE, scanned between

1 and 5 days after birth. Surviving infants were examined at 1 year of age. Again, the Lac/NAA ratio in the thalamus was found to be the most predictive of moderate/severe disability, with a cutoff value of 0.24 having a sensitivity of 0.85, specificity of 0.88, and area under the ROC curve of 0.96. In a smaller cohort of 14 noncooled neonates, the ratios of Lac/Cr and Lac/NAA within the first 4 days of life were significantly different for the babies who died compared with those who survived birth asphyxia.[41] The investigators found that an Lac/NAA more than 2 SD greater than the mean (cutoff value not reported in the paper) on early MRS combined with moderate to severe abnormalities on early neurologic examination had a sensitivity, specificity, PPV, and NPV of 100%, although both tests were performed on only 6 infants. Maximum Lac/NAA more than 2 SD greater than the mean alone also performed well to predict later outcomes, with a sensitivity of 0.79, specificity of 0.93, PPV of 0.92, and NPV of 0.81.

Like MRI, MRS seems to still be valuable in the hypothermia era. Corbo and colleagues[42] evaluated 38 infants with birth asphyxia, half of whom were cooled. There were lower levels of Lac in the infants treated with hypothermia, but the NAA ratios were not different between the 2 groups. Lac was present in the occipital gray matter in 31.6% of the noncooled neonates and 10.5% of the cooled neonates. Follow-up was not performed in this study. Ancora and colleagues[29] followed 20 babies to 2 years of age who were treated for HIE with selective head cooling and had MRI in the neonatal period. NAA/Cr in the basal ganglia (value $\leq$0.67) had a PPV of 1.0 and NPV of 0.93 to predict poor outcomes (death or severe CP at 2 years of age), and other MRS predictors from the basal ganglia had reasonable predictive accuracy as well.

With the variety of imaging predictors available, several investigators have attempted to increase the predictive power by combining them. In a series of 19 noncooled infants with HIE and scanned with MRI and MRS between day 3 and day 7 of life, Goergen and colleagues[22] found that either an Lac/NAA of 0.25 or greater or bilateral DWI signal abnormality in the PLIC (agreed on by 3 radiologists) had a sensitivity and specificity of 1.0 to predict poor outcomes (death or any Bayley score <70 at 2 years). Despite a small sample size, this study is important because it combines quantitative and qualitative MRI data. In a larger cohort, Alderliesten and colleagues[43] improved outcome prediction by combining the MRI score (based on T1 and T2 imaging) with the ADC on DWI or MRS. Sensitivity, specificity, PPV, and NPV were not calculated; but the area under the curve (AUC) was 0.85 for MRI score plus Lac/NAA ratio, and AUC was 0.93 for MRI score plus basal ganglia ADC.

AMPLITUDE-INTEGRATED ELECTROENCEPHALOGRAM

The term *aEEG* refers to the raw EEG signal that has been amplified, passed through a filter to minimize artifacts, and time compressed. Most modern aEEG machines have the ability to use a single-channel (3 electrodes) or 2-channel (5 electrodes) aEEG for recording, and most also have the option of displaying the raw EEG trace. One study showed that the 2-channel tracing was more sensitive to detect cerebral injury than the single channel.[44] Two main classification systems for aEEG have been developed, using either voltage or pattern to determine the background (see **Table 1**).[45,46] Although both classifications have been used in predictive studies and have been shown to perform similarly,[47] in 2 studies the pattern method was found to be more sensitive than the voltage method.[48,49] The presence, absence, and time to recovery of sleep-wake cycling, seen as smooth sinusoidal variations mostly in the lower margin of the aEEG tracing, has also been evaluated as a prognostic indicator.

Medications, such as sedatives and anticonvulsants, can alter the aEEG tracing, usually by suppressing the background[50,51]; caution should be used in the interpretation of the aEEG tracing for at least 60 minutes after administration of these medications. Artifacts due to electrical interference and movement/shivering are also common in the aEEG tracing and may lead to incorrect classification of the background.[52–54] Hypothermia at the temperatures used in current practice (33.5°C) should not affect the EEG trace.[55]

Early studies on the predictive value of aEEG concluded that the aEEG tracing at or before 6 hours of life was an excellent predictor of later poor outcomes. A meta-analysis of 8 studies published before the widespread adoption of therapeutic hypothermia found a pooled sensitivity of 0.91 for aEEG to predict poor outcomes, although time at aEEG and age at outcome determination were variable in this meta-analysis.[56] However, since therapeutic hypothermia has become standard of care, the predictive value of aEEG seems to have decreased. This decrease is likely because hypothermia may improve later outcomes even in infants with a very abnormal initial tracing.

Time to recovery of background seems to be important; even infants with a severely abnormal background pattern (burst suppression) in the first 6 hours of life had a good likelihood of survival without significant disability if the pattern normalized within the first 24 hours of life.[57] Another study had similar findings: the more quickly the aEEG pattern normalizes in the first 72 hours, the more likely the infant had a better outcome.[58] In infants treated with hypothermia, only those who had aEEG abnormalities persisting at or beyond 24 hours showed poor neurologic outcomes at 1 year of age.[59] Another study also found that the recovery time to normal background was the best predictor of poor outcomes and that, in cooled infants, if background had recovered by 48 hours, outcomes were likely to be good (vs 24 hours in noncooled infants).[49]

Time of onset of sleep-wake cycles (SWC) also may be predictive of later outcomes. Even in infants with absent SWC initially, onset of SWC within the first 36 hours of life was associated with normal outcomes, whereas those who never had normal SWC were more likely to have significant disability at 18 to 22 months.[60] Another study had similar findings in cooled babies, demonstrating that all infants who developed SWC by 72 hours of life had a good outcome and that nondevelopment of SWC resulted in a PPV of 0.73 for a poor outcome.[61] Finally, a third study showed that both infants treated with hypothermia and those in the standard group who never developed SWC almost invariably had poor outcomes.[49]

NEAR-INFRARED SPECTROSCOPY

NIRS is a method of noninvasively monitoring tissue oxygenation. The early monitors attempted to use changes in oxygenated and deoxygenated hemoglobin as measures of cerebral oxygenation, but it was difficult to use these as long-term measures.[62] In the newer NIRS devices, the cerebral tissue oxygenation index (TOI) and the regional cerebral oxygen saturation ($rScO_2$) can be used to estimate changes in cerebral oxygen saturation. Fractional cerebral tissue extraction (FTOE) can also be calculated, which represents the balance between oxygen delivery and oxygen consumption. Several investigators have attempted to use NIRS measurements for both short- and long-term outcomes in infants after birth asphyxia with mixed success. One study showed that infants with HIE (n = 12) who had a poor outcome (death, CP, or global delays at 12 months) had a higher level of cerebral oxygenation using TOI at 12 hours of age than those with a normal outcome.[63] Another study had

---

Box 1
Amplitude-integrated electroencephalography classification systems

Classification by voltage[a,45]

Normal (upper >10 µV, lower >5 µV)

Moderately abnormal (upper >10 µV, lower ≤5 µV)

Severely abnormal/suppressed (upper <10 µV, lower <5 µV)

Classification by pattern[b,46]

Continuous normal voltage

Discontinuous voltage

Burst suppression

Continuous low voltage

Flat tracing

[a] The first method uses voltage of the upper and lower margin of the aEEG signal to classify amplitude as normal, moderately abnormal, or severely abnormal.
[b] The second method distinguishes 5 different patterns. For purposes of outcome prediction, burst suppression, continuous low voltage, and flat tracing are considered significantly abnormal, whereas normal and discontinuous are considered normal/mildly abnormal.

---

similar findings in 22 term neonates with HIE, whereby in the first day of life the TOI was 80.1% in infants with abnormal outcomes at 1 year versus 74.7% in infants with normal 1-year outcomes (P = .04). In a third study of 18 term infants with birth asphyxia, the rSO_2 increased to supranormal values after 24 hours in those infants with an adverse outcome at 5 years of age. A larger study (n = 39) in the era of therapeutic hypothermia again demonstrated that cerebral oxygenation was higher in neonates with an adverse outcome and calculated the predictive values of an $rSCO_2$ more than 77% (**Box 1**).[64]

In a more recent series, 18 infants with HIE undergoing therapeutic hypothermia had NIRS monitoring in the first 72 hours of life.[65] No relationship was found between cerebral rSO_2 and outcome at all time points. Taken together, these studies suggest that infants with birth asphyxia and a later adverse outcome have higher cerebral oxygenation in the first 12 to 48 hours of life. It is unclear whether this hyperperfusion/hyperoxygenation contributes to the injury or represents a compensatory mechanism,[66] and larger studies need to be undertaken to determine the best NIRS variable and cutoff value.

SUMMARY

There have been significant advances in our understanding of neonatal hypoxic-ischemic brain injury over the past years. Despite the introduction of therapeutic hypothermia, the rate of death and severe disability remains high. It is critical to develop new techniques to predict long-term outcomes. MRI, particularly advanced MR techniques, and aEEG seem to provide some insights about prognosis; but their accuracy and ability to predict the full range of neurodevelopment, rather than just death or severe disability, need further refinement. A more collaborative approach among researchers, including sharing of MR measurements and standardization of clinical protocols, would help us achieve this goal.

<hr>

Best practices

What is the current practice?

Currently, most centers perform MRI between 3 and 10 days of life, although some centers still use CT as a primary imaging modality.

What changes in current practice are likely to improve outcomes?

All infants with birth asphyxia and an initial abnormal neurologic examination should have an MRI with MRS and DWI at 3 to 7 days of life (days 3–5 preferred), interpreted by a pediatric neuroradiologist.

The aEEG is also a useful tool for prognosis, with particular emphasis on recovery of background and SWCs.

After reviewing the examination, neuroimaging, and aEEG findings, a meeting should be held with the family, pediatric neurologist, and neonatologist to discuss likely outcomes and need for further neurodevelopmental monitoring and early intervention.

Further research should focus on using more advanced neuroimaging techniques to refine the prediction of outcomes.

<hr>

REFERENCES

1. Ferriero DM. Neonatal brain injury. N Engl J Med 2004;351:1985–95.
2. Barnette AR, Horbar JD, Soll RF, et al. Neuroimaging in the evaluation of neonatal encephalopathy. Pediatrics 2014;133:e1508–17.
3. Hall P, Adami HO, Trichopoulos D, et al. Effect of low doses of ionising radiation in infancy on cognitive function in adulthood: Swedish population based cohort study. BMJ 2004;328:19.
4. Cowan F, Rutherford M, Groenendaal F, et al. Origin and timing of brain lesions in term infants with neonatal encephalopathy. Lancet 2003;361:736–42.
5. Miller SP, Ramaswamy V, Michelson D, et al. Patterns of brain injury in term neonatal encephalopathy. J Pediatr 2005;146:453–60.
6. Chau V, Poskitt KJ, Sargent MA, et al. Comparison of computer tomography and magnetic resonance imaging scans on the third day of life in term newborns with neonatal encephalopathy. Pediatrics 2009;123:319–26.
7. Rutherford M, Counsell S, Allsop J, et al. Diffusion-weighted magnetic resonance imaging in term perinatal brain injury: a comparison with site of lesion and time from birth. Pediatrics 2004;114:1004–14.
8. Barkovich AJ, Miller SP, Bartha A, et al. MR imaging, MR spectroscopy, and diffusion tensor imaging of sequential studies in neonates with encephalopathy. AJNR Am J Neuroradiol 2006;27:533–47.
9. Gano D, Chau V, Poskitt KJ, et al. Evolution of pattern of injury and quantitative MRI on days 1 and 3 in term newborns with hypoxic-ischemic encephalopathy. Pediatr Res 2013;74:82–7.
10. Myers RE. Two patterns of perinatal brain damage and their conditions of occurrence. Am J Obstet Gynecol 1972;112:246–76.
11. Sie LT, van der Knaap MS, Oosting J, et al. MR patterns of hypoxic-ischemic brain damage after prenatal, perinatal or postnatal asphyxia. Neuropediatrics 2000;31: 128–36.

12. McKinstry RC, Miller JH, Snyder AZ, et al. A prospective, longitudinal diffusion tensor imaging study of brain injury in newborns. Neurology 2002;59:824–33.
13. Barkovich AJ, Westmark KD, Bedi HS, et al. Proton spectroscopy and diffusion imaging on the first day of life after perinatal asphyxia: preliminary report. AJNR Am J Neuroradiol 2001;22:1786–94.
14. Rutherford MA, Pennock JM, Counsell SJ, et al. Abnormal magnetic resonance signal in the internal capsule predicts poor neurodevelopmental outcome in infants with hypoxic-ischemic encephalopathy. Pediatrics 1998;102:323–8.
15. Thayyil S, Chandrasekaran M, Taylor A, et al. Cerebral magnetic resonance biomarkers in neonatal encephalopathy: a meta-analysis. Pediatrics 2010;125: e382–95.
16. Hayes BC, Ryan S, McGarvey C, et al. Brain magnetic resonance imaging and outcome after hypoxic ischaemic encephalopathy. J Matern Fetal Neonatal Med 2016;29:777–82.
17. Bednarek N, Mathur A, Inder T, et al. Impact of therapeutic hypothermia on MRI diffusion changes in neonatal encephalopathy. Neurology 2012;78:1420–7.
18. Rutherford M, Ramenghi LA, Edwards AD, et al. Assessment of brain tissue injury after moderate hypothermia in neonates with hypoxic-ischaemic encephalopathy: a nested substudy of a randomised controlled trial. Lancet Neurol 2010;9: 39–45.
19. Cheong JL, Coleman L, Hunt RW, et al. Prognostic utility of magnetic resonance imaging in neonatal hypoxic-ischemic encephalopathy: substudy of a randomized trial. Arch Pediatr Adolesc Med 2012;166:634–40.
20. Pappas A, Shankaran S, McDonald SA, et al. Cognitive outcomes after neonatal encephalopathy. Pediatrics 2015;135:e624–34.
21. van Laerhoven H, de Haan TR, Offringa M, et al. Prognostic tests in term neonates with hypoxic-ischemic encephalopathy: a systematic review. Pediatrics 2013;131:88–98.
22. Goergen SK, Ang H, Wong F, et al. Early MRI in term infants with perinatal hypoxic-ischaemic brain injury: interobserver agreement and MRI predictors of outcome at 2 years. Clin Radiol 2014;69:72–81.
23. Miller SP, Vigneron DB, Henry RG, et al. Serial quantitative diffusion tensor MRI of the premature brain: development in newborns with and without injury. J Magn Reson Imaging 2002;16:621–32.
24. Mukherjee P, Miller JH, Shimony JS, et al. Diffusion-tensor MR imaging of gray and white matter development during normal human brain maturation. AJNR Am J Neuroradiol 2002;23:1445–56.
25. Beaulieu C. The basis of anisotropic water diffusion in the nervous system - a technical review. NMR Biomed 2002;15:435–55.
26. Drobyshevsky A, Song SK, Gamkrelidze G, et al. Developmental changes in diffusion anisotropy coincide with immature oligodendrocyte progression and maturation of compound action potential. J Neurosci 2005;25:5988–97.
27. Ward P, Counsell S, Allsop J, et al. Reduced fractional anisotropy on diffusion tensor magnetic resonance imaging after hypoxic-ischemic encephalopathy. Pediatrics 2006;117:e619–30.
28. Hunt RW, Neil JJ, Coleman LT, et al. Apparent diffusion coefficient in the posterior limb of the internal capsule predicts outcome after perinatal asphyxia. Pediatrics 2004;114:999–1003.
29. Ancora G, Testa C, Grandi S, et al. Prognostic value of brain proton MR spectroscopy and diffusion tensor imaging in newborns with hypoxic-ischemic encephalopathy treated by brain cooling. Neuroradiology 2013;55:1017–25.

30. Bonifacio SL, Saporta A, Glass HC, et al. Therapeutic hypothermia for neonatal encephalopathy results in improved microstructure and metabolism in the deep gray nuclei. AJNR Am J Neuroradiol 2012;33:2050–5.

31. Alderliesten T, de Vries LS, Khalil Y, et al. Therapeutic hypothermia modifies perinatal asphyxia-induced changes of the corpus callosum and outcome in neonates. PLoS One 2015;10:e0123230.

32. Tusor N, Wusthoff C, Smee N, et al. Prediction of neurodevelopmental outcome after hypoxic-ischemic encephalopathy treated with hypothermia by diffusion tensor imaging analyzed using tract-based spatial statistics. Pediatr Res 2012; 72:63–9.

33. Glenn OA, Ludeman NA, Berman JI, et al. Diffusion tensor MR imaging tractography of the pyramidal tracts correlates with clinical motor function in children with congenital hemiparesis. AJNR Am J Neuroradiol 2007;28:1796–802.

34. Massaro AN, Evangelou I, Fatemi A, et al. White matter tract integrity and developmental outcome in newborn infants with hypoxic-ischemic encephalopathy treated with hypothermia. Dev Med Child Neurol 2015;57:441–8.

35. Barkovich AJ, Raybaud C. Pediatric neuroimaging. 5th edition. Philadelphia: Lippincott Williams & Wilkins; 2012.

36. Shanmugalingam S, Thornton JS, Iwata O, et al. Comparative prognostic utilities of early quantitative magnetic resonance imaging spin-spin relaxometry and proton magnetic resonance spectroscopy in neonatal encephalopathy. Pediatrics 2006;118:1467–77.

37. Cheong JL, Cady EB, Penrice J, et al. Proton MR spectroscopy in neonates with perinatal cerebral hypoxic-ischemic injury: metabolite peak-area ratios, relaxation times, and absolute concentrations. AJNR Am J Neuroradiol 2006;27:1546–54.

38. van Doormaal PJ, Meiners LC, ter Horst HJ, et al. The prognostic value of multivoxel magnetic resonance spectroscopy determined metabolite levels in white and grey matter brain tissue for adverse outcome in term newborns following perinatal asphyxia. Eur Radiol 2012;22:772–8.

39. Roelants-Van Rijn AM, Van Der Grond J, De Vries LS, et al. Value of (1)h-MRS using different echo times in neonates with cerebral hypoxia-ischemia. Pediatr Res 2001;49:356–62.

40. Amess PN, Penrice J, Wylezinska M, et al. Early brain proton magnetic resonance spectroscopy and neonatal neurology related to neurodevelopmental outcome at 1 year in term infants after presumed hypoxic-ischaemic brain injury. Dev Med Child Neurol 1999;41:436–45.

41. Brissaud O, Chateil JF, Bordessoules M, et al. Chemical shift imaging and localised magnetic resonance spectroscopy in full-term asphyxiated neonates. Pediatr Radiol 2005;35:998–1005.

42. Corbo ET, Bartnik-Olson BL, Machado S, et al. The effect of whole-body cooling on brain metabolism following perinatal hypoxic–ischemic injury. Pediatr Res 2012;71:85–92.

43. Alderliesten T, de Vries LS, Benders MJ, et al. MR imaging and outcome of term neonates with perinatal asphyxia: value of diffusion-weighted MR imaging and (1) H MR spectroscopy. Radiology 2011;261:235–42.

44. Lavery S, Shah DK, Hunt RW, et al. Single versus bihemispheric amplitude-integrated electroencephalography in relation to cerebral injury and outcome in the term encephalopathic infant. J Paediatr Child Health 2008;44:285–90.

45. al Naqeeb N, Edwards AD, Cowan FM, et al. Assessment of neonatal encephalopathy by amplitude-integrated electroencephalography. Pediatrics 1999;103: 1263–71.

46. Hellstrom-Westas L, Rosen I. Continuous brain-function monitoring: state of the art in clinical practice. Semin Fetal Neonatal Med 2006;11:503–11.
47. Shellhaas RA, Gallagher PR, Clancy RR. Assessment of neonatal electroencephalography (EEG) background by conventional and two amplitude-integrated EEG classification systems. J Pediatr 2008;153:369–74.
48. Shany E, Goldstein E, Khvatskin S, et al. Predictive value of amplitude-integrated electroencephalography pattern and voltage in asphyxiated term infants. Pediatr Neurol 2006;35:335–42.
49. Thoresen M, Hellstrom-Westas L, Liu X, et al. Effect of hypothermia on amplitude-integrated electroencephalogram in infants with asphyxia. Pediatrics 2010;126: e131–9.
50. Bernet V, Latal B, Natalucci G, et al. Effect of sedation and analgesia on postoperative amplitude-integrated EEG in newborn cardiac patients. Pediatr Res 2010; 67:650–5.
51. Hellstrom-Westas L. Midazolam and amplitude-integrated EEG. Acta Paediatr 2004;93:1153–4.
52. Hagmann CF, Robertson NJ, Azzopardi D. Artifacts on electroencephalograms may influence the amplitude-integrated EEG classification: a qualitative analysis in neonatal encephalopathy. Pediatrics 2006;118:2552–4.
53. Marics G, Cseko A, Vasarhelyi B, et al. Prevalence and etiology of false normal aEEG recordings in neonatal hypoxic-ischaemic encephalopathy. BMC Pediatr 2013;13:194.
54. Sarkar S, Barks JD, Donn SM. Should amplitude-integrated electroencephalography be used to identify infants suitable for hypothermic neuroprotection? J Perinatol 2008;28:117–22.
55. Horan M, Azzopardi D, Edwards AD, et al. Lack of influence of mild hypothermia on amplitude integrated-electroencephalography in neonates receiving extracorporeal membrane oxygenation. Early Hum Dev 2007;83:69–75.
56. Spitzmiller RE, Phillips T, Meinzen-Derr J, et al. Amplitude-integrated EEG is useful in predicting neurodevelopmental outcome in full-term infants with hypoxic-ischemic encephalopathy: a meta-analysis. J Child Neurol 2007;22:1069–78.
57. van Rooij LG, Toet MC, Osredkar D, et al. Recovery of amplitude integrated electroencephalographic background patterns within 24 hours of perinatal asphyxia. Arch Dis Child Fetal Neonatal Ed 2005;90:F245–51.
58. ter Horst HJ, Sommer C, Bergman KA, et al. Prognostic significance of amplitude-integrated EEG during the first 72 hours after birth in severely asphyxiated neonates. Pediatr Res 2004;55:1026–33.
59. Hallberg B, Grossmann K, Bartocci M, et al. The prognostic value of early aEEG in asphyxiated infants undergoing systemic hypothermia treatment. Acta Paediatr 2010;99:531–6.
60. Osredkar D, Toet MC, van Rooij LG, et al. Sleep-wake cycling on amplitude-integrated electroencephalography in term newborns with hypoxic-ischemic encephalopathy. Pediatrics 2005;115:327–32.
61. Cseko AJ, Bango M, Lakatos P, et al. Accuracy of amplitude-integrated electroencephalography in the prediction of neurodevelopmental outcome in asphyxiated infants receiving hypothermia treatment. Acta Paediatr 2013;102:707–11.
62. Toet MC, Lemmers PM. Brain monitoring in neonates. Early Hum Dev 2009;85: 77–84.
63. Ancora G, Maranella E, Grandi S, et al. Early predictors of short term neurodevelopmental outcome in asphyxiated cooled infants. A combined brain amplitude

integrated electroencephalography and near infrared spectroscopy study. Brain Dev 2013;35:26–31.

64. Lemmers PM, Zwanenburg RJ, Benders MJ, et al. Cerebral oxygenation and brain activity after perinatal asphyxia: does hypothermia change their prognostic value? Pediatr Res 2013;74:180–5.

65. Shellhaas RA, Kushwaha JS, Plegue MA, et al. An evaluation of cerebral and systemic predictors of 18-month outcomes for neonates with hypoxic ischemic encephalopathy. J Child Neurol 2015;30:1526–31.

66. Greisen G. Cerebral blood flow and oxygenation in infants after birth asphyxia. Clinically useful information? Early Hum Dev 2014;90:703–5.

67. Ferrari F, Todeschini A, Guidotti I, et al. General movements in full-term infants with perinatal asphyxia are related to basal ganglia and thalamic lesions. J Pediatr 2011;158:904–11.

68. Twomey E, Twomey A, Ryan S, et al. MR imaging of term infants with hypoxic-ischaemic encephalopathy as a predictor of neurodevelopmental outcome and late MRI appearances. Pediatr Radiol 2010;40:1526–35.

69. Ancora G, Soffritti S, Lodi R, et al. A combined a-EEG and MR spectroscopy study in term newborns with hypoxic-ischemic encephalopathy. Brain Dev 2010;32:835–42.

70. Liauw L, van Wezel-Meijler G, Veen S, et al. Do apparent diffusion coefficient measurements predict outcome in children with neonatal hypoxic-ischemic encephalopathy? AJNR Am J Neuroradiol 2009;30:264–70.

71. Vermeulen RJ, van Schie PE, Hendrikx L, et al. Diffusion-weighted and conventional MR imaging in neonatal hypoxic ischemia: two-year follow-up study. Radiology 2008;249:631–9.

72. L'Abee C, de Vries LS, van der Grond J, et al. Early diffusion-weighted MRI and 1H-magnetic resonance spectroscopy in asphyxiated full-term neonates. Biol Neonate 2005;88:306–12.

73. Belet N, Belet U, Incesu L, et al. Hypoxic-ischemic encephalopathy: correlation of serial MRI and outcome. Pediatr Neurol 2004;31:267–74.

74. Khong PL, Tse C, Wong IY, et al. Diffusion-weighted imaging and proton magnetic resonance spectroscopy in perinatal hypoxic-ischemic encephalopathy: association with neuromotor outcome at 18 months of age. J Child Neurol 2004;19:872–81.

75. Biagioni E, Mercuri E, Rutherford M, et al. Combined use of electroencephalogram and magnetic resonance imaging in full-term neonates with acute encephalopathy. Pediatrics 2001;107:461–8.

76. Groenendaal F, van der Grond J, van Haastert IC, et al. Findings in cerebral proton spin resonance spectroscopy in newborn infants with asphyxia, and psychomotor development. Ned Tijdschr Geneeskd 1996;140:255–9 [in Dutch].

77. Murray DM, Boylan GB, Ryan CA, et al. Early EEG findings in hypoxic-ischemic encephalopathy predict outcomes at 2 years. Pediatrics 2009;124:e459–67.

78. Toet MC, Lemmers PM, van Schelven LJ, et al. Cerebral oxygenation and electrical activity after birth asphyxia: their relation to outcome. Pediatrics 2006;117:333–9.

79. Toet MC, Hellstrom-Westas L, Groenendaal F, et al. Amplitude integrated EEG 3 and 6 hours after birth in full term neonates with hypoxic-ischaemic encephalopathy. Arch Dis Child Fetal Neonatal Ed 1999;81:F19–23.

80. Eken P, Toet MC, Groenendaal F, et al. Predictive value of early neuroimaging, pulsed Doppler and neurophysiology in full term infants with hypoxic-ischaemic encephalopathy. Arch Dis Child Fetal Neonatal Ed 1995;73:F75–80.

81. van Lieshout HB, Jacobs JW, Rotteveel JJ, et al. The prognostic value of the EEG in asphyxiated newborns. Acta Neurol Scand 1995;91:203–7.
82. Thornberg E, Ekstrom-Jodal B. Cerebral function monitoring: a method of predicting outcome in term neonates after severe perinatal asphyxia. Acta Paediatr 1994;83:596–601.
83. Prechtl HF, Ferrari F, Cioni G. Predictive value of general movements in asphyxiated full-term infants. Early Hum Dev 1993;35:91–120.

Birth Asphyxia and Hypoxic-Ischemic Brain Injury in the Preterm Infant

Abbot R. Laptook, MD

KEYWORDS

- Hypoxia-ischemia • Asphyxia • Preterm infants • Therapeutic hypothermia
- Neuroprotection

KEY POINTS

- Identifying perinatal hypoxic-ischemic/asphyxial events in preterm infants is more challenging compared with infants ≥36 weeks' gestation.
- For the more mature preterm infant, extrapolation of criteria used in infants ≥36 weeks' gestation to identify perinatal hypoxia-ischemia may be feasible.
- For the extreme preterm infant, identification of perinatal hypoxia-ischemia that is linked to early childhood outcome is difficult given the many morbidities of prematurity; this will limit a targeted approach for neuroprotective treatments.
- A major knowledge gap is whether the neuropathology of hypoxic-ischemic injury among moderate and late preterm infants is similar to extreme preterm infants (arrest of pre-oligodendrocyte maturation) or term infants (selective neuronal necrosis) or a combination of the 2.

Identification of infants ≥36 weeks' gestation with perinatal hypoxia-ischemia or asphyxia has allowed investigation of potential neuroprotective treatments. Therapeutic hypothermia is the first therapy demonstrated to be efficacious for infants ≥36 weeks' gestation with hypoxia-ischemia or asphyxia. Multiple randomized trials demonstrated that relatively small reductions in core temperature alone or a combination of reduced head and core temperature (therapeutic hypothermia) reduces death or disability at 18 months.[1–5] Disability was typically severe and could be any of cognitive, motor, or sensory deficits. Neuroprotective effects of therapeutic hypothermia persist even at 6 to 7 years of age.[6,7] The importance of this therapy extends beyond the benefits provided to infants and their families; it signifies that hypoxic-ischemic brain injury is modifiable and has accelerated testing other potential neuroprotective

Disclosure: The author has no financial relationship with a commercial entity producing healthcare related products and/or services.
Department of Pediatrics, Women and Infants Hospital of Rhode Island, 101 Dudley Street, Providence, RI 02905, USA
E-mail address: alaptook@wihri.org

Clin Perinatol 43 (2016) 529–545
http://dx.doi.org/10.1016/j.clp.2016.04.010
0095-5108/16/$ – see front matter © 2016 Elsevier Inc. All rights reserved.

interventions either with or without therapeutic hypothermia.[8] Two National Institutes of Health Consensus conferences on therapeutic hypothermia have provided the neonatal community with guidance on dissemination and gaps in knowledge of this new therapy.[9,10]

It has been widely recommended that centers that offer therapeutic hypothermia follow studied protocols to ensure appropriate use in clinical practice. Analysis of therapeutic hypothermia implementation in the United Kingdom using the TOBY registry suggests consistency with prior clinical trials.[11] However, there is evidence of drift from evidence-based recommendations; in the TOBY registry, hypothermia treatment was provided to 2.8% of infants who were less than 36 weeks' gestation.[11] Similarly, 5.8% of infants in the Vermont Oxford Registry for encephalopathy between 2006 and 2011 were less than 36 weeks' gestation and received hypothermia treatment.[12] Outcomes of preterm infants undergoing hypothermia were not provided from either registry. In the absence of data from clinical trials, it is likely that therapies tested in more mature infants will be extended to preterm infants.

The objective of this report was to provide an overview of perinatal hypoxic-ischemic or asphyxial brain injury in preterm infants. Available information for preterm infants is contrasted with more mature infants ($\geq$36 weeks' gestation). Hypoxic-ischemic brain injury is examined with advancing maturation from extreme to moderate to late preterm infants.

TERMINOLOGY

In clinical practice, the terms hypoxia-ischemia and asphyxia are often used interchangeably. Technically there are important differences. Hypoxia is a low content of oxygen in the blood, whereas ischemia represents a reduction in tissue blood flow. Ischemia in turn can be partial or complete in extent, and can be focal or global in distribution. Hypoxia and ischemia are often combined because each component may result in the other. In contrast, asphyxia indicates an impairment of gas exchange and is characterized by anoxia and extremes of hypercarbia. In the clinical setting, asphyxia is more commonly partial in severity, resulting in hypoxia and more moderate increases in CO_2 tension; ischemia may result if asphyxia is prolonged or severe. The potential modulating effect of hypercapnia is frequently overshadowed by hypoxia and ischemia.[13,14] Translating this potential broad range of physiologic perturbations into robust, easily applied, clinical criteria that distinguish asphyxia from hypoxia-ischemia is not possible with present tools. For these reasons, no attempt will be made to distinguish hypoxia-ischemia and asphyxia in this review of the preterm infant.

CRITERIA FOR THE DIAGNOSIS OF HYPOXIA-ISCHEMIA

For infants $\geq$36 weeks' gestation, a tiered set of criteria have emerged to diagnose hypoxia-ischemia shortly after birth. This includes identification of an event that can impair fetal gas exchange or objective evidence of altered fetal gas exchange. The newborn in turn needs to manifest biologic effects of impaired gas exchange. The latter is done by demonstrating the presence of encephalopathy because links between perinatal hypoxia-ischemia/asphyxia and childhood neurodevelopmental deficits almost always include the presence of neonatal encephalopathy. Different scoring systems for encephalopathy have been used with or without modification.[15,16] All trials of therapeutic hypothermia have used a tiered approach to establish a diagnosis of hypoxia-ischemia. As a first step, infants need to demonstrate clinical or biochemical indicators of impaired placental-fetal gas exchange. If the latter is present, infants then need to manifest moderate or severe encephalopathy. Finally, in selected trials, a neuro-physiological correlate of clinical encephalopathy was ascertained[1,3,4] (Table 1). With this tiered approach, a rate of death or disability of 63% was reported among noncooled infants of the hypothermia trials.[17]

There are limitations to a tiered approach for the diagnosis of hypoxia-ischemia among preterm infants that are more problematic with decreasing gestational age. Although the presence of profound fetal acidemia (eg, umbilical artery pH <7.0) is an objective measure, other potential indicators of impaired placental gas exchange at birth may be affected by morbidities of prematurity. For example, low Apgar scores or the need for intubation/resuscitation at birth may reflect physiologic attributes of prematurity rather than a hypoxic-ischemic event. Apgar scores are characteristically lower among preterm compared with term infants, given inherent hypotonia, depressed reflex irritability, and difficulty initiating effective respiratory efforts.[18] The use of intubation and mechanical ventilation at birth is frequent in extremely and moderately preterm infants and may not indicate respiratory depression due to hypoxia-ischemia. Successful transition at birth requires initiation of ventilation, establishment of a functional residual capacity, and increases in pulmonary blood flow. To accomplish this, preterm infants need an adequate respiratory effort, surfactant sufficiency, proper levels of end-expiratory pressure, a normal pulmonary vascular response, and adequate cardiac and neuro-muscular function. Preterm infants with surfactant deficiency are just 1 example of morbidities of prematurity that make it difficult to determine if delivery room events (intubation and mechanical ventilation, low Apgar scores) reflect preterm disease processes, transitional physiology, or potential hypoxia-ischemia.

Central to the criteria of clinically important hypoxia-ischemia among term infants is encephalopathy. Encephalopathy is a clinical syndrome of brain dysfunction and has many etiologies, including hypoxia-ischemia. Encephalopathy is characterized by a depressed state of consciousness (lethargy, stupor, or coma), abnormal muscle tone (hypotonia or flaccidity), decreased spontaneous movement, loss of primitive reflexes (suck and Moro), and inability to initiate or sustain respiratory drive. Examination of preterm infants in the absence of hypoxia-ischemia is notable for many similar findings. Furthermore, the neurologic examination of extreme, moderate, and late preterm infants shows a maturation toward that of the term infant.[19] It may be feasible to recognize encephalopathy in more mature preterm infants following the presence of umbilical cord metabolic acidosis, but the impact of prematurity on the assessment

Table 1		
Criteria for inclusion in trials of therapeutic hypothermia		
Term	Criteria	Examples
Tier 1[a]	Potential impaired fetal gas exchange	History of an acute perinatal event, fetal acidemia, prolonged low Apgar scores, need for resuscitation
Tier 2	Clinical evidence of impaired brain function	Sarnat stage, HIE score (Thompson score), clinical seizures
Tier 3	Neurophysiological evidence of brain dysfunction	Amplitude-integrated EEG, full-montage EEG

Abbreviations: EEG, electroencephalogram; HIE, hypoxic-ischemic encephalopathy.
   [a] Infants need to manifest tier 1 criteria before evaluation for tier 2, and manifest tier 2 criteria before evaluation for tier 3.

of encephalopathy has not been critically evaluated.[20] It is important to distinguish encephalopathy among term infants, a clinical syndrome, from the label "encephalopathy of prematurity."[21] The latter denotes the dominant neuropathological lesion among extreme preterm infants: periventricular leukomalacia (PVL) and its associated distant neuronal and axonal deficits. These deficits can result in extensive involvement of cerebral cortex, thalamus, basal ganglia, and white matter. The encephalopathy of prematurity highlights the underlying pathology and clinical manifestations found during early childhood (motor, cognitive, attentional, and behavioral deficits).

An important distinction between term and preterm infants is the timing of hypoxic-ischemic events. In term infants, recognizable hypoxic-ischemic events occur predominantly before or during birth and represent the primary diagnosis secondary to impaired fetal gas exchange. A 2-hit hypothesis is recognized whereby the in utero environment (eg, placental pathology) and/or fetal characteristics (eg, small for gestational age) may increase the risk for a hypoxic-ischemic perinatal event.[22] More infrequent are isolated intrapartum events (eg, abuptio placenta, cord accidents, ruptured uterus).[23] With identification of remote and proximal risk factors among term infants, pathways culminating in neonatal encephalopathy may be more complex than a straightforward 2-hit hypothesis.[24] The risk for hypoxia-ischemia among preterm infants also may reflect intrapartum events, but in contrast, may also reflect cardiopulmonary disorders of prematurity that tend to be most severe in the first days following birth. The latter make it difficult to easily identify and time hypoxic-ischemic/asphyxial events. Preterm infants also are at risk for hypoxic-ischemic events remote from delivery secondary to morbidities, such as late-onset sepsis, necrotizing enterocolitis, nosocomial pneumonias, apnea and bradycardia, and symptomatic anemia (**Fig. 1**). These events increase the risk for repeated episodes of hypoxia-ischemia among preterm compared with term infants.

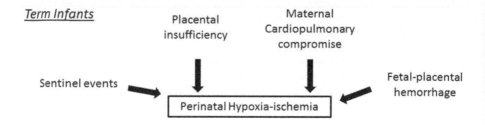

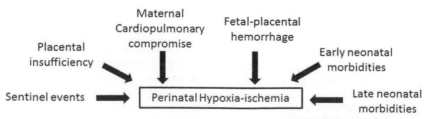

Fig. 1. Events that may lead to hypoxia-ischemia in the term infant primarily are encountered before or during birth. Extreme preterm infants may also be subjected to hypoxia-ischemia from early neonatal morbidities and subsequently from later encountered morbidities.

Given the limitations of easily identifying hypoxia-ischemia/asphyxia among preterm infants and the overlap of the preterm infant's neurologic examination with encephalopathy, other tools are needed to confirm neurologic dysfunction. Amplitude-integrated electroencephalogram (aEEG) was used as inclusion criteria in some hypothermia trials. It provides correlates with the background activity of a full-montage EEG, and the pattern among term infants with hypoxic-ischemic encephalopathy was associated with neurodevelopmental outcome at 12 to 18 months.[25,26] Prematurity, however, is associated with maturational changes of aEEG[27] and may pose challenges to define abnormalities among preterm infants. With decreasing gestational age, the aEEG is more discontinuous and the voltage of the lower border is reduced, both potential indicators of abnormality in more mature infants. Posing further challenges, there is remarkable heterogeneity of the aEEG pattern among preterm infants of the same gestational age[28] (**Fig. 2**). Serum biomarkers that indicate dysfunction of the neurovascular unit (glial fibrillary acidic protein, ubiquitin carboxylase-terminal hydrolase, neuron-specific enolase, and S100ß) and a general inflammatory response (interleukin 6, 1ß, 10) have shown promise as indicators of adverse outcome following hypoxia-ischemia/asphyxia in term infants.[29,30] Similar work for preterm infants represents an important area of investigation.

NEUROPATHOLOGY OF HYPOXIC-ISCHEMIC BRAIN INJURY
Term Infants

The neuropathology of hypoxic-ischemic/asphyxial brain injury differs as a function of gestational age. Hypoxic-ischemic injury among term infants is dominated by selective neuronal necrosis, followed by parasagittal cerebral injury and least commonly

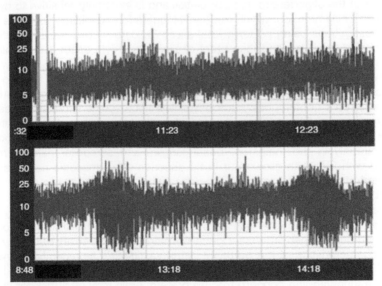

Fig. 2. aEEG recordings within the first 72 hours following birth from 2 late preterm infants born between 34⁰ and 34⁶ weeks. The top panel shows an immature pattern with a lower border predominantly at or below 5 microvolts and without cycles (intermittent broadening of the pattern). The lower panel shows a mature pattern with an elevated lower border during noncycle activity and 2 intervals of cycles. (*From* Sommers R, Tucker R, Harini C, et al. Neurological maturation of late preterm infants at 34 wk assessed by amplitude integrated electroencephalogram. Pediatr Res 2013;74:705–11.)

focal ischemic necrosis in a vascular distribution.[19] The distribution of these lesions follow patterns observed in asphyxial brain injury of the near-term monkey fetus.[31,32] With total or complete asphyxia, the neuropathology primarily affected the thalamus and brainstem. Partial prolonged asphyxia was associated with a greater distribution of neuropathology and included the basal ganglia, parasagittal aspects of the cerebrum, and with milder extents of asphyxia, cerebral white matter involvement. The parasagittal injury involved the paracentral cerebral cortex and associated white matter and represents a watershed injury between major vascular arteries. Different combinations of these injuries may occur depending on duration, severity, repetitiveness, and susceptibility of the affected fetus; thus, injury can span the spectrum from isolated focal white matter injury to hemispheric devastation. Although uncommon, some autopsy reviews indicate the presence of PVL.[33]

Preterm Infants

In contrast, the major hypoxic-ischemic lesion of the preterm infant is PVL representing injury to the cerebral white matter. Preterm infants thought to be at greatest risk for PVL are those born between 23 and 32 weeks' gestation, although systematic imaging among moderate and late preterm infants is not available. PVL is a spectrum from the classic focal cystic variety to diffuse noncystic white matter injury. Interestingly, PVL with focal macrocysts detectable by sonography has declined[34] and PVL is dominated by the diffuse variety that can be detected by MRI but not sonography. Diffuse PVL may or may not have microcysts that cannot be visualized with conventional imaging. The predominant pathology underlying PVL is an arrest in the lineage of oligodendrocytes at the pre-oligodendrocyte stage and results in reduced brain myelination.[35,36] For the extreme preterm infant (<29 weeks' gestation), the pre-oligodendrocyte represents most of the oligodendrocyte population and is extremely sensitive to hypoxia-ischemia and inflammation, which represent triggers for the initiation of white matter injury. Investigations using preterm fetal sheep indicate that ischemia is critical for the initiation of the injury and the extent of oligodendrocyte death is determined by the cell type; pre-oligodendrocytes are exquisitely sensitive to ischemia, whereas earlier and later oligodendrocytes are more resistant.[37,38] When injury is more extensive, all cell types are affected including oligodendrocytes, glia and axons resulting in cysts. Based on a contemporary autopsy series, microscopic necrosis represents a small percentage of diffuse PVL and contributes little to overall myelination defects.[39] However, PVL with microcysts (focal necrosis) is associated with remote neuronal loss most commonly in the thalamus, basal ganglia, and cerebellar dentate nucleus compared with PVL with gliosis but in the absence of microscopic necrosis.[40] The involvement of gray matter lesions with diffuse white matter injury has prompted the term "encephalopathy of prematurity" by Volpe.[21]

Intracranial hemorrhage (ICH) may also represent a hypoxic-ischemic injury occurring primarily in extreme preterm infants (<29 weeks' gestation). ICH is a hemorrhagic lesion initiated in the periventricular germinal matrix; the propensity to bleed reflects inherent characteristics of the germinal matrix vasculature as recently reviewed by Ballabh.[41] However, deranged cerebral hemodynamics may contribute to ICH. There has been a longstanding concern that the preterm brain may be at risk for hypoxic-ischemic injury due to uncertainties regarding minimum values of systemic blood pressure to maintain organ perfusion, limited ability to assess myocardial performance, and inadequate cerebral blood flow autoregulation. These concerns are greatest during the initial days following birth when morbidities of prematurity tend to be of highest acuity. Derangements of autoregulation have been demonstrated in the past and are most prevalent among sicker preterm infants.[42,43] Recent work has examined near infrared spectroscopy (a surrogate of cerebral blood flow) in preterm infants in response to natural oscillations of blood pressure. A dampening of blood pressure oscillations by the cerebral vasculature was observed, indicating an intact autoregulatory response, but this ability was progressively reduced with decreasing gestational age and among infants with an ICH.[44] Limited autoregulation could increase the vulnerability of the brain to altered systemic blood pressure, venous pressure, and blood gases.

A major gap in knowledge is the neuropathology of hypoxic-ischemic injury among moderate and late preterm infants; is it primarily selective neuronal necrosis or an arrest of maturation of the pre-oligodendrocyte or some combination of the two (**Table 2**)? There are limited data on this issue. The neuropathology of late preterm brains has been examined in a small cohort (n = 16) and compared with infants of less than 34 weeks (n = 25).[45] Late preterm infants demonstrated focal periventricular necrosis and diffuse reactive gliosis with microglial activation in the surrounding white matter. Gray matter lesions occurred in approximately a third of infants with PVL and were most frequent in the thalamus, globus pallidus, and cerebellar dentate nucleus. Clinical data regarding the hypoxic-ischemic events were limited. This demonstrates that PVL occurs in late preterm infants but is not informative regarding the neuropathology in the presence of identifiable hypoxic-ischemic or sentinel events.

IMAGING HYPOXIC-ISCHEMIC/ASPHYXIAL BRAIN INJURY
Term Infants

Imaging of hypoxic-ischemic brain injury among term infants is consistent with patterns of neuropathology. MRI is the imaging mode of choice for selective neuronal necrosis and detects abnormal signal in the basal ganglia, thalami, and posterior limb of the internal capsule, loss of gray-white matter differentiation in the cerebral hemispheres, and highlighting of the cerebral cortex (**Fig. 3**). Miller and colleagues[46] reported on MRIs acquired from 173 term infants (median age, 6 days) with neonatal encephalopathy identified between 1994 and 2000. Predominant patterns of injury were basal ganglia-thalamic in 25%, watershed in 45%, and normal in 30%. The basal ganglia-thalamic pattern included infants with total brain injury (basal ganglia-thalamic, watershed with cortical injury beyond the watershed pattern). Okereafor and colleagues[47] described MRI findings of 48 infants with encephalopathy between 1992 and 2005 who had evidence of an acute hypoxic event before birth. The predominant abnormality was lesions of the basal ganglia-thalamic region with or without

Table 2
Predominant neuropathology of hypoxic-ischemia in extreme preterm versus term infants

Gestational Age Group	Primary Cell Type Affected	Common Pattern(s) of Injury	Affected Regions
Extreme preterm	Pre-oligodendrocyte (arrested lineage)	Periventricular ± remote gray matter	Diffuse white matter ± thalamus, basal ganglia, hippocampus, cerebellum, brainstem
Term	Neuron (selective necrosis)	Basal ganglia-thalamic Watershed Diffuse hemispheric	Basal ganglia Thalamus PLIC Intervascular white matter Cortical gray/white

Abbreviation: PLIC, posterior limb of the internal capsule.

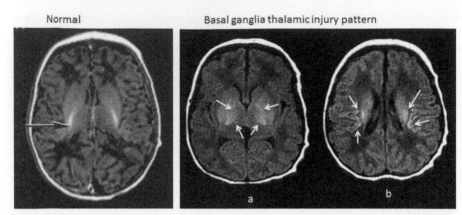

Fig. 3. The left panel displays an MRI T1-weighted axial image at the level of the basal ganglia and thalamus from a healthy infant. The arrow indicates the posterior limb of the internal capsule, which displays increased signal intensity indicating myelination. The right panel is from an infant with hypoxia-ischemia. (a) Abnormal signal intensity in the basal ganglia and thalamus (*arrows*), and decreased signal intensity in the posterior limb of the internal capsule. (b) Abnormal signal intensity in the medial thalamus and cortical ribbon (*arrows*).

white matter damage. These investigators suggested that basal ganglia-thalamic lesions are the imaging signature of a hypoxic-ischemic sentinel event. Brainstem involvement is less common and presumably reflects high mortality associated with this lesion. Imaging data from randomized trials of hypothermia consistently note abnormalities in the basal ganglia-thalamic region, white matter, cortex and posterior limb of the internal capsule.[48,49] Shankaran and colleagues[50] developed a pattern of injury hierarchy progressing from isolated cerebral lesions, to abnormalities of the basal ganglia-thalamic regions with or without other lesions, to hemispheric devastation.

Preterm Infants

MRI is often acquired at term equivalent age when performed among extreme preterm infants. MRI can visualize white matter signal abnormalities and other features of diffuse PVL, including loss of volume, cysts, enlarged ventricles, thinning of the corpus callosum, and delayed myelination (**Fig. 4**).[51,52] These are presumably the markers of hypoxic-ischemic brain injury in preterm infants. When imaged at term equivalent, the findings represent an evolved lesion, whereas those described for term infants represent an evolving lesion unless imaged remote from delivery. Clinical MRI is typically performed at 1.5 or 3.0 T and will not be able to detect microscopic cysts.[53] Serial MRI has been performed in a cohort of infants less than 30 weeks starting shortly after birth with follow-up scans based on clinical stability though 36 weeks postmenstrual age.[54] Abnormalities on early imaging was dominated by destructive lesions (ICH, ventricular dilatation), whereas the predominant abnormality at or beyond 36 weeks was diffuse excessive high signal intensity within the white matter. Consistent with the neuropathology, white matter injury in preterm infants is associated with injury to other brain regions. Inder and colleagues[55] demonstrated associations between diffuse white matter injury and reduced volume of cerebral gray matter, deep nuclear gray matter, myelinated white matter, and an increase in cerebral volume. The precise incidence of white matter injury among preterm infants across advancing gestational

Normal   Diffuse PVL

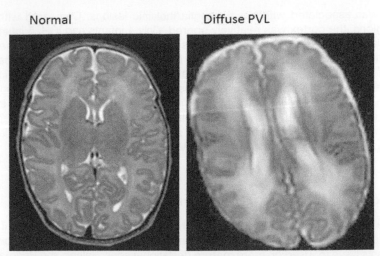

Fig. 4. Both panels display T2-weighted axial images from preterm infants acquired at term equivalent age. On the left is a normal brain for reference. On the right is an example of diffuse excessive high signal intensity of the white matter in the frontal and posterior regions.

age is unclear given the logistics of acquiring MRIs. Some reports suggest that diffuse PVL is common; among 167 infants less than 30 weeks' gestation undergoing MRI at term equivalent (representing a high proportion of eligible infants), mild, moderate, and severe white matter abnormalities were detected in 51%, 17%, and 4%, respectively.[56] Other reports have not confirmed such a high occurrence; differences may reflect recruitment strategies and resultant acuity of illness.[57] The incidence of diffuse PVL in the more mature preterm infant (33–36 weeks) is unclear. Recent cohorts indicate that white matter abnormality (diffusion tensor imaging), a smaller brain size, and an immature gyral pattern are more common among moderate and late preterm infants compared with term controls when imaged at 38 to 44 weeks.[58,59] The clinical correlates of these observations are unclear.

Preterm Infants with Sentinel Events

There are limited imaging data of preterm infants with a well-characterized hypoxic-ischemic event at birth. Barkovich and colleagues[60] described 5 infants between 27 and 32 weeks after profound asphyxia imaged with different modalities (MRI, computed tomography, and ultrasound). Four had cardiac arrest at birth and 1 had an in utero insult remote from delivery. Similar patterns of injury were displayed and included involvement of the thalami, basal ganglia, and cerebellum and a relative sparing of the cortex. Remote from the injury, there was a reduced cerebral hemispheric white matter and shrunken basal ganglia, thalami, brainstem, and cerebellum. A larger series of preterm infants accumulated over 15 years (n = 55, 26–36 weeks' gestation) reported on MRI at less than 6 weeks postnatal age after a presumed diagnosis of hypoxic-ischemic encephalopathy (clinical criteria and need for major resuscitation at birth).[61] Major sites of injury were basal ganglia and thalamic (57%, typically severe in extent), white matter injury (89% mostly mild in extent and diffuse), brainstem (44%), and cortex (58%, mostly mild); different combinations of involved regions were observed in individual infants. Severe white matter injury was uncommon and when present was associated with basal ganglia/thalamic lesions. Compared with other brain regions, the cortex was relatively spared. Only 4 infants had ICH, 5 infants had extra-axial hemorrhage, and cystic PVL was not observed. Consistent with the brainstem imaging abnormalities, preterm infants (n = 68, 28–35 weeks) with a clinical diagnosis of hypoxia-ischemia at birth have altered brainstem functional integrity evidenced by brainstem auditory evoked response.[62] In spite of methodological limitations, these data suggest that a *profound* asphyxia or hypoxic-ischemic sentinel event in a preterm infant leads to abnormalities that differed from PVL and approximated the term brain injury pattern. A less severe hypoxic-ischemic/asphyxia event may trigger the more common noncystic PVL.

INCIDENCE OF HYPOXIA-ISCHEMIA/ASPHYXIA AMONG PRETERM INFANTS

Because it is difficult to identify hypoxia-ischemia/asphyxia among preterm infants at or soon after birth, studies that examined the incidence of these events among preterm infants have focused on more mature gestational ages. Salhab and Perlman[20] reported moderate and severe encephalopathy among infants 31 to 36 weeks' gestation with severe fetal acidemia; the incidence of encephalopathy was 1.4 per 1000 live births. Schmidt and Walsh[63] reported the incidence of hypoxic-ischemic encephalopathy based on fulfilling 5 criteria (sentinel event, cord or initial postnatal pH lower than 7.0, 5-minute Apgar score less than 6, encephalopathy, and absence of other etiology for the encephalopathy) among preterm infants 32 to 36 weeks' gestation; the incidence of encephalopathy was much higher at 9 cases per 1000 live births. Chalak and colleagues[64] reviewed all infants with perinatal acidosis among infants with a gestational age of 33 to 35 weeks and then applied the National Institute of Child Health and Human Development Neonatal Research Network Hypothermia trial criteria.[2] Moderate or severe encephalopathy was found in 5 cases per 1000 live births. **Table 3** provides more detail on each of these studies. All of these investigations were single-center studies. In 2 of the 3 reports, placental abruption was the most common cause for preterm delivery.[20,63] In the reports that used fetal acidemia to trigger a review for encephalopathy, cord blood gases were sent from 97% of deliveries. It is unclear how the features of prematurity were accounted for in assessment of encephalopathy in each report. In addition, these studies were retrospective and the detail of the neurologic assessments, interexaminer variability, timing of neurologic assessments, differences in gestational age, and the absence of standardized data collection may contribute to the wide differences among the studies. There are no available data for the incidence of hypoxia-ischemia/asphyxia among extreme preterm infants.

Table 3
Estimates of the incidence of perinatal hypoxia-ischemia among preterm infants

Authors	GA, wk	Years Reviewed	Total Infants in the GA Window	Screening Criteria	Rate per 1000 Live Births
Salhab[20]	31–36	1993–2002	5533	UA pH <7.0	1.4
Schmidt[63]	32–36	2002–2008	1325	Apgar <6 at 5 min	9.0
Chalak[64]	33–35	2005–2008	1305	UA pH ≤7.15 or BD ≥10 mEq/L	5.0

Abbreviations: BD, base deficit; GA, gestational age; UA, umbilical artery.

IS THERAPEUTIC HYPOTHERMIA A VIABLE TREATMENT OPTION FOR PRETERM INFANTS?

Therapeutic hypothermia is the only therapy demonstrated to be efficacious for hypoxic-ischemic/asphyxial brain injury among infants ≥36 weeks' gestation based on 5 randomized trials. One of these trials and a smaller pilot trial enrolled infants ≥35 weeks.[5,65] Based on personal communication with the investigators, only 7 infants born between 35[0] and 35[6] weeks were randomized in these 2 trials. The Committee on the Fetus and Newborn of the American Academy of Pediatrics concluded in a report on hypothermia and neonatal encephalopathy that data regarding the efficacy of therapeutic hypothermia for infants less than 35 weeks' gestation are lacking.[66] However, the risks and benefits of therapeutic hypothermia for infants 35[0] to 35[6] weeks cannot be determined with limited enrollees in randomized trials and further study is justified.

There is biologic rationale for considering therapeutic hypothermia as a treatment option for preterm infants. Investigators in New Zealand studied preterm fetal sheep at 103 to 104 days (approximately 0.7 gestation, term 147 days) subjected to complete umbilical cord occlusion for 25 minutes followed 90 minutes later by either 70 hours of cerebral hypothermia or normothermia.[67] Hypothermia was achieved by circulating cool water through a coil affixed to the head in utero. Brain assessment following a 3-day recovery indicated that hypothermia was associated with less neuronal loss in the basal ganglia and hippocampus, a reduction in the loss of immature oligodendrocytes in the periventricular white matter, and evidence of suppressed apoptosis and inflammation compared with normothermic animals. These are important results, as they demonstrate that hypothermia may provide neuroprotection for oligodendrocytes, the critical target for brain injury in extreme preterm infants. Furthermore, hypothermia provides protection for brain regions frequently part of the injury pattern in term infants. Given these results, interest in offering therapeutic hypothermia to the preterm population is not surprising. Some editorials have suggested that it would not be unreasonable to offer therapeutic hypothermia to encephalopathic infants as early as 33 weeks' gestation in the presence of hypoxia-ischemia at birth (eg, placental abruption).[68] As mentioned earlier, registry data indicate that hypothermia is being provided to some infants less than 36 weeks' gestation.[11,12]

Two reports provide detail regarding therapeutic hypothermia in preterm infants. Smit and colleagues[69] reported on hypothermia treatment for infants from a single center that did not fulfill cooling criteria as used in randomized trials. This included 6 infants of a gestational age between 34[0] and 35[4] weeks. All infants survived and 25% had a mental developmental and psychomotor index less than 70 on the Bayley Scales of Infant Development, second edition. No information was provided regarding the condition at birth and 1 infant developed a pulmonary hemorrhage in association with inhaled nitric oxide use for pulmonary hypertension on day 6. Walsh and colleagues[70] reported a pilot study of cooling 4 infants between 32 to 35 weeks with hypoxic-ischemic encephalopathy. Given concerns of prolonged exposure to hypothermia in preterm infants, the feasibility of head cooling to achieve brain hypothermia was examined. Infants fulfilled 6 criteria to warrant a diagnosis of hypoxic-ischemic encephalopathy and receive cooling treatment. Abruptio placenta occurred in 3 of 4 mothers and all infants had cord umbilical artery pH values less than 6.9. The water temperature circulating through the cooling cap could not be reduced sufficiently without decreases in rectal temperature, prompting addition of a heating mattress to minimize drops in rectal temperature; unfortunately, plots of infant temperatures were not included. One infant developed a grade III ICH and a pulmonary hemorrhage on day 3 of life. Outcomes were poor; 1 infant died in the first week of life, and of the survivors, 2 had severe cognitive deficits and cerebral palsy and 1 infant had moderate cerebral palsy and a cognitive score of 90. The investigators concluded that hypothermia should not be provided to preterm infants outside of a clinical trial.

It appears likely that in the absence of evidence, hypothermia treatment will increasingly be extended to preterm infants based on the hypothermia trials in infants ≥36 weeks' gestation. In view of this knowledge gap, the National Institute of Child Health and Development Neonatal Research Network has initiated a randomized trial of whole-body cooling (target esophageal temperature of 33.5°C for 72 hours) compared with normothermia (target esophageal temperature of 36.5–37.3°C for 72 hours) initiated within 6 hours of birth for infants born between 33^0 and 35^6 weeks' gestation (clinicaltrials.gov NCT01793129). The primary outcome is death or moderate/severe disability assessed at 18 months of age. Enrollment opened in June 2015 and the projected sample size is 168 infants. This study is purposely targeted at the more mature preterm infant, given the challenges previously discussed.

An important aspect of extending hypothermia or any neuroprotective therapy to preterm infants will be safety. Avoidance of hypothermia in preterm infants is a fundamental principle in neonatal care based on increased mortality of infants nursed in cooler compared with warmer environments over the first 5 days after birth.[71] Hypothermia is associated with a broad spectrum of effects that may have important implications on morbidities of preterm infants.[72] More mature moderate and late preterm infants have a low frequency of ICH, although precise data are not available because screening is not routine at these gestational ages.[73] The effects of hypothermia on the coagulation cascade and platelet function could increase ICH, especially in the setting of hypoxia-ischemia.[74] Hypothermia shifts the hemoglobin-oxygen dissociation curve to the left and reduces tissue oxygen availability. This could impair oxygenation among preterm infants with severe respiratory morbidities. Serum concentrations of drugs used in the care of critically ill infants may be elevated either due to temperature-associated effects on hepatic drug metabolizing enzymes[75] or to altered hepatic/renal function secondary to injury.[76] Hypothermia is also associated with immune suppression and may place preterm infants at greater risk for nosocomial infection.

NEUROPROTECTION FOR HYPOXIA-ISCHEMIA/ASPHYXIA IN EXTREME PRETERM INFANTS

There are multiple reasons why neuroprotective strategies for extreme preterm infants will differ from moderate and late preterm infants. Hypoxic-ischemic events are probably most frequent around the time of birth or in the first days after birth coincident with serious morbidities of prematurity and associated hemodynamic instability. Even with this knowledge, it is difficult to determine the impact of putative hypoxic-ischemic events because sensitive and specific markers of brain injury are not available and remain a focus of research. Not all morbidities of prematurity with adverse effects on the brain reflect hypoxia-ischemia; inflammation, drug toxicity, nutritional deficits, and deficient endogenous repair mechanisms may also contribute to brain injury. The neurologic examination of extreme preterm infants has few distinctive findings to identify neurologic dysfunction and more robust markers are needed to identify brain injury. Finally, the preterm brain remains vulnerable to injury from many morbidities that may occur during a prolonged hospitalization, including late-onset sepsis, necrotizing enterocolitis, apnea and bradycardia, evolving bronchopulmonary dysplasia, and suboptimal nutrition. Thus, an easily identifiable, timed insult triggering evaluation for an intervention in the hours after birth (eg, therapeutic hypothermia) is probably not realistic for most extreme preterm infants.

In contrast to moderate and late preterm infants, there is a stronger rationale for providing neuroprotective therapies to all or the highest-risk infants within specific gestational age ranges. A broad approach to neuroprotection acknowledges the high rates of neurodevelopmental impairment among extreme preterm infants,[77] limited ability to time an insult, and predict vulnerability to hypoxic-ischemic events. Consistent with this approach are widely used therapies evaluated in extreme preterm infants based on birth weight or gestational age. For example, caffeine therapy was evaluated in a randomized, blinded trial among infants with a birth weight of 500 to 1250 g and whose clinician considered them candidates for this treatment: caffeine improved survival without neurodevelopmental impairment at 18 months corrected age.[78] Other interventions provided at birth or on the first day reduce ICH (delayed cord clamping, prophylactic indomethacin) but remain controversial due to lack of (indomethacin) or uncertainty of (delayed cord clamping) improved neurodevelopmental outcome in early childhood.[79,80] Ongoing trials are using a broad approach to neuroprotection. The PENUT trial (NCT 01378273) is examining recombinant human erythropoietin from 48 hours of age to 32 weeks corrected age in a placebo-controlled randomized trial for infants between 24 and 27 weeks' gestation.

SUMMARY

Birth asphyxia is a modifiable process, as demonstrated by randomized trials of therapeutic hypothermia in infants ≥36 weeks' gestation with evidence of hypoxia-ischemia/asphyxia. Extending investigation to preterm infants is well justified; however, there are many challenges. Identifying perinatal hypoxic-ischemic/asphyxial events in preterm infants is more challenging compared with infants ≥36 weeks' gestation. For the more mature preterm infant, extrapolation of criteria used in infants ≥36 weeks' gestation may be feasible although with some caveats. For the extreme preterm infant, different criteria will be needed to complement evidence of impaired placental-fetal gas exchange because the clinical examination provides little insight into the presence or absence of neurologic dysfunction unless a condition is extreme. Neuroprotective therapies extended over longer time intervals may be appropriate for extreme preterm infants at risk of injury from multiple morbidities of prematurity. Important questions remain that have implications for the efficacy of potential neuroprotective strategies. Chief among them is whether the neuropathology of hypoxic-ischemic brain injury of moderate and late preterm infants more closely approximates diffuse white matter injury of extreme preterm infants or selective neuronal necrosis of term infants. It also remains unclear whether the incidence of ICH is increased in the setting of hypoxia-ischemia among preterm infants. Therapeutic hypothermia may have applications in selected cohorts of moderate and late preterm infants but probably will not be applicable to the extreme preterm infant. Whatever therapies emerge as potential candidate neuroprotective treatments, a comprehensive assessment of safety will be critical.

REFERENCES

1. Gluckman PD, Wyatt JS, Azzopardi D, et al. Selective head cooling with mild systemic hypothermia after neonatal encephalopathy: multicentre randomised trial. Lancet 2005;365:663–70.
2. Shankaran S, Laptook AR, Ehrenkranz RA, et al. Whole-body hypothermia for neonates with hypoxic-ischemic encephalopathy. N Engl J Med 2005;353:1574–84.

3. Azzopardi DV, Strohm B, Edwards AD, et al. Moderate hypothermia to treat perinatal asphyxial encephalopathy. N Engl J Med 2009;361:1349–58.

4. Simbruner G, Mittal RA, Rohlmann F, et al. Systemic hypothermia after neonatal encephalopathy: outcomes of neo.nEURO.network RCT. Pediatrics 2010;126: e771–8.

5. Jacobs SE, Morley CJ, Inder TE, et al. Whole-body hypothermia for term and near-term newborns with hypoxic-ischemic encephalopathy: a randomized controlled trial. Arch Pediatr Adolesc Med 2011;165:692–700.

6. Shankaran S, Pappas A, McDonald SA, et al. Childhood outcomes after hypothermia for neonatal encephalopathy. N Engl J Med 2012;366:2085–92.

7. Azzopardi D, Strohm B, Marlow N, et al. Effects of hypothermia for perinatal asphyxia on childhood outcomes. N Engl J Med 2014;371:140–9.

8. Robertson NJ, Tan S, Groenendaal F, et al. Which neuroprotective agents are ready for bench to bedside translation in the newborn infant? J Pediatr 2012; 160:544–52.e4.

9. Higgins RD, Raju TN, Perlman J, et al. Hypothermia and perinatal asphyxia: executive summary of the National Institute of Child Health and Human Development workshop. J Pediatr 2006;148:170–5.

10. Higgins RD, Raju T, Edwards AD, et al. Hypothermia and other treatment options for neonatal encephalopathy: an executive summary of the Eunice Kennedy Shriver NICHD workshop. J Pediatr 2011;159:851–8.e1.

11. Azzopardi D, Strohm B, Linsell L, et al. Implementation and conduct of therapeutic hypothermia for perinatal asphyxial encephalopathy in the UK–analysis of national data. PLoS One 2012;7:e38504.

12. Pfister RH, Edwards EM, Soll RF, et al. Do infants treated with hypothermic therapy in routine practice meet the eligibility criteria from the original randomized trials? E-PAS2013:1400.1.

13. Corbett RJ, Sterett R, Laptook AR. Evaluation of potential effectors of agonal glycolytic rate in developing brain measured in vivo by 31p and 1h nuclear magnetic resonance spectroscopy. J Neurochem 1995;64:322–31.

14. Vannucci RC, Towfighi J, Heitjan DF, et al. Carbon dioxide protects the perinatal brain from hypoxic-ischemic damage: an experimental study in the immature rat. Pediatrics 1995;95:868–74.

15. Sarnat HB, Sarnat MS. Neonatal encephalopathy following fetal distress. A clinical and electroencephalographic study. Arch Neurol 1976;33:696–705.

16. Thompson CM, Puterman AS, Linley LL, et al. The value of a scoring system for hypoxic ischaemic encephalopathy in predicting neurodevelopmental outcome. Acta Paediatr 1997;86:757–61.

17. Jacobs SE, Berg M, Hunt R, et al. Cooling for newborns with hypoxic ischaemic encephalopathy. Cochrane Database Syst Rev 2013;(1):CD003311.

18. Catlin EA, Carpenter MW, Brann BS, et al. The Apgar score revisited: influence of gestational age. J Pediatr 1986;109:865–8.

19. Volpe JJ. Neurology of the newborn. 5th edition. Philadelphia: Saunders Elsevier; 2008.

20. Salhab WA, Perlman JM. Severe fetal acidemia and subsequent neonatal encephalopathy in the larger premature infant. Pediatr Neurol 2005;32:25–9.

21. Volpe JJ. Brain injury in premature infants: a complex amalgam of destructive and developmental disturbances. Lancet Neurol 2009;8:110–24.

22. Badawi N, Kurinczuk JJ, Keogh JM, et al. Antepartum risk factors for newborn encephalopathy: the Western Australian case-control study. BMJ 1998;317: 1549–53.

23. Badawi N, Kurinczuk JJ, Keogh JM, et al. Intrapartum risk factors for newborn encephalopathy: the Western Australian case-control study. BMJ 1998;317:1554–8.
24. American College of Obstetricians and Gynecologists, American Academy of Pediatrics. Neonatal encephalopathy and neurologic outcome. 2nd edition. Washington, DC: American College of Obstetricians and Gynecologists; 2014.
25. Hellstrom-Westas L, Rosen I, Svenningsen NW. Predictive value of early continuous amplitude integrated EEG recordings on outcome after severe birth asphyxia in full term infants. Arch Dis Child Fetal Neonatal Ed 1995;72:F34–8.
26. al Naqeeb N, Edwards AD, Cowan FM, et al. Assessment of neonatal encephalopathy by amplitude-integrated electroencephalography. Pediatrics 1999;103: 1263–71.
27. Kuint J, Turgeman A, Torjman A, et al. Characteristics of amplitude-integrated electroencephalogram in premature infants. J Child Neurol 2007;22:277–81.
28. Sommers R, Tucker R, Harini C, et al. Neurological maturation of late preterm infants at 34 wk assessed by amplitude integrated electroencephalogram. Pediatr Res 2013;74:705–11.
29. Mir IN, Chalak LF. Serum biomarkers to evaluate the integrity of the neurovascular unit. Early Hum Dev 2014;90:707–11.
30. Orrock JE, Panchapakesan K, Vezina G, et al. Association of brain injury and neonatal cytokine response during therapeutic hypothermia (TH) in newborns with hypoxic-ischemic encephalopathy (hie). Pediatr Res 2016;79(5):742–7.
31. Myers RE. Two patterns of perinatal brain damage and their conditions of occurrence. Am J Obstet Gynecol 1972;112:246–76.
32. Myers RE. Four patterns of perinatal brain damage and their conditions of occurrence in primates. Adv Neurol 1975;10:223–34.
33. Eken P, Jansen GH, Groenendaal F, et al. Intracranial lesions in the full-term infant with hypoxic ischaemic encephalopathy: ultrasound and autopsy correlation. Neuropediatrics 1994;25:301–7.
34. Hamrick SE, Miller SP, Leonard C, et al. Trends in severe brain injury and neurodevelopmental outcome in premature newborn infants: the role of cystic periventricular leukomalacia. J Pediatr 2004;145:593–9.
35. Back SA, Riddle A, McClure MM. Maturation-dependent vulnerability of perinatal white matter in premature birth. Stroke 2007;38:724–30.
36. Volpe JJ, Kinney HC, Jensen FE, et al. The developing oligodendrocyte: key cellular target in brain injury in the premature infant. Int J Dev Neurosci 2011; 29:423–40.
37. Riddle A, Luo NL, Manese M, et al. Spatial heterogeneity in oligodendrocyte lineage maturation and not cerebral blood flow predicts fetal ovine periventricular white matter injury. J Neurosci 2006;26:3045–55.
38. McClure MM, Riddle A, Manese M, et al. Cerebral blood flow heterogeneity in preterm sheep: lack of physiologic support for vascular boundary zones in fetal cerebral white matter. J Cereb Blood Flow Metab 2008;28:995–1008.
39. Buser JR, Maire J, Riddle A, et al. Arrested preoligodendrocyte maturation contributes to myelination failure in premature infants. Ann Neurol 2012;71:93–109.
40. Pierson CR, Folkerth RD, Billiards SS, et al. Gray matter injury associated with periventricular leukomalacia in the premature infant. Acta Neuropathol 2007; 114:619–31.
41. Ballabh P. Pathogenesis and prevention of intraventricular hemorrhage. Clin Perinatol 2014;41:47–67.
42. Lou HC, Lassen NA, Friis-Hansen B. Impaired autoregulation of cerebral blood flow in the distressed newborn infant. J Pediatr 1979;94:118–21.

43. Pryds O. Control of cerebral circulation in the high-risk neonate. Ann Neurol 1991; 30:321–9.
44. Vesoulis ZA, Liao SM, Trivedi SB, et al. A novel method for assessing cerebral autoregulation in preterm infants using transfer function analysis. Pediatr Res 2016; 79(3):453–9.
45. Haynes RL, Sleeper LA, Volpe JJ, et al. Neuropathologic studies of the encephalopathy of prematurity in the late preterm infant. Clin Perinatol 2013;40:707–22.
46. Miller SP, Ramaswamy V, Michelson D, et al. Patterns of brain injury in term neonatal encephalopathy. J Pediatr 2005;146:453–60.
47. Okereafor A, Allsop J, Counsell SJ, et al. Patterns of brain injury in neonates exposed to perinatal sentinel events. Pediatrics 2008;121:906–14.
48. Rutherford M, Ramenghi LA, Edwards AD, et al. Assessment of brain tissue injury after moderate hypothermia in neonates with hypoxic-ischaemic encephalopathy: a nested substudy of a randomised controlled trial. Lancet Neurol 2010;9: 39–45.
49. Cheong JL, Coleman L, Hunt RW, et al. Prognostic utility of magnetic resonance imaging in neonatal hypoxic-ischemic encephalopathy: substudy of a randomized trial. Arch Pediatr Adolesc Med 2012;166:634–40.
50. Shankaran S, Barnes PD, Hintz SR, et al. Brain injury following trial of hypothermia for neonatal hypoxic-ischaemic encephalopathy. Arch Dis Child Fetal Neonatal Ed 2012;97:F398–404.
51. Inder TE, Wells SJ, Mogridge NB, et al. Defining the nature of the cerebral abnormalities in the premature infant: a qualitative magnetic resonance imaging study. J Pediatr 2003;143:171–9.
52. Rutherford MA, Supramaniam V, Ederies A, et al. Magnetic resonance imaging of white matter diseases of prematurity. Neuroradiology 2010;52:505–21.
53. Back SA. Cerebral white and gray matter injury in newborns: new insights into pathophysiology and management. Clin Perinatol 2014;41:1–24.
54. Dyet LE, Kennea N, Counsell SJ, et al. Natural history of brain lesions in extremely preterm infants studied with serial magnetic resonance imaging from birth and neurodevelopmental assessment. Pediatrics 2006;118:536–48.
55. Inder TE, Warfield SK, Wang H, et al. Abnormal cerebral structure is present at term in premature infants. Pediatrics 2005;115:286–94.
56. Woodward LJ, Anderson PJ, Austin NC, et al. Neonatal MRI to predict neurodevelopmental outcomes in preterm infants. N Engl J Med 2006;355:685–94.
57. Hintz SR, Barnes PD, Bulas D, et al. Neuroimaging and neurodevelopmental outcome in extremely preterm infants. Pediatrics 2015;135:e32–42.
58. Kelly CE, Cheong JL, Gabra Fam L, et al. Moderate and late preterm infants exhibit widespread brain white matter microstructure alterations at term-equivalent age relative to term-born controls. Brain Imaging Behav 2016;10(1): 41–9.
59. Walsh JM, Doyle LW, Anderson PJ, et al. Moderate and late preterm birth: effect on brain size and maturation at term-equivalent age. Radiology 2014;273: 232–40.
60. Barkovich AJ, Hajnal BL, Vigneron D, et al. Prediction of neuromotor outcome in perinatal asphyxia: evaluation of MR scoring systems. AJNR Am J Neuroradiol 1998;19:143–9.
61. Logitharajah P, Rutherford MA, Cowan FM. Hypoxic-ischemic encephalopathy in preterm infants: antecedent factors, brain imaging, and outcome. Pediatr Res 2009;66:222–9.

62. Jiang ZD, Brosi DM, Chen C, et al. Impairment of perinatal hypoxia-ischemia to the preterm brainstem. J Neurol Sci 2009;287:172–7.
63. Schmidt JW, Walsh WF. Hypoxic-ischemic encephalopathy in preterm infants. J Neonatal Perinatal Med 2010;3:277–84.
64. Chalak LF, Rollins N, Morriss MC, et al. Perinatal acidosis and hypoxic-ischemic encephalopathy in preterm infants of 33 to 35 weeks' gestation. J Pediatr 2012; 160:388–94.
65. Eicher DJ, Wagner CL, Katikaneni LP, et al. Moderate hypothermia in neonatal encephalopathy: efficacy outcomes. Pediatr Neurol 2005;32:11–7.
66. Committee on Fetus and Newborn. Hypothermia and neonatal encephalopathy. Pediatrics 2014;133:1146–50.
67. Bennet L, Roelfsema V, George S, et al. The effect of cerebral hypothermia on white and grey matter injury induced by severe hypoxia in preterm fetal sheep. J Physiol 2007;578:491–506.
68. Austin T, Shanmugalingam S, Clarke P. To cool or not to cool? Hypothermia treatment outside trial criteria. Arch Dis Child Fetal Neonatal Ed 2013;98:F451–3.
69. Smit E, Liu X, Jary S, et al. Cooling neonates who do not fulfil the standard cooling criteria—short- and long-term outcomes. Acta Paediatr 2015;104:138–45.
70. Walsh WF, Butler D, Schmidt JW. Report of a pilot study of cooling four preterm infants 32-35 weeks gestation with HIE. J Neonatal-Perinatal Med 2015;8:47–51.
71. Silverman WA, Fertig JW, Berger AP. The influence of the thermal environment upon the survival of newly born premature infants. Pediatrics 1958;22:876–86.
72. Schubert A. Side effects of mild hypothermia. J Neurosurg Anesthesiol 1995;7:139–47.
73. Laptook AR. Neurologic and metabolic issues in moderately preterm, late preterm, and early term infants. Clin Perinatol 2013;40:723–38.
74. Rohrer MJ, Natale AM. Effect of hypothermia on the coagulation cascade. Crit Care Med 1992;20:1402–5.
75. Roka A, Melinda KT, Vasarhelyi B, et al. Elevated morphine concentrations in neonates treated with morphine and prolonged hypothermia for hypoxic ischemic encephalopathy. Pediatrics 2008;121:e844–9.
76. Liu X, Borooah M, Stone J, et al. Serum gentamicin concentrations in encephalopathic infants are not affected by therapeutic hypothermia. Pediatrics 2009;124:310–5.
77. Hintz SR, Kendrick DE, Wilson-Costello DE, et al. Early-childhood neurodevelopmental outcomes are not improving for infants born at <25 weeks' gestational age. Pediatrics 2011;127:62–70.
78. Schmidt B, Roberts RS, Davis P, et al. Long-term effects of caffeine therapy for apnea of prematurity. N Engl J Med 2007;357:1893–902.
79. Schmidt B, Davis P, Moddemann D, et al. Long-term effects of indomethacin prophylaxis in extremely-low-birth-weight infants. N Engl J Med 2001;344:1966–72.
80. Tarnow-Mordi WO, Duley L, Field D, et al. Timing of cord clamping in very preterm infants: more evidence is needed. Am J Obstet Gynecol 2014;211:118–23.

The Role of the Neurointensive Care Nursery for Neonatal Encephalopathy

Hannah C. Glass, MDCM, MAS[a,b,c],*, David H. Rowitch, MD, PhD[d,e]

KEYWORDS

- Neurocritical care • Infant • Critical care • Therapeutic hypothermia
- Neonatal seizures • Cerebral palsy • Neonatal encephalopathy
- Hypoxic-ischemic encephalopathy

KEY POINTS

- In neonatal neurocritical "brain-focused" care units, all bedside providers maintain constant awareness of the neurologic complications of critical illnesses, and the impact of management on the developing brain.
- Neonatal encephalopathy is the commonest condition treated by a neonatal neurocritical care service.
- A neurocritical care approach may mitigate adverse outcomes among neonates with HIE by preventing secondary brain injury, rapid recognition and treatment of neurologic complications, consistent management using guidelines and protocols, and use of optimized teams at dedicated referral centers.

INTRODUCTION

Neonatal encephalopathy due to intrapartum events is estimated to occur in 1 to 2 per 1000 live births in high-income countries.[1] Outcomes following neonatal encephalopathy due to birth asphyxia include death and neurologic disabilities, such as cerebral palsy, epilepsy, and cognitive impairment.

Disclosures: The authors have no financial conflicts of interest to disclose. H.C. Glass is supported by the NINDS K23NS066137 and the Neonatal Brain Research Institute.
[a] Department of Neurology, Benioff Children's Hospital, University of California San Francisco, 675 Nelson Rising Lane, Room 494, Box 0663, San Francisco, CA 94158, USA; [b] Department of Pediatrics, Benioff Children's Hospital, University of California San Francisco, San Francisco, CA, USA; [c] Department of Epidemiology & Biostatistics, University of California San Francisco, San Francisco, CA, USA; [d] Department of Paediatrics, University of Cambridge, Cambridge, UK; [e] Department of Pediatrics and Neurological Surgery, University of California San Francisco, San Francisco, CA, USA
* Corresponding author. Department of Neurology, University of California San Francisco, 675 Nelson Rising Lane, Room 494, Box 0663, San Francisco, CA 94158.
E-mail address: Hannah.Glass@ucsf.edu

Clin Perinatol 43 (2016) 547–557
http://dx.doi.org/10.1016/j.clp.2016.04.011
0095-5108/16/$ – see front matter © 2016 Elsevier Inc. All rights reserved.

perinatology.theclinics.com

Neonatal neurocritical care has emerged over the past decade as a subspecialty that involves a culture change toward a "brain-focused" approach with all bedside providers (physicians, nurses, respiratory technologists, and trainees) maintaining constant awareness of the potential neurologic complications of critical illnesses, as well as the impact of management on the developing or injured brain. Several important advances have prompted this culture change, including increased survival from critical illness, as well as the advent of digital neurophysiology monitoring and safe, high-resolution MRI. Conditions cared for in a neurocritical care unit include neonatal encephalopathy (and hypoxic-ischemic encephalopathy [HIE]), seizures, intracranial hemorrhage, ischemic stroke, and intracranial infection, among others. A neurocritical care approach to monitoring, diagnosis, and treatment of neurologic conditions has been shown to improve outcomes among adults.[2,3] In neonates, a neurocritical care approach may mitigate adverse outcomes among neonates with HIE by preventing secondary brain injury; rapid recognition and treatment of neurologic complications, like seizures; early identification of HIE mimics, like neonatal-onset epileptic encephalopathies; consistent management using guidelines and protocols; and use of optimized teams at dedicated referral centers, although long-term outcome studies are needed to show the benefits of this management.

Neonatal encephalopathy is the commonest condition treated by a neurocritical care service.[4,5] Neonates with HIE require rapid implementation of neuroprotection with hypothermia, have high rates of multiorgan failure, and neurologic signs and symptoms, such as encephalopathy, seizures, and brain injury. Therefore, this condition lends itself to the neurocritical care approach. In principle, a neurointensive care nursery (NICN) can lessen adverse outcomes as a result of prevention of secondary brain injury through attention to basic physiology, earlier recognition and treatment of neurologic complications, such as seizures, consistent management using guidelines and protocols, and use of optimized teams at dedicated referral centers, as discussed later in this article.[6] Moreover, the NICN can also serve as an ideal platform for research. Early diagnosis will allow interventions during critical neuroplasticity windows,[7–9] high-intensity therapies,[10] and patient stratification for novel interventions. For example, recent early phase safety studies have evaluated hypothermia combined with administration of potential biological (eg, erythropoietin[11,12]), inhaled (eg, Xenon[13]) and cell-based (eg, cord blood stem cells[14]) therapeutics.

Establishing a Neurointensive Care Nursery

The neurocritical care approach involves a culture shift for the entire neonatal intensive care unit (NICU) toward brain-focused care, such that providers at every level are continually aware of the potential neurologic complications of critical illnesses and the impact of their management strategies on the developing brain. From the time of birth through patient discharge, the neonatal neurocritical care team serves to prevent secondary injury, implement neuroprotective strategies, including therapeutic hypothermia, manage neurologic complications, optimize developmental care, and establish outpatient developmental services and high-risk follow-up.

To establish an NICN, a leadership team (with representatives from neonatology, neurology, and nursing) must work together to establish a program for the following core functions of the unit:

- Training and education for all providers, including physicians, nurses, nurse practitioners, and respiratory therapists

- Local guidelines for management of neonatal encephalopathy (including resuscitation, implementation, and maintenance of hypothermia and use of extracorporeal membrane oxygenation), as well as neurologic monitoring and treatment of complications, including use of electroencephalogram (EEG) amplitude–integrated EEG (aEEG), seizure treatment, and brain imaging using MRI
- Ensuring adequate resources, equipment, and training for brain monitoring, imaging, and application of hypothermia
- Community outreach and education to foster timely referrals

Current NICNs are closed units, with the neonatologist acting as the physician of record and the neurologist acting as a consultant with an active role in decision-making and communication with the family. The NICN itself may have a dedicated or specific area within the NICU, or else operate "virtually" with a team that can operate at any bedside.

Role of the neonatologist
The neonatologist typically acts as the physician of record and identifies neonates who are eligible for hypothermia and consultation by the NICN team. Neonatologists will perform the initial resuscitation and manage the patient with close attention to physiologic homeostasis with a focus on cardiopulmonary support, maintaining normal electrolyte and glucose levels, and temperature control to minimize secondary brain injury (**Table 1**).

Role of the neurologist
The neurologist takes an early active role from the time of the initial presentation of neurologic signs or symptoms. For neonates with encephalopathy due to birth asphyxia, the neurologist is notified at the time of referral or admission. At most centers, the neonatologist makes the decision of whether or not to initiate cooling therapy, conferring with the neurologist as needed. The neurologist then serves to document a detailed neurologic examination, as well as guide the initial investigation and management decisions, including rapid implementation of hypothermia (if not initiated at the referral center or during transport). The neurologist will often consider other causes of neonatal encephalopathy, such as congenital brain anomalies, intracranial infection

Table 1	
Preventing secondary brain injury	
Parameter	**Approach**
Temperature	• Avoid hyperthermia (associated with worse outcomes in term neonates with encephalopathy[16])
Ventilation/ oxygenation	• Maintain normocarbia/permissive mild hypercapnia • Avoid hypoxemia including transfer to extracorporeal membrane oxygenation if needed in cases of severe persistent pulmonary hypertension • Avoid rapid shifts in carbon dioxide tension • Both hypocarbia and hypercarbia can impact cerebral blood flow
Blood pressure	• Maintain normal blood pressure to support cerebral blood flow • Cerebral autoregulation may be impaired[17]
Glucose	• Maintain normoglycemia • Hypoglycemia is associated with both de novo brain injury and worse outcome in the setting of existing brain injury[18–20]

or hemorrhage, inborn errors of metabolism, neonatal-onset epilepsy, and other genetic conditions, and plan additional investigations accordingly.

At the time of admission, the neurologist serves to coordinate with the neurophysiology service for application and interpretation of EEG, and urgent cranial imaging if needed (eg, suspicion for hemorrhage). Along with the neonatologist, the neurologist manages the patient and communicates with the family during the period of critical illness. The neurologist is key in providing guidance for seizure therapy and coordinating with the neuroradiologist to ensure appropriate imaging protocols. Finally, the neurologist perspective is especially important when discussing prognosis and neurologic follow-up with the family, and the neurologist assists with planning outpatient services, such as physical and occupational therapy or Early Start program, especially if the child is expected to have a long-term disabling neurologic condition.

Role of the specialized neurointensive bedside neonatal intensive care unit nurse

The bedside nurse has a vital role in the NICN program.[15] Didactic and hands-on education to care for neonates with neurologic conditions distinguishes the specialized neurologic nurse from the general NICU nursing pool. The nurse learns to recognize neurologic signs and symptoms, as well as interpret the aEEG so the physician can be alerted at the first sign of clinical or electrographic seizure, or worsening of encephalopathy. The bedside nurse can help to optimize care by quickly setting up the cooling blanket and EEG/aEEG machine, which allows for faster treatment. In addition, nurses learn to adhere to management guidelines and anticipate next steps in care, safely transport critically ill neonates to the MR scanner, and communicate effectively with families.

Preventing Secondary Injury

Perinatal asphyxia puts the neonate at risk for end-organ failure, which can lead to cardiopulmonary instability, inadequate brain perfusion, and hypoglycemia. Hypotension, hypoxemia, hypocarbia, hyperthermia, and hypo/hyperglycemia can exacerbate brain injury and so these parameters must be carefully monitored and actively managed by all members of the neurocritical care team from the time of birth (see **Table 1**).

Implementing Therapeutic Hypothermia

Neonatal encephalopathy is the most common condition managed by a neurocritical care service, and therapeutic hypothermia is among the most common treatments.[5,21] Several randomized controlled trials have shown that treatment with hypothermia leads to lower rates of death or disability at 18 to 24 months of age (Relative risk (RR) 0.75, 95% confidence interval 0.68–0.83), and the benefit appears to be sustained through school age.[22–24]

Treatment of neonatal encephalopathy in the setting of a specialized NICN can offer the following benefits:

1. Quicker onset of cooling by an experienced team
2. Rapid, around-the-clock detection and treatment of seizures
3. High-quality brain imaging
4. Counseling for parents by experienced physicians and nurses
5. Timely and accurate diagnosis of conditions that can mimic HIE, such as neonatal-onset epilepsies, inborn errors of metabolism, and congenital central and peripheral nervous system disorders

Screening tools, such as the hypothermia toolkit by the California Perinatal Quality Care Collaborative can help outlying centers to quickly identify neonates who may benefit from hypothermia (**Fig. 1**).[25] Both animal and human studies show that early

Goal timeline

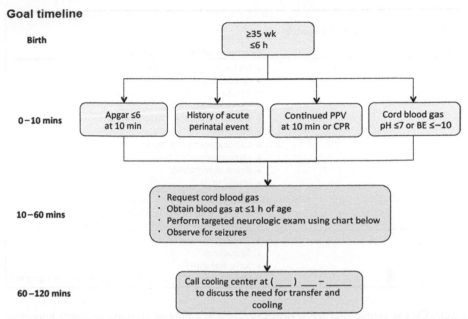

Fig. 1. Screening criteria for evaluation of risk for neonatal encephalopathy. BE, base excess; CPR, cardiopulmonary resuscitation; PPV, positive pressure ventilation.

initiation of therapy is associated with improved outcomes, and so rapid implementation of hypothermia is critical.[26–28] Implementation of hypothermia at the referral center or by the transport team is safe. Use of a portable servo-controlled cooling device on transport provides more stable temperature management with a higher percentage of temperatures within the target range as compared with neonates who are passively cooled.[29]

Guidelines and protocols that are site specific and endorsed by neonatology, neurology, and nursing can help to standardize the approach to implementation of therapeutic hypothermia (**Table 2**).

Managing Neurologic Complications

Although recent reports suggest that the burden of seizures among neonates undergoing hypothermia is lower than for neonates who are not cooled, the risk remains approximately 50%.[30–32] Neonates with encephalopathy due to perinatal asphyxia should receive neurophysiology monitoring using continuous, video EEG and/or a simplified montage aEEG monitoring for bedside use. Continuous neurophysiology monitoring is important to evaluate dynamic change in background brain activity and degree of encephalopathy, as well as seizures. Clinical indicators such as resuscitation parameters and degree of encephalopathy do not appear to be associated with risk of seizures. An abnormal initial EEG background (ie, excessively discontinuous, burst suppression, depressed and undifferentiated, or extremely low voltage) is associated with greater than 60% seizure risk. Neonates with a normal initial EEG background have the lowest risk of seizures (~10%).[30] The EEG and aEEG recordings also provide important prognostic information that can be used to start counseling parents regarding risk of disability and goals of care. Early normal or mildly abnormal

Table 2 Guidelines for therapeutic hypothermia	
Guideline	Examples of Guideline Contents
Therapeutic hypothermia	• Inclusion/exclusion criteria • Resuscitation and transport procedures • Temperature monitoring and management • Cardiopulmonary support • Use of extracorporeal membrane oxygenation • Sedation • Laboratory/blood work • Hydration/nutrition • Brain monitoring • Imaging • Skin care
Seizures	• Monitoring modality and duration • First, second, and third-line antiseizure agents
Imaging	• Timing • Sequences • Safe transport • Use of magnetic resonance–compatible equipment

EEG/aEEG is reassuring for a good prognosis, whereas an early severely abnormal EEG/aEEG (eg, burst suppression, depressed and undifferentiated, extremely low voltage, or status epilepticus at the onset of recording) is associated with a poor prognosis and brain injury if it persists beyond 24 to 36 hours of life.[33,34]

aEEG and full-montage EEG can be recorded by using the same system. The aEEG can be displayed at the bedside for the neurocritical care team and the full-montage EEG sent to remote servers for access in the neurophysiology laboratory or personal device. The limited montage of the aEEG can be easily applied at the time of admission so that the bedside nurse and neonatology team can quickly assess the degree of encephalopathy and for the presence of seizures. The full-montage EEG is applied as soon as a technician is available. The aEEG is then available as a screening tool for the bedside neurocritical care team and yet the EEG is available to the neurophysiologist as the gold standard to confirm presence or absence of seizures and detect seizures that are not visible on the aEEG recording.[35]

Neonates undergoing hypothermia are at high risk for brain injury. MRI is an important tool to assess the location and severity of injury, and to rule out other causes of encephalopathy (eg, dysgenesis).[36,37] Furthermore, moderate-severe injury on MRI is associated with a high risk of death or disability.[38] The neurocritical care team should be prepared to safely take a critically ill neonate to the MRI scanner. Resources for safe transport include MRI-compatible incubators, ventilators, and cardiopulmonary monitoring equipment, as well as skilled staff who have completed training and mock codes in the MRI suite. The optimal timing of MRI may depend on the resources of the neurocritical care team. Because the appearance of the injury evolves over time, neonates at a given center should be imaged within a standard time frame. Imaging neonates just after cooling has ended (day 4–6) offers several advantages:

1. Lower need for sedation, as the neonate often remains encephalopathic
2. Serves as a good turning point between the neurocritical care phase of the admission and convalescence
3. MRI can be performed before discharge home

At some centers, the second week of life is the preferred timing for imaging, as there are rare reports that the brain injury can evolve over this time period. To mitigate issues related to timing of imaging, it is our practice to repeat imaging in a neonate whose early scan is normal but who remains encephalopathic after the first 5 to 7 days after birth or if the results of ancillary testing are discordant (ie, very abnormal neurologic examination or EEG results and/or difficulty establishing feeding and with a normal MRI).

Palliative Care

Unfortunately, therapeutic hypothermia does not prevent death or developmental disabilities in all patients with neonatal encephalopathy due to birth asphyxia; approximately 50% have adverse outcome.[39] When a neonate has multiorgan failure that is not compatible with life, and/or is expected to develop severe and permanent developmental disabilities, the neurocritical care team may wish to discuss the option of transition to a palliative approach. Using information from the neurologic examination, EEG and aEEG, and MRI, an experienced team can predict those children who are likely to suffer severe disabilities, and counsel the family accordingly.[40] The entire neurocritical care team, including the neonatologist, neurologist, and bedside nurse must work together to provide a consistent message to the family and provide compassionate supportive care.

Compassion fatigue and burn out are common among bedside providers who frequently care for children with adverse outcomes. All members of the team should be given the option to request a different patient assignment in case of ethical concerns or compassion fatigue. An important aspect of the NICN is to provide specialized neurologic nurses with adequate breaks, psychological support, and a safe space to debrief difficult cases, as well as updates on children with good outcomes.

Optimizing Developmental Care

Once the neonate with encephalopathy has recovered from the critical illness, the focus of the neurocritical care team should turn toward achieving oral feeds and optimizing developmental outcomes. Inpatient services include consultation with physical and occupational therapists, as well as lactation consultants. Neonates with neurologic disorders may need assistance with state regulation, positioning, and oral feeding readiness and preparation, as well as optimizing tone, strength, and ability to take in external stimuli. The family also should learn about developmentally appropriate exercises (eg, upright positioning, tummy time, language exposure, and early exposure to fine motor tasks). Enriched environments can provide the intensive, repetitive, task-specific interventions that are needed for improved outcomes.[7,8,41,42]

Outpatient Developmental Services and Neurologic Care

Survivors of neonatal encephalopathy due to perinatal asphyxia are at high risk for long-term disabilities, including cerebral palsy, epilepsy, and intellectual disabilities. A neonatal neurointensive care program should make provisions for outpatient care by a neurologist and/or high-risk infant program. The American Academy of Pediatrics recommends that longitudinal neurodevelopmental outcome be monitored in all neonates who undergo hypothermia.[43] Although practically speaking, this means follow-up until 18 to 24 months of age, this is inadequate to capture major learning milestones. Consideration of follow-up through age 6 is encouraged to better evaluate the ultimate impact of neonatal neurointensive care interventions.

SUMMARY/DISCUSSION

Neonates with encephalopathy are often critically ill with multiorgan failure. They are at high risk for brain injury and seizures, which can lead to death or long-term disabilities. A NICN can optimally support neonates by providing brain-focused care from the time of resuscitation through discharge home. Members of the neurocritical care team include a neonatologist, neurologist, and specialized bedside nurse. Guidelines and protocols can help to standardize care and optimize therapies. Early recognition and treatment of neurologic complications, such as seizures, as well as prevention of secondary brain injury through attention to basic physiology can minimize brain injury. Finally, experienced teams at dedicated referral centers provide the specialized care that children and parents need, which includes close follow-up to address late-emerging issues.

Best practices

What is the current practice?

Therapeutic hypothermia is standard of care for neonates with encephalopathy due to perinatal asphyxia who would have fulfilled inclusion and exclusion criteria for the clinical trials.

Best Practice/Guideline/Care Path Objective(s)

Neonates with encephalopathy should be quickly identified and transferred to a center with experience in management of multiorgan failure, neurologic complications, and therapeutic hypothermia.

What changes in current practice are likely to improve outcomes?

1. Careful attention to basic physiology, including temperature regulation, glucose homeostasis, oxygenation, and blood pressure support to prevent secondary injury;

2. Use of protocols and/or guidelines;

3. Early recognition and treatment of neurologic complications;

4. Management by an experienced, multidisciplinary neurocritical care team in a dedicated referral unit.

Major Recommendations
- Establish an experienced team of neonatologists, neurologists, and bedside nurses to manage neonates with encephalopathy due to perinatal asphyxia.
- Establish guidelines to manage implementation of therapeutic hypothermia, brain monitoring, seizure treatment, and brain imaging.

Summary Statement

A NICN can optimally support neonates with encephalopathy due to birth asphyxia by providing brain-focused care from the time of resuscitation through discharge home.

REFERENCES

1. Lee AC, Kozuki N, Blencowe H, et al. Intrapartum-related neonatal encephalopathy incidence and impairment at regional and global levels for 2010 with trends from 1990. Pediatr Res 2013;74(Suppl 1):50–72.

2. Egawa S, Hifumi T, Kawakita K, et al. Impact of neurointensivist-managed intensive care unit implementation on patient outcomes after aneurysmal subarachnoid hemorrhage. J Crit Care 2015;32:52–5.
3. Josephson SA, Douglas VC, Lawton MT, et al. Improvement in intensive care unit outcomes in patients with subarachnoid hemorrhage after initiation of neurointensivist co-management. J Neurosurg 2010;112:626–30.
4. Glass HC, Bonifacio SL, Shimotake T, et al. Neurocritical care for neonates. Curr Treat Options Neurol 2011;13:574–89.
5. Mulkey SB, Swearingen CJ. Advancing neurologic care in the neonatal intensive care unit with a neonatal neurologist. J Child Neurol 2014;29:31–5.
6. Rincon F, Mayer SA. Neurocritical care: a distinct discipline? Curr Opin Crit Care 2007;13:115–21.
7. Shepherd RB. Cerebral palsy in infancy. New York: Churchill Livingstone Elsevier; 2014.
8. Morgan C, Novak I, Badawi N. Enriched environments and motor outcomes in cerebral palsy: systematic review and meta-analysis. Pediatrics 2013;132:e735–46.
9. Novak I. Evidence-based diagnosis, health care, and rehabilitation for children with cerebral palsy. J Child Neurol 2014;29:1141–56.
10. Kolb B, Muhammad A. Harnessing the power of neuroplasticity for intervention. Front Hum Neurosci 2014;8:377.
11. Wu YW, Bauer LA, Ballard RA, et al. Erythropoietin for neuroprotection in neonatal encephalopathy: safety and pharmacokinetics. Pediatrics 2012;130:683–91.
12. Rogers EE, Bonifacio SL, Glass HC, et al. Erythropoietin and hypothermia for hypoxic-ischemic encephalopathy. Pediatr Neurol 2014;51:657–62.
13. Azzopardi D, Robertson NJ, Bainbridge A, et al. Moderate hypothermia within 6 h of birth plus inhaled xenon versus moderate hypothermia alone after birth asphyxia (TOBY-Xe): a proof-of-concept, open-label, randomised controlled trial. Lancet Neurol 2015. [Epub ahead of print].
14. Cotten CM, Murtha AP, Goldberg RN, et al. Feasibility of autologous cord blood cells for infants with hypoxic-ischemic encephalopathy. J Pediatr 2014;164: 973–9.e1.
15. Glass HC, Rogers EE, Peloquin S, et al. Interdisciplinary approach to neurocritical care in the intensive care nursery. Semin Pediatr Neurol 2014;21:241–7.
16. Wyatt JS, Gluckman PD, Liu PY, et al. Determinants of outcomes after head cooling for neonatal encephalopathy. Pediatrics 2007;119:912–21.
17. Kasdorf E, Perlman JM. Strategies to prevent reperfusion injury to the brain following intrapartum hypoxia-ischemia. Semin Fetal Neonatal Med 2013;18: 379–84.
18. Wong DS, Poskitt KJ, Chau V, et al. Brain injury patterns in hypoglycemia in neonatal encephalopathy. AJNR Am J Neuroradiol 2013;34:1456–61.
19. Tam EW, Haeusslein LA, Bonifacio SL, et al. Hypoglycemia is associated with increased risk for brain injury and adverse neurodevelopmental outcome in neonates at risk for encephalopathy. J Pediatr 2012;161:88–93.
20. Filan PM, Inder TE, Cameron FJ, et al. Neonatal hypoglycemia and occipital cerebral injury. J Pediatr 2006;148:552–5.
21. Glass HC, Bonifacio SL, Peloquin S, et al. Neurocritical care for neonates. Neurocrit Care 2010;12:421–9.
22. Jacobs SE, Berg M, Hunt R, et al. Cooling for newborns with hypoxic ischaemic encephalopathy. Cochrane Database Syst Rev 2013;(1):CD003311.
23. Azzopardi D, Strohm B, Marlow N, et al. Effects of hypothermia for perinatal asphyxia on childhood outcomes. N Engl J Med 2014;371:140–9.

24. Shankaran S. Outcomes of hypoxic-ischemic encephalopathy in neonates treated with hypothermia. Clin Perinatol 2014;41:149–59.
25. California Perinatal Quality Care Collaborative, 2015. Early screening and identification of candidates for neonatal therapeutic hypothermia toolkit. 2015. Available at: https://www.cpqcc.org/qi-tool-kits/early-screening-and-identification-candidates-neonatal-therapeutic-hypothermia-toolkit. Accessed January 13, 2016.
26. Azzopardi DV, Strohm B, Edwards AD, et al. Moderate hypothermia to treat perinatal asphyxial encephalopathy. N Engl J Med 2009;361:1349–58.
27. Thoresen M, Tooley J, Liu X, et al. Time is brain: starting therapeutic hypothermia within three hours after birth improves motor outcome in asphyxiated newborns. Neonatology 2013;104:228–33.
28. Gunn AJ, Thoresen M. Hypothermic neuroprotection. NeuroRx 2006;3:154–69.
29. Akula VP, Joe P, Thusu K, et al. A randomized clinical trial of therapeutic hypothermia mode during transport for neonatal encephalopathy. J Pediatr 2015;166(4): 856–61.e1–2.
30. Glass HC, Wusthoff CJ, Shellhaas RA, et al. Risk factors for EEG seizures in neonates treated with hypothermia: a multicenter cohort study. Neurology 2014;82: 1239–44.
31. Low E, Boylan GB, Mathieson SR, et al. Cooling and seizure burden in term neonates: an observational study. Arch Dis Child Fetal Neonatal Ed 2012;97: F267–72.
32. Wusthoff CJ, Dlugos DJ, Gutierrez-Colina A, et al. Electrographic seizures during therapeutic hypothermia for neonatal hypoxic-ischemic encephalopathy. J Child Neurol 2011;26:724–8.
33. Nash KB, Bonifacio SL, Glass HC, et al. Video-EEG monitoring in newborns with hypoxic-ischemic encephalopathy treated with hypothermia. Neurology 2011;76: 556–62.
34. Thoresen M, Hellstrom-Westas L, Liu X, et al. Effect of hypothermia on amplitude-integrated electroencephalogram in infants with asphyxia. Pediatrics 2010;126: e131–9.
35. Glass HC, Wusthoff CJ, Shellhaas RA. Amplitude-integrated electroencephalography: the child neurologist's perspective. J Child Neurol 2013;28: 1342–50.
36. Mrelashvili A, Bonifacio SL, Rogers EE, et al. Outcome after therapeutic hypothermia in term neonates with encephalopathy and a syndromic diagnosis. J Child Neurol 2015;30:1453–8.
37. Felix JF, Badawi N, Kurinczuk JJ, et al. Birth defects in children with newborn encephalopathy. Dev Med Child Neurol 2000;42:803–8.
38. Rutherford M, Ramenghi LA, Edwards AD, et al. Assessment of brain tissue injury after moderate hypothermia in neonates with hypoxic-ischaemic encephalopathy: a nested substudy of a randomised controlled trial. Lancet Neurol 2010;9: 39–45.
39. Tagin MA, Woolcott CG, Vincer MJ, et al. Hypothermia for neonatal hypoxic ischemic encephalopathy: an updated systematic review and meta-analysis. Arch Pediatr Adolesc Med 2012;166:558–66.
40. Bonifacio SL, deVries LS, Groenendaal F. Impact of hypothermia on predictors of poor outcome: how do we decide to redirect care? Semin Fetal Neonatal Med 2015;20(2):122–7.
41. Damiano DL. Activity, activity, activity: rethinking our physical therapy approach to cerebral palsy. Phys Ther 2006;86:1534–40.

42. Novak I, McIntyre S, Morgan C, et al. A systematic review of interventions for children with cerebral palsy: state of the evidence. Dev Med Child Neurol 2013;55: 885–910.
43. Committee on Fetus and Newborn, Papile LA, Baley JE, et al. Hypothermia and encephalopathy. Pediatrics 2014;133:1146–50.

Long-Term Cognitive Outcomes of Birth Asphyxia and the Contribution of Identified Perinatal Asphyxia to Cerebral Palsy

CrossMark

Athina Pappas, MD[a],*, Steven J. Korzeniewski, PhD[b]

KEYWORDS

- Neonatal encephalopathy • Hypoxic ischemic encephalopathy • Newborn
- Cognitive outcome • Cerebral palsy

KEY POINTS

- Neonatal encephalopathy (NE) contributes to significant cognitive impairment among survivors who do and do not develop cerebral palsy (CP).
- A watershed MRI pattern of brain injury may predict worse cognitive outcomes even among the nondisabled survivors of NE who manifest no functional motor deficits or evidence of CP.
- Despite therapeutic hypothermia for NE, cognitive and learning deficits continue to occur and merit comprehensive assessment through school age.
- A better understanding of the extent of brain injury as it relates to cognitive impairment may lead to targeted interventions to improve childhood outcomes.
- A common misconception is that a vast majority of infants with CP have NE attributed to hypoxic ischemic encephalopathy (HIE) and intrapartum events; evidence indicates that fewer than 12% of children who are diagnosed with CP were exposed to perinatal asphyxia.

INTRODUCTION

NE among survivors of presumed perinatal asphyxia is recognized as an important cause of CP and neuromotor impairment. Recent studies suggest that moderate to severe NE contributes to a wide range of neurodevelopmental and cognitive

---

Disclosure statement: The authors have nothing to disclose.
[a] Department of Pediatrics, St. John Hospital and Medical Center, NICU CCB-5, Wayne State University School of Medicine, 22101 Moross, Detroit, MI 48236, USA; [b] Hutzel Women's Hospital, Perinatology Research Branch (NICHD/NIH), 4 Brush - Office 4817, 3990 John R. Street, Detroit, MI 48201, USA
* Corresponding author.
E-mail address: apappas@med.wayne.edu

Clin Perinatol 43 (2016) 559–572
http://dx.doi.org/10.1016/j.clp.2016.04.012   **perinatology.theclinics.com**
0095-5108/16/$ – see front matter © 2016 Elsevier Inc. All rights reserved.

impairments among survivors with and without CP.[1–6] Neonates who have severe encephalopathy at birth more often develop disabling neurologic and cognitive deficits, whereas those who survive moderate encephalopathy typically have more variable outcomes, with milder neuromotor impairments and a wider range of lesser cognitive deficits. Nearly 1 of 4 (23%) neonates who are treated with hypothermia has or develops CP.[7] Although NE only accounts for an estimated 10% of all CP cases, it seems to play a role in 25% of those who are born at term, although in many such births there is no evidence of intrapartum perinatal sentinel events.[8,9] Although some consider hypoxia-ischemia resulting from peripartum asphyxia to be the sole cause of what is called NE,[10] single-cause attribution is inherently problematic.[11] The inability to directly measure cerebral oxygen, the limited performance of its surrogate biomarkers in discriminating children who do and do not develop NE, and evidence that multiple antecedents contribute to umbilical artery acidemia in term infants strongly suggest a multifactorial origin,[12] one that might involve subtypes in which the underlying pathobiology is not fundamentally hypoxic or ischemic[13,14] — hence, the preference for NE over the term, HIE.[12] Nevertheless, this article uses these 2 terms interchangeably. The focus of this article is to review the long-term cognitive outcomes of children presumably exposed to birth asphyxia and to describe what is known about its contribution to CP.

COGNITIVE OUTCOMES AT 18 TO 24 MONTHS AFTER PRESUMED HYPOXIC ISCHEMIC ENCEPHALOPATHY IN THE ERA OF THERAPEUTIC HYPOTHERMIA

Few data are available on the cognitive outcomes of 18-month-old to 24-month-old children after presumed HIE, in large part because earlier developmental instruments did not specifically test cognition. The major randomized controlled trials of hypothermia for HIE assessed developmental outcomes using the Bayley Scales of Infant Development, Second Edition (BSID-II).[15–21] Cognitive and language outcomes were evaluated by way of the mental developmental index (MDI) component, not separately. As in other subscales of the BSID-II, scores range from 50 to 150, with a mean of 100 and an SD of 15, and significant mental delay is denoted by a score less than 70 (representative of 2 SDs below the mean). At 18 to 24 months, the prevalence of significant mental developmental delay after hypothermia for presumed HIE ranges from 23% to 30% (**Tables 1** and **2**).[15–22] Two hypothermia trials report mean MDI scores[14,19] for neonates who were cooled, ranging between 80.2 (SD 20.2) and 90.4 (SD 25.2).[7]

Smaller observational studies explored early childhood cognitive outcomes specifically. Jary and colleagues[23] investigated 18-month neurodevelopmental outcomes for 61 term infants treated with therapeutic hypothermia and compared BSID-II and Bayley Scales of Infant and Toddler Development, Third Edition (BSID-III), assessments among those who survived. The mean and median BSID-III cognitive scores were higher than the BSID-II MDI scores (mean 102 [SD 12.3] versus 91 [SD 17]; median 100 [range 65–125] versus 93 [range 50–121]). Severe disability cutoff thresholds less than 70 also revealed differences between the 2 assessments. Among the 10 neonates who had an MDI score less than 70, only 3 had cognitive and language composite scores less than 70. Chalak and colleagues[24] reported BSID-III outcomes in another prospective cohort study of neonates treated with whole-body hypothermia for HIE (n = 62). The median BSID-III cognitive composite score was 85 (with an interquartile range of 70–90). Only 8% of infants had scores less than 70 and 34% had scores of 70 to 84; hence, a vast majority of children scored within the reported normal range for the BSID-III. Studies comparing BSID-II and BSID-III cognitive and language

Table 1
Outcomes at 18 to 24 months after therapeutic hypothermia

Outcomes Among all Trial Participants Randomized to Hypothermia

Study	Death or Neurodevelopmental Impairment			Death			Major Neurodevelopmental Impairment (Among All)		
	N	Total	%	N	Total	%	N	Total	%
Gunn et al,[22] 1998	7	18	39	3	18	17	4	18	22
CoolCap study,[53] 2005	59	108	55	36	108	33	23	108	21
NICHD trial,[16] 2005	45	102	44	24	102	24	21	102	21
TOBY trial,[36] 2009	74	163	45	42	163	26	32	163	20
neo.nEURO study,[19] 2010	27	53	51	20	53	38	7	53	13
Zhou study,[20] 2010	31	100	31	20	100	20	11	100	11
ICE study,[18] 2011	55	107	51	27	108	25	28	107	26
All	298	651	46	172	652	26	126	651	19

Outcomes Among Survivors Randomized to Hypothermia

Study	Major Neurodevelopmental Impairment			Mental Developmental Index Less Than 2 SD Below Mean			Cerebral Palsy		
	N	Total	%	N	Total	%	N	Total	%
Gunn et al,[22] 1998	4	15	27	3	13	23	3	15	20
CoolCap study,[53] 2005	23	72	32	21	70	30	23	72	32
NICHD trial,[16] 2005	21	78	27	19	75	25	15	77	19
TOBY trial,[36] 2009	32	120	27	28	115	24	33	120	28
neo.nEURO study,[19] 2010	7	33	21	—	—	—	4	32	13
Zhou study,[20] 2010	11	80	14	—	—	—	10	80	13
ICE study,[18] 2011	28	80	35	17	73	23	21	79	27
All	126	478	26	88	346	25	109	475	23

Table 2
Bayley Scales of Infant and Toddler Development, Third Edition, outcomes for 18-month-old to 24-month-old children with hypoxic ischemic encephalopathy treated with hypothermia

Study	N	BSID-III Cognitive Composite Median Score	BSID-III Language Composite Median Score	BSID-III Motor Composite Median Score
Jary et al,[51] 2013	61	100 (range 65–125)	97 (range 68–135)	103 (range 76–124)
Chalak et al,[52] 2014	62	85 (IQR 70–90)	83 (IQR 74–91)	85 (IQR 73–97)

Abbreviation: IQR, interquartile (25–75) range.

scores in typically developing term and preterm infants reported mean cognitive composite scores ranging between 104 and 108.9 and mean language composite scores ranging between 108.2 and 109 in normally developing term infants.[25,26] This is an important consideration for those interpreting developmental test scores for high-risk neonates, because most normally developing children score above the reported mean of the test instrument; moreover, the relationship between cognitive and MDI scores is not a simple offset, because cognitive scores are reported to be increasingly higher than MDI at lower scores.[27] Dichotomization of outcomes into normal and abnormal presents impairment as an all-or-nothing phenomenon and might well overlook the true cognitive deficits of children with more subtle impairments that have an impact on school readiness and performance. Accurate assessment of the spectrum of cognitive functioning among the survivors of presumed HIE is important in appraising the impact of perinatal interventions, in selecting children for referral to early-intervention and support services, and in counseling parents and families on potential long-term problems.

COGNITIVE OUTCOMES AT SCHOOL AGE IN THE PREHYPOTHERMIA ERA

Many reports of school-aged cognitive outcomes of neonates after HIE involve survivors born in the prehypothermia era (**Table 3**).[6,28–33] Difficulty in assimilating the neurocognitive outcomes reported across studies lies in the varied definitions of HIE, differential staging of NE, and differing definitions of long-term outcomes. Nonetheless, these studies generate the bedrock of evidence used to inform current work in this field and provide important information about the spectrum of neurocognitive outcomes after presumed perinatally acquired hypoxic ischemic brain injury. In general, neonates who have mild encephalopathy defined using the Sarnat criteria[34] are reported to have normal developmental outcomes, whereas those with severe encephalopathy more often have or develop spastic quadriplegic or dyskinetic CP with severe cognitive dysfunction. By contrast, children with moderate encephalopathy are reported to have more variable outcomes that may be missed in early childhood or deemed insignificant if not compared with normally developing controls. For a comprehensive review of early studies on cognitive outcomes at school age prior to hypothermia, please see the work of van Handel and colleagues[35] and Dilenge and colleagues.[36]

Robertson and colleagues[28,30] studied the school-aged outcomes of 2 consecutive birth cohorts of children diagnosed with mild to severe HIE in the newborn period, comparing them with those of age-matched controls without HIE. The study participants were born in Alberta, Canada, between 1974 and 1979 and were assessed at 5.5 and 8 years of age. All survivors with severe HIE at birth were disabled at school age with multiple handicaps (CP, severe vision, or hearing impairment; IQ >3 SDs below the mean; or a known seizure disorder), whereas fewer than 20% of survivors with moderate HIE were disabled and only 8% had multiple disabilities. At 5.5 years, compared with controls or children with mild encephalopathy, nondisabled survivors with moderate encephalopathy had lower IQ scores and lower scores for quantitative language, auditory memory, letter recognition, and visual-motor integration. At 8 years, children with moderate to severe encephalopathy had significantly lower IQ, visual-motor integration, and receptive vocabulary scores compared with children with mild or no encephalopathy. Nondisabled survivors of moderate NE were similar to healthy controls with respect to perceptual motor skills and receptive vocabulary but showed delays in school-related activities, including reading, spelling, and arithmetic. These children were likely to be 1 grade level behind their healthy age-matched peers.

Marlow and colleagues[31] evaluated the neurocognitive and behavioral outcomes of a group of school-aged children from the former Trent region in the United Kingdom who suffered from moderate to severe HIE in the neonatal period; 65 of 130 eligible children born between 1992 and 1994 were assessed at the age of 7 years along with 49 comparison children who attended mainstream schools. The comparison children were selected from the same school and were matched for gender, ethnic group, first language, and age. Cognitive assessments included the British Ability Scales: Second Edition (BAS-II) school-aged battery and A Developmental Neuropsychological Assessment (NEPSY), a scale designed to assess the neuropsychological performance of children with acquired brain injury (attention/executive function, language, sensorimotor function, visuospatial processing, memory, and learning). Disability (classified according to the World Health Organization[37]) was more common in children who had a history of severe encephalopathy than among those who had moderate encephalopathy (42% vs 6%); 15 children overall had major disability, including CP. Among the 50 children who had no major disability, general cognitive ability scores were lowest for those with a history of severe encephalopathy (mean IQ difference from peers −11.3 points; 95% CI, −19.0 to −3.6). Cognitive ability scores on the BAS-II were similar between children who had moderate HIE at birth and their school-aged peers. Neuropsychological testing with the NEPSY derived similar results, with more memory and attention/executive function deficits among children who had a history of severe HIE. Despite no significant differences in developmental quotients among children with moderate encephalopathy and their school-aged peers, those with a history of HIE still had more special educational needs and lower achievement on assessments of national curriculum attainment.

COGNITIVE OUTCOMES AT SCHOOL AGE IN THE THERAPEUTIC HYPOTHERMIA ERA

The outcomes of neonates who received therapeutic hypothermia are considerably improved in terms of survival and neuromotor disabilities, including CP, yet some cognitive impairment continues to occur. Two trials report long-term cognitive outcomes of neonates randomized to therapeutic hypothermia.[17,38]

National Institute of Child Health and Human Development Trial

The National Institute of Child Health and Human Development (NICHD) trial of whole-body hypothermia randomized 208 neonates with moderate to severe NE to hypothermia or supportive care.[16] Participants were followed to 6 to 7 years and evaluated for cognitive, attention and executive function, visuospatial processing, neurologic outcome, and physical and psychosocial health.[38] IQ scores were measured with the Wechsler Preschool and Primary Scale of Intelligence – Third Edition (WPPSI-III)

Table 3
School-aged cognitive outcomes prior to therapeutic hypothermia

Study	N^a	Definition of Asphyxia	Follow-up Duration	Outcome Measures	Results
Robertson and Finer,[28] 1988	127	Altered consciousness with altered muscle tone or primitive reflexes after 1 h of age (mild or moderate HIE), together with 1 or more of fetal distress, Apgar <5, neonatal resuscitation	5.5 y	Stanford-Binet Intelligence Scales	NE without major disability (CP, severe vision or hearing impairment, IQ >3 SDs below the mean or a known seizure disorder) • Mild NE: mean IQ ± SD = 106 ± 12[b] • Moderate NE: mean IQ ± SD = 99 ± 18 • Control: mean IQ ± SD = 108 ± 14 • Term NICU graduates (no encephalopathy): Mean IQ ± SD = 105 ± 15
Shankaran et al,[29] 1991	14	Three of • Fetal distress • Meconium • Need for intubation • Abnormal tone and/or seizures at <24 h	5 y	McCarthy Scales of Children's Abilities	• Stages of encephalopathy not distinguished (mild–severe) • 64% of participants: 1 SD below mean • 86% of participants: 2 SD below mean

Robertson et al,[30] 1989	145	Altered consciousness with altered muscle tone or primitive reflexes after 1 h of age (mild, moderate, or severe HIE), together with 1 or more of: fetal distress, Apgar <5, neonatal resuscitation	8 y	WISC	• Mild HIE outcomes similar to controls
					• Moderate and severe HIE significantly lower scores compared with controls, even nondisabled survivors
					• Mean IQ ± SD:
					  ○ Mild HIE (nonimpaired): 106 ± 13, n = 56
					  ○ Moderate HIE (total): 95 ± 23, n = 84
					  ○ Moderate HIE (nonimpaired): 102 ± 17, n = 66[c]
					  ○ Moderate HIE (impaired): 68 ± 27, n = 18
					  ○ Severe HIE (impaired): 48 ± 21, n = 5

Barnett et al,[31] 2002	33	1-min Apgar <5 or neurologic abnormalities within 48 h of birth	5.5–6.5 y	WPPSI-R	• Childhood survivors without CP:
					  ○ Mean FSIQ ± SD = 107.3 ± 14.9
					  ○ Mean VIQ ± SD = 105.9 ± 16.9
					  ○ Mean PIQ ± SD = 104.7 ± 15.5
					  ○ Mild NE: mean IQ ± SD = 109.7 ± 14.6 (N = 1: 76, remainder >90)
					  ○ Moderate NE: mean IQ ± SD = 106.2 ± 11.8

Study	N	Definition	Age	Test	Outcomes
Barnett et al,[32] 2004	53	Convulsions or neurologic abnormalities within 48 h of birth (abnormal tone, feeding, or altered level of consciousness)	5.5–6.5 y	WPPSI-R	• Stages of encephalopathy not distinguished (mild–severe) • 85% of participants who could be tested with IQ ≥85 • Mean IQ ± SD (range) = 102 ± 16 (69–139)
Marlow et al,[33] 2005	50	Neurologic abnormalities within 1 wk lasting >24 h. Moderate NE: abnormal consciousness, difficulty maintaining respirations of central origin, abnormal tone and reflexes. Severe NE: ventilation for more than 24 h; 2 or more anticonvulsants; comatose or stuporous	7 y	BAS-II	• Mean general cognitive score ± SD: ○ Comparison group: 114 ± 13.8 ○ Moderate NE: 112.3 ± 11.3 ○ Severe NE: 102.7 ± 13.2 ○ Academic special needs: 14% comparison children, 26% moderate encephalopathy and 79% severe encephalopathy
Perez et al,[6] 2013	57	At least 1 criterion in these 3 groups: 1. Intrauterine asphyxia- bradycardia, limited beat-to-beat variability, late decelerations, or meconium-stained amniotic fluid 2. Perinatal asphyxia: Apgar score <5 at 5 min or <6 at 10 min, umbilical cord pH <7.1 and base deficit ≤10 mmol/L 3. Postpartum encephalopathy first 48 h	11 y	WISC-R (German version)	• Mean IQ (range) for children without major disability: ○ Full-scale IQ score: 95.3 (62–120) ○ Verbal IQ score: 98.2 (63–123) ○ Performance IQ score: 94.9 (66–118) ○ Full-scale IQ score <85: 24.6% ○ Full-scale IQ score <70: 5.3%

Stanford-Binet Intelligence Scales: mean = 100; SD = 16.
McCarthy Scales of Children's Abilities: mean = 100; SD = 16.
WISC: mean = 100; SD = 15.
WPPSI-R: mean = 100; SD = 15.
General cognitive score: mean = 100; SD = 15.
Stages of encephalopathy are not always classified according to the classification system of Sarnat.
Abbreviations: FSIQ, full-scale IQ; NICU, neonatal ICU; PIQ, performance IA; VIQ, verbal IQ.
[a] Number who underwent cognitive assessment.
[b] Mild NE not significantly below comparison group.
[c] Despite IQ in normal range, even nondisabled survivors of moderate NE approximately 1 grade level behind healthy age-matched controls (delays in school-related activities, such as reading, spelling, and arithmetic).

or the Wechsler Intelligence Scale for Children IV (WISC-IV). Higher cognitive functions not typically assessed with IQ or achievement tests were evaluated with the NEPSY. Death or an IQ score below 70 was the primary outcome and was available for 190 of 208 (91%) trial participants. The primary outcome occurred in 46/97 (47%) of children randomized to hypothermia compared with 58/93 (62%) of children randomized to supportive care ($P = .06$). IQ scores were subnormal (<85) in approximately half of the participants randomized to hypothermia, and 27% of these children had IQ less than 70. Higher cognitive function (eg, attention and executive function and visuospatial processing) could be examined only among the nondisabled survivors who functioned at a level that permitted formal assessment; these domains did not differ significantly between the hypothermia and control groups. Overall, 96% of survivors with CP had an IQ less than 70; 9% of children without CP had an IQ less than 70, and 31% had an IQ of 70 to 84[5]; 32% of the hypothermia-treated children who were functioning at a level that permitted formal neurodevelopmental or IQ testing required special educational services.[5]

Total Body Hypothermia for Neonatal Encephalopathy Trial

In the Total Body Hypothermia for Neonatal Encephalopathy (TOBY) trial, 325 newborns with NE randomized to therapeutic hypothermia were followed to 6 to 7 years of age and assessed for neurocognitive function. The primary outcome of the study was survival with an IQ score greater than or equal to 85. IQ testing was performed with the WPPSI-III or the WISC-IV. Additionally, children were assessed for attention and executive function, visuospatial processing, sensorimotor function, and memory and learning. These cognitive abilities were evaluated with the NEPSY–Second Edition and the Working Memory Test Battery for Children. Outcome data were available for 86% of trial participants: 184 survivors and 96 children who died before 6 to 7 years of age; 75 of 145 children in the hypothermia group (52%) compared with 52 of 132 (39%) in the control group survived with an IQ greater than or equal to 85. There was no significant difference in the results of the other psychometric assessments, with the exception of attention and executive function scores, which were higher in the hypothermia group. Although the mean difference in academic achievement scores was not significant between the 2 groups, the use of special educational resources was lower in the hypothermia group. **Table 4** displays the mean IQ scores for the various Wechsler intelligence subscales for participants of the NICHD and TOBY trials.

COGNITIVE OUTCOMES IN ADOLESCENCE (11–19 YEARS)

A few studies report cognitive outcomes in adolescence, and each enrolled infants born prior to the introduction of hypothermia. Perez and colleagues[6] assessed the long-term outcomes of 57 prospectively enrolled children with NE without subsequent major disability (defined as an IQ <55 or severe CP, Palisano and colleagues[39] grade 4 or 5) who were followed to a mean age of 11.2 years. Cognitive outcome was assessed with the German version of the WISC–Revised (WISC-R). Mean full-scale IQ was 95.3 (range 62–120); 24.6% of children had an IQ score less than 85, and 5.3% of children had an IQ score less than 70.

Lindstrom and colleagues[4] assessed the teenage cognitive and behavioral outcomes of term infants born in Sweden in 1985 with moderate neonatal HIE who survived with no significant neurologic impairment. Of 56 surviving children who could be assessed at 15 to 19 years of age, the parents of 13 declined participation; 28 of the 43 remaining children did not have CP or major neurologic impairment and were included in the study; siblings (n = 15) served as controls. Teens who had a history

Table 4
Cognitive outcomes, 6-year to 7-year, of children treated with hypothermia for hypoxic ischemic encephalopathy

Study	NICHD Trial Hypothermia Group, N = 63	NICHD Trial Control Group, N = 47	Difference in Means	TOBY Trial Hypothermia Group, N = 98	TOBY Trial Control Group, N = 86	Difference in Means
Full-scale IQ score						
Mean (± SD)	89.9 ± 23.3[a]	75.3 ± 24.4[a]	14.6	103.6 ± 14.4	98.5 ± 18.9	5.1
Missing data (n)	—	—		18	25	
Verbal IQ score						
Mean (± SD)	85.9 ± 19.1	86.4 ± 13.7	0.5	105.2 ± 15.6	101.1 ± 17.3	4.0
Missing data (n)	8	11		21	25	
Performance IQ score						
Mean (± SD)	91.3 ± 17.3	90.5 ± 16.3	0.8	101.1 ± 15.0	96.7 ± 19.0	4.4
Missing data (n)	8	11		19	22	
Processing speed score						
Mean (± SD)	93.2 ± 17.2	92.4 ± 17.0	0.8	98.7 ± 12.4	95.3 ± 18.7	3.4
Missing data (n)	8	11		25	31	

The WPPSI-III or the WISC-IV was used to assess cognitive outcomes. The NICHD trial reported detailed cognitive outcomes in a secondary study of all children followed at 18 to 22 months and at school age; 30 children were lost to follow-up (12 in the hypothermia group and 18 in the control group).

[a] Nineteen children were deemed so severely impaired as to preclude psychometric evaluation and were assigned a full-scale IQ of 39; functional outcomes in these children were assessed with the Pediatric Evaluation of Disability Inventory. No scores were imputed for verbal IQ, performance IQ, or processing speed. In the TOBY trial, 43 children were lost to follow-up and an additional 41 children were unable to complete IQ testing (37 with severe physical impairment and 4 who would not cooperate). No scores were imputed for the severely disabled children, although they were all deemed as having subnormal IQ.

of HIE had definite cognitive dysfunction more often than the siblings without HIE (20/28 [71%] versus 2/15 [13%]). Problems with short-term memory, time-perception, orientation, and behavior (assessed by parental report) also were more common among the teens with a history of moderate HIE.

MRI PATTERNS OF BRAIN INJURY ASSOCIATED WITH COGNITIVE IMPAIRMENT

Specific MRI patterns of neonatal brain injury predict worse cognitive outcomes among the survivors of NE: deep gray nuclei involvement (a basal ganglia/thalamus pattern) is associated with severe neuromotor and cognitive outcomes, whereas cerebral white matter injury (a watershed pattern) is associated with cognitive impairment in the absence of CP or functional motor deficits.[1,40,41] Miller and colleagues[41] were among the first to report this association in 174 neonates with NE at 30 months: among neonates with and without neuromotor impairment, those with a predominantly basal ganglia injury pattern had the most severe cognitive and motor outcomes, whereas neonates with a mostly watershed injury pattern had cognitive impairment that was less severe and did not demonstrate significant neuromotor impairment. The same group examined the association between neonatal brain injury patterns and domain-specific cognitive functions at 4 years of age among neonates without functional motor deficits (n = 64).[3] Children were evaluated with a 5-point neuromotor score and the Wechsler Preschool and Primary Scale of Intelligence–Revised (WPPSI-R). An increasing watershed pattern was associated with greater deficits in verbal IQ. In an elegant study of 68 prospectively enrolled children with HIE and neonatal MRI who were followed to a mean age of 11.2 years, watershed injury pattern on neonatal MRI correlated with both full-scale and verbal IQ scores.[6] Neonatal MRI pattern failed to correlate with motor performance in children without major disability.

CONTRIBUTION OF PERINATAL ASPHYXIA TO CEREBRAL PALSY

A common misconception is that a vast majority of children with CP have NE attributed to HIE and intrapartum events. The idea that difficult labor and reduced blood flow to the fetal brain around birth is a major contributor is as old as CP itself; it was first proposed by Little in his initial description of the disorder in 1862.[42] Despite the enduring popularity, strong evidence opposes this view. Perhaps the most authoritative information comes from the National Collaborative Perinatal Project (NCPP), a study of approximately 50,000 children born from 1959 to 1966 and followed to age 7 years. The NCPP conclusively showed that clinical indicators of birth asphyxia (eg, fetal bradycardia, low Apgar score, and delayed time to first breath) occurred in only a minority of children who had CP.[43] For example, approximately 70% of children in the NCPP who had CP had Apgar scores of 7 or more at 5 minutes and 80% of the children who survived after having Apgar scores of 0 to 3 at 10 minutes or later were free of major handicap at early school age.[44] Moreover, despite apparent improvements in Apgar scores, a tremendous increase in cesarean section deliveries, and significant advances in perinatal care over the past 20 to 30 years, the prevalence of CP has remained remarkably steady in developed countries, ranging between 1.5 and 3 per 1000 live births from 1950 to 2000,[45] although more recent US estimates suggest an increasing prevalence among school-aged children.[46–49]

Estimates of the fraction of children with CP who were exposed to birth asphyxia range widely, from below 3% to more than 50% in studies published between 1986 and 2010[50]; these estimates, however, are biased by heterogeneity in definitions of both asphyxia and CP. Studies that excluded nonasphyxial causes from their CP definition and used only clinically recognized actual asphyxia events to define birth asphyxia found that 12% or less of children who had CP were exposed. This is generally consistent with a Western Australian population-based study that found just 10% of all children with CP and 24% of those who were born at term had NE.[8] It is important, however, to understand that most (69%) children who have NE do not have intrapartum risk factors, and only an estimated 5% of affected children have intrapartum risk factors exclusively.[9]

SUMMARY

Severe NE with abnormal neurologic findings defined via the Sarnat criteria is an important mediator of the relationship between birth asphyxia and CP.[51] Absent such neonatal neurologic abnormalities, it is unlikely for a case of CP to be attributable to any peripartum metabolic abnormality.[52] Evidence indicates that birth asphyxia and/or NE contributes to only a small fraction of CP cases overall, probably less than approximately 10%, as was originally proposed by the NCPP investigators.[43] Moderate NE may be associated with milder neuromotor impairments or CP and a wider range of lesser cognitive deficits that might be missed in early childhood or deemed insignificant if not compared with normally developing controls. In the same vein, it is important to recognize that most children who have NE are not exposed to birth asphyxia[9]; strong evidence provides support in favor of a multifactorial origin that might involve subtypes involving neither hypoxia nor ischemia, hence the preference for the term NE over HIE.[12]

REFERENCES

1. Gonzalez FF, Miller SP. Does perinatal asphyxia impair cognitive function without cerebral palsy? Arch Dis Child Fetal Neonatal Ed 2006;91:F454–9.
2. Miller SP, Newton N, Ferriero DM, et al. Predictors of 30-month outcome after perinatal depression: role of proton MRS and socioeconomic factors. Pediatr Res 2002;52:71–7.
3. Steinman KJ, Gorno-Tempini ML, Glidden DV, et al. Neonatal watershed brain injury on magnetic resonance imaging correlates with verbal IQ at 4 years. Pediatrics 2009;123:1025–30.
4. Lindstrom K, Lagerroos P, Gillberg C, et al. Teenage outcome after being born at term with moderate neonatal encephalopathy. Pediatr Neurol 2006;35:268–74.
5. Pappas A, Shankaran S, McDonald SA, et al. Cognitive outcomes after neonatal encephalopathy. Pediatrics 2015;135:e624–34.
6. Perez A, Ritter S, Brotschi B, et al. Long-term neurodevelopmental outcome with hypoxic-ischemic encephalopathy. J Pediatr 2013;163:454–9.
7. Jacobs SE, Berg M, Hunt R, et al. Cooling for newborns with hypoxic ischaemic encephalopathy. Cochrane Database Syst Rev 2013;(1):CD003311.
8. Badawi N, Felix JF, Kurinczuk JJ, et al. Cerebral palsy following term newborn encephalopathy: a population-based study. Dev Med Child Neurol 2005;47: 293–8.
9. Badawi N, Kurinczuk JJ, Keogh JM, et al. Intrapartum risk factors for newborn encephalopathy: the Western Australian case-control study. BMJ 1998;317:1554–8.
10. Volpe JJ. Neonatal encephalopathy: an inadequate term for hypoxic-ischemic encephalopathy. Ann Neurol 2012;72:156–66.
11. Leviton A. Single-cause attribution. Dev Med Child Neurol 1987;29:805–7.
12. Leviton A. Why the term neonatal encephalopathy should be preferred over neonatal hypoxic-ischemic encephalopathy. Am J Obstet Gynecol 2013;208: 176–80.

13. McIntyre S, Badawi N, Blair E, et al. Does aetiology of neonatal encephalopathy and hypoxic-ischaemic encephalopathy influence the outcome of treatment? Dev Med Child Neurol 2015;57(Suppl 3):2–7.

14. Marret S. Causes and pathways of cerebral palsy following neonatal encephalopathy in children born at term. Dev Med Child Neurol 2016;58:118–20.

15. Gluckman PD, Wyatt JS, Azzopardi D, et al. Selective head cooling with mild systemic hypothermia after neonatal encephalopathy: multicentre randomised trial. Lancet 2005;365:663–70.

16. Shankaran S, Laptook AR, Ehrenkranz RA, et al. Whole-body hypothermia for neonates with hypoxic-ischemic encephalopathy. N Engl J Med 2005;353: 1574–84.

17. Azzopardi DV, Strohm B, Edwards AD, et al. Moderate hypothermia to treat perinatal asphyxial encephalopathy. N Engl J Med 2009;361:1349–58.

18. Jacobs SE, Morley CJ, Inder TE, et al. Whole-body hypothermia for term and near-term newborns with hypoxic-ischemic encephalopathy: a randomized controlled trial. Arch Pediatr Adolesc Med 2011;165:692–700.

19. Simbruner G, Mittal RA, Rohlmann F, et al. Systemic hypothermia after neonatal encephalopathy: outcomes of neo.nEURO.network RCT. Pediatrics 2010;126: e771–8.

20. Zhou WH, Cheng GQ, Shao XM, et al. Selective head cooling with mild systemic hypothermia after neonatal hypoxic-ischemic encephalopathy: a multicenter randomized controlled trial in China. J Pediatr 2010;157:367–72, 372.e1–3.

21. Jacobs S. Whole-body hypothermia for neonatal hypoxic-ischemic encephalopathy reduces mortality into childhood. J Pediatr 2012;161:968–9.

22. Gunn AJ, Gluckman PD, Gunn TR. Selective head cooling in newborn infants after perinatal asphyxia: a safety study. Pediatrics 1998;102:885–92.

23. Jary S, Whitelaw A, Walloe L, et al. Comparison of Bayley-2 and Bayley-3 scores at 18 months in term infants following neonatal encephalopathy and therapeutic hypothermia. Dev Med Child Neurol 2013;55:1053–9.

24. Chalak LF, DuPont TL, Sanchez PJ, et al. Neurodevelopmental outcomes after hypothermia therapy in the era of Bayley-III. J Perinatol 2014;34:629–33.

25. Anderson PJ, De Luca CR, Hutchinson E, et al, Victorian infant Collaborative Group. Underestimation of developmental delay by the new Bayley-III scale. Arch Pediatr Adolesc Med 2010;164:352–6.

26. Serenius F, Kallen K, Blennow M, et al. Neurodevelopmental outcome in extremely preterm infants at 2.5 years after active perinatal care in Sweden. JAMA 2013;309:1810–20.

27. Moore T, Johnson S, Haider S, et al. Relationship between test scores using the second and third editions of the Bayley Scales in extremely preterm children. J Pediatr 2012;160:553–8.

28. Robertson CM, Finer NN. Educational readiness of survivors of neonatal encephalopathy associated with birth asphyxia at term. J Dev Behav Pediatr 1988;9: 298–306.

29. Shankaran S, Woldt E, Koepke T, et al. Acute neonatal morbidity and long-term central nervous system sequelae of perinatal asphyxia in term infants. Early Hum Dev 1991;25:135–48.

30. Robertson CM, Finer NN, Grace MG. School performance of survivors of neonatal encephalopathy associated with birth asphyxia at term. J Pediatr 1989;114: 753–60.

31. Barnett A, Mercuri E, Rutherford M, et al. Neurological and perceptual-motor outcome at 5-6 years of age in children with neonatal encephalopathy: relationship with neonatal brain MRI. Neuropediatrics 2002;33:242–8.
32. Barnett AL, Guzzetta A, Mercuri E, et al. Can the Griffiths scales predict neuromotor and perceptual-motor impairment in term infants with neonatal encephalopathy? Arch Dis Child 2004;89:637–43.
33. Marlow N, Rose AS, Rands CE, et al. Neuropsychological and educational problems at school age associated with neonatal encephalopathy. Arch Dis Child Fetal Neonatal Ed 2005;90:F380–7.
34. Sarnat HB, Sarnat MS. Neonatal encephalopathy following fetal distress. A clinical and electroencephalographic study. Arch Neurol 1976;33:696–705.
35. van Handel M, Swaab H, de Vries LS, et al. Long-term cognitive and behavioral consequences of neonatal encephalopathy following perinatal asphyxia: a review. Eur J Pediatr 2007;166:645–54.
36. Dilenge ME, Majnemer A, Shevell MI. Long-term developmental outcome of asphyxiated term neonates. J Child Neurol 2001;16:781–92.
37. WHO. International classification of impairments, disabilities, and handicaps: a manual of classification relating to the consequences of disease. Geneva (Switzerland): WHO; 1982.
38. Shankaran S, Pappas A, McDonald SA, et al. Childhood outcomes after hypothermia for neonatal encephalopathy. N Engl J Med 2012;366:2085–92.
39. Palisano R, Rosenbaum P, Walter S, et al. Development and reliability of a system to classify gross motor function in children with cerebral palsy. Dev Med Child Neurol 1997;39:214–23.
40. Mercuri E, Ricci D, Cowan FM, et al. Head growth in infants with hypoxic-ischemic encephalopathy: correlation with neonatal magnetic resonance imaging. Pediatrics 2000;106:235–43.
41. Miller SP, Ramaswamy V, Michelson D, et al. Patterns of brain injury in term neonatal encephalopathy. J Pediatr 2005;146:453–60.
42. Little WJ. On the incidence of abnormal parturition, difficult labour, premature birth and asphyxia neonatorum on the mental and physical condition of the child, especially in relation to deformities. Trans Obstetrical Soc (London) 1862;3:293–344.
43. Nelson KB, Ellenberg JH. Antecedents of cerebral palsy. Multivariate analysis of risk. N Engl J Med 1986;315:81–6.
44. Nelson KB, Ellenberg JH. Apgar scores as predictors of chronic neurologic disability. Pediatrics 1981;68:36–44.
45. Paneth N, Hong T, Korzeniewski S. The descriptive epidemiology of cerebral palsy. Clin Perinatol 2006;33:251–67.
46. Yeargin-Allsopp M, Van Naarden Braun K, Doernberg NS, et al. Prevalence of cerebral palsy in 8-year-old children in three areas of the United States in 2002: a multisite collaboration. Pediatrics 2008;121:547–54.
47. Arneson CL, Durkin MS, Benedict RE, et al. Prevalence of cerebral palsy: autism and developmental disabilities Monitoring network, three sites, United States, 2004. Disabil Health J 2009;2:45–8.
48. Kirby RS, Wingate MS, Van Naarden Braun K, et al. Prevalence and functioning of children with cerebral palsy in four areas of the United States in 2006: a report from the Autism and Developmental Disabilities Monitoring Network. Res Dev Disabil 2011;32:462–9.
49. Van Naarden Braun K, Christensen D, Doernberg N, et al. Trends in the prevalence of autism spectrum disorder, cerebral palsy, hearing loss, intellectual

disability, and vision impairment, metropolitan Atlanta, 1991-2010. PLoS One 2015;10:e0124120.

50. Ellenberg JH, Nelson KB. The association of cerebral palsy with birth asphyxia: a definitional quagmire. Dev Med Child Neurol 2013;55:210–6.

51. Paneth N, Korzeniewski S, Hong T. The role of the intrauterine and perinatal environment in cerebral palsy. NeoReviews 2005;6:e133–40.

52. Collins M, Paneth N. The relationship of birth asphyxia to later motor disability. In: Donn SM, Sinha SK, Chiswick ML, editors. Birth asphyxia and the brain: basic science and clinical implications. Armonk (NY): Futura Publishing; 2002. p. 23–47.

53. Guillet R, Edwards AD, Thoresen M, et al. Seven-to eight-year follow-up of the CoolCap trial of head cooling for neonatal encephalopathy. Pediatr Res 2012; 71(2):205–9.

Neonatal Resuscitation in Low-Resource Settings

Sara K. Berkelhamer, MD[a],*, Beena D. Kamath-Rayne, MD, MPH[b],
Susan Niermeyer, MD, MPH[c]

KEYWORDS

- Neonatal resuscitation • Birth asphyxia • Intrapartum-related events
- Low-income countries • Low resource • Resuscitation education

KEY POINTS

- Simplified resuscitation programs reduce fresh stillbirth and early neonatal mortality rates in low-resource settings (LRSs) where the burden of death is greatest.
- Goals set by the Every Newborn Action Plan call for national and global efforts to improve coverage and quality of neonatal resuscitation.
- The science of resuscitation demonstrates that more than 95% of babies will respond to simple steps of drying, stimulation, warmth, suctioning if needed, and bag-mask ventilation.
- Despite notable progress, barriers remain in access to resuscitation equipment, presence of a skilled provider at birth, and quality assurance in resuscitation training.
- Future efforts to advance neonatal resuscitation in LRSs need to consider preservice education, skills retention through refresher training or low-dose, high-frequency practice, as well as expansion of health information systems and quality improvement initiatives.

INTRODUCTION

Almost all newborn deaths occur in low-income and middle-income countries (LMICs) where access to health care, including resuscitation at birth, is limited. Data from the last 2 decades starkly contrast the 31 million neonatal deaths in South and East Asian LMICs and 21 million in African LMICs with the 1 million neonatal deaths occurring in high-income countries.[1] Estimates suggest almost one-fourth of neonatal deaths can be attributed to intrapartum-related events or what is commonly referred to as birth asphyxia.[2,3] As a result, an estimated 720,000 deaths each year are thought to result from intrapartum-related events, although definitive causes cannot be confirmed.[4]

Disclosure: The authors have no financial obligations or affiliations to disclose.
[a] Department of Pediatrics, University at Buffalo, SUNY, 219 Bryant Street, Buffalo, NY 14222, USA; [b] Department of Pediatrics, Cincinnati Children's Hospital Medical Center, 3333 Burnet Avenue, MLC 7009, Cincinnati, OH 45229, USA; [c] Department of Pediatrics, University of Colorado, 13121 East 17th Avenue, Mail Stop 8402, Aurora, CO 80045, USA
* Corresponding author.
E-mail address: saraberk@buffalo.edu

Clin Perinatol 43 (2016) 573–591
http://dx.doi.org/10.1016/j.clp.2016.04.013   **perinatology.theclinics.com**

Notably, studies suggest that the systematic implementation of low-cost and effective newborn resuscitation programs in low-resource settings (LRSs) has the potential to avert nearly 200,000 of these intrapartum-related deaths each year.[5,6] In addition, an estimated 1.3 million intrapartum stillbirths occur annually; these deaths are potentially preventable by improved care during labor and at the time of delivery.[7]

Frequently quoted studies imply that 10% of infants require some support or stimulation at birth although only 3% to 6% of newborns require positive-pressure ventilation to initiate spontaneous respirations. An even smaller proportion (<1%) requires advanced care, including chest compression or medications (**Fig. 1**).[5,8–10] However, these estimates are biased towards care in resourced or facility settings where high rates of prenatal care, fetal monitoring, and cesarean delivery reduce the prevalence and impact of intrauterine hypoxia. These data may greatly underestimate the need in low-resource environments where the burden of neonatal morbidity and mortality is highest.[11–13] Studies from rural home deliveries in Zambia suggest 16% to 21% of infants require stimulation at birth, whereas unpublished data from community settings in Bangladesh imply even higher rates of need for intervention.[11]

Although reduction of neonatal mortality calls for primary prevention through improved fetal monitoring and obstetric care, resuscitation and stabilization of nonbreathing infants alone have the potential to save lives.[6] Studies have shown that even simple measures, including appropriate stimulation, clearing of the airway, and avoidance of hypothermia can reduce mortality.[13,14] The addition of assisted ventilation when clinically indicated represents a simple and critical intervention to reduce both morbidity and mortality associated with birth asphyxia.[15] Growing recognition of the burden of prematurity has included estimates implicating preterm birth as the direct cause of 35% of neonatal deaths.[16] In partnership with access to special care, resuscitation education has potential to reduce this burden by supporting preterm infants who are at greatest risk of breathing problems at birth.

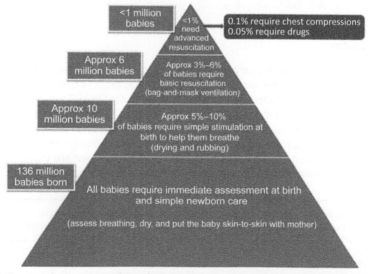

Fig. 1. Estimate of annual number of all newborns who require assistance to breathe at birth and varying levels of neonatal resuscitation. (*From* Lee AC, Cousens S, Wall SN, et al. Neonatal resuscitation and immediate newborn assessment and stimulation for the prevention of neonatal deaths: a systematic review, meta-analysis and Delphi estimation of mortality effect. BMC Public Health 2011;11(Suppl 3):S12.)

Significant progress has been made over the past decade with respect to development and distribution of educational programming and equipment for newborn resuscitation. However, numerous challenges remain in providing every infant, regardless of where they are born, access to optimal care and a chance of survival. With 50% of births in LMICs occurring in the home, possibly far from a health care facility, the challenges to making sustainable changes in neonatal resuscitation coverage are formidable.[15] Additional barriers include, but are not limited to, ineffective educational systems and programming, inadequate equipment and personnel, insufficient data monitoring, and limited political and social support to improve current care.[17,18]

These barriers exist despite heightened awareness of neonatal mortality as the single largest contributor to under-5 mortality, the target of Millennium Developmental Goal (MDG) 4. The commitment to reducing the global burden of neonatal mortality under the Sustainable Development Goals was renewed in 2014 by the World Health Organization (WHO), United Nations Children's Emergency Fund (UNICEF), and multiple global partners as the Every Newborn Action Plan (ENAP).[19] ENAP defines an ambitious agenda to end preventable newborn deaths and stillbirths by 2035. Targets include the continued and accelerated reduction in national neonatal mortality rates to 10 or fewer per 1000 live births, with an average worldwide neonatal mortality rate of 7 per 1000 by 2035 and reduction in stillbirths to 10 or fewer per 1000 total births.[19] Critical to achieving these goals will be attention to equity gaps through expanded access to resuscitation programming and equipment as well as an ongoing national and global commitment to providing skilled care at all deliveries, whether they occur in a health care facility, community setting or home.

Several publications have reviewed the status of newborn resuscitation in LRSs.[11,15,17,20,21] This article summarizes the status as of 2016, with attention to the impact of recent updates to the WHO and the International Liaison Committee on Resuscitation (ILCOR) guidelines, updates to educational programming, and the current status of resuscitation equipment. Barriers to achieving goals established for 2035 are acknowledged and strategies for accelerating progress and improving quality of resuscitative care are discussed.

CURRENT RESUSCITATION GUIDELINES AND IMPLICATION FOR CARE IN LOW-RESOURCE SETTINGS

Recent updates to recommendations on resuscitative care include the 2012 WHO Basic Newborn Resuscitation guidelines and the 2015 ILCOR Consensus on Science and Treatment Recommendations.[22,23] Although overlap of these recommendations exists, the objective of the WHO guidelines is "to ensure that newborns in resource-limited settings who require resuscitation are effectively resuscitated."[23] In contrast, the ILCOR rigorously evaluates the evidence underlying both basic and advanced resuscitation practices in resource-intensive and resource-limited settings. Updated or newly emphasized WHO and ILCOR recommendations follow, with discussion of their relevance to LRSs.

Attendance of Skilled Provider at Birth

Both WHO and ILCOR suggest that every birth should be attended by a person trained in resuscitation. Surveys from LMICs identify significant gaps in access to skilled personnel.[15,24] Although 72% of deliveries worldwide are attended by a skilled provider, only 67% and 48% of women in South East Asia and sub-Saharan Africa give birth with skilled personnel present.[25] Challenges remain most acute in assuring presence of skilled providers in nonfacility settings. Multicountry and wealth-based analysis demonstrates that more than half of births occur at home, with rates of home delivery approaching 90% for the poorest women in sub-Saharan Africa, South Asia, and South East Asia (**Fig. 2**).[26]

The heightened emphasis on adequate preparation for birth in the 2015 ILCOR updates may affect resource distribution and support task shifting in LRSs. Approaches may include basic resuscitation training of alternative cadres, including traditional birth attendants (TBAs) or community-based midwives. TBAs are relatively common in many health care systems, with approximately 50% of home deliveries in sub-Saharan Africa attended by a TBA.[26]

Although successful models of training TBAs in newborn resuscitation exist,[12,27–29] the approach remains controversial. Some countries have actively discouraged resuscitation training of home birth attendants in an effort to encourage deliveries in a hospital setting and to assure standardized obstetric and newborn care. Arguments are made that efforts to extend resuscitation training should instead be focused on transition towards facility-based deliveries.

However, transition to facility-based deliveries may overwhelm health care systems and increase risks of facility-acquired infections.[30,31] In addition, this approach may be unrealistic in remote LRSs where access and transportation barriers are common. The safety of home births, even in low-risk, well-resourced settings, remains a concern. A 2010 meta-analysis and more recent studies have demonstrated a 2-fold to 3-fold higher rate of perinatal or neonatal mortality with home deliveries.[32,33]

Management of the Airway

A major change in ILCOR 2015 guidelines is the approach to management of meconium. Routine intubation for tracheal suctioning is no longer suggested as insufficient data exist to continue this practice. In contrast, WHO guidelines recommend endotracheal suctioning for nonbreathing infants born with meconium, although the quality of evidence is rated as very low.

Both ILCOR and WHO specifically discourage the use of suctioning in spontaneously breathing infants and routine oral suctioning with meconium. Updated guidelines state that suctioning should be limited to infants with obvious airway obstruction. Concerns remain that high rates of unnecessary suctioning occur in resuscitation of newborns in LRSs and can cause bradycardia or trauma.[34] A study published in 2011 reported that unnecessary suctioning was used in 94.9% of deliveries in a hospital setting.[35] Ongoing educational efforts need to thoughtfully address overuse and highlight risks associated with excessive or aggressive suctioning.

Umbilical Cord Management

Delayed cord clamping (DCC) results in improved iron status in infancy after term birth as well as improved cardiovascular stability and reduced need for transfusion among preterm infants.[36,37] These advantages become particularly valuable in LMICs where rates of maternal iron deficiency are high and a safe blood supply may not be readily available. Performing DCC of the newborn infant while on the mother's abdomen may also promote thermal stability and early initiation of breastfeeding. ILCOR recommendations suggest DCC for preterm infants who do not require resuscitation at birth. These guidelines align with WHO recommendations from 2012 that advocate clamping no earlier than 1 minute after birth for both term and preterm babies who do not require positive pressure ventilation.[23] Although recent data on cord milking suggests it may serve as an appropriate alternative to delayed clamping,[38–40] insufficient evidence to support widespread use of this practice currently exists.

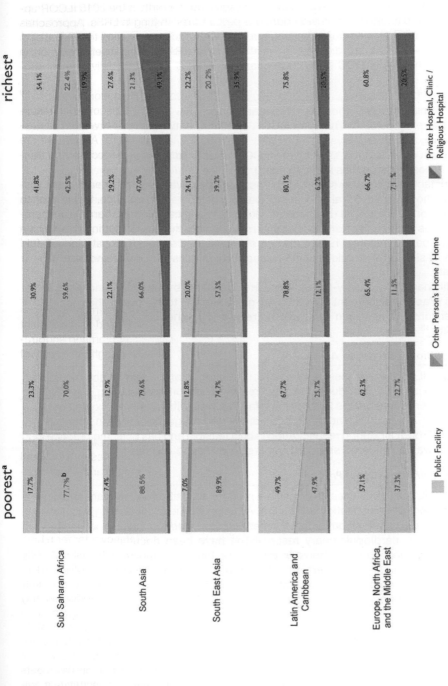

Fig. 2. Place of birth by region. Data from 23 countries identify that home birth occurred in more than half of deliveries and is most common among the poor. [a] 'Poorest' and 'richest' refer to an aggregate of country-weighted wealth quintiles for each region and are only approximations of true regional wealth quintiles. [b] Percentages for all Locations by quintile can be found in Spreadsheet SI. (*From* Montagu D, Yamey G, Visconti A, et al. Where do poor women in developing countries give birth? A multi-country analysis of demographic and health survey data. PLoS One 2011;6(2):e17155.)

In addition, both ILCOR and WHO state that there is insufficient evidence to recommend DCC when resuscitation is indicated. However, animal data and some observational or retrospective studies in birth cohorts indicate the physiologic benefits of cord clamping after the onset of respiration. This sequence of events allows the newborn to benefit from placental transfusion during a period of relative systemic hypoperfusion due to decreased pulmonary vascular resistance with increased pulmonary blood flow.[41–43] Numerous studies are currently in progress to address evidence gaps regarding the role of DCC when resuscitation is needed.

Thermal Support

Hypothermia elevates the risk of neonatal mortality, with a documented dose-response relationship.[44] The 2015 ILCOR recommendations emphasize thermal support during and after delivery.

Although options addressed by the ILCOR include radiant warmers or thermal mattresses, these approaches are both resource-intensive and risk hyperthermia. Skin-to-skin contact remains the safest and most cost-effective mode of providing thermal support; however, cultural and social barriers continue to limit widespread use in some regions. Traditional dress may make positioning the infant a challenge and privacy issues persist. In addition, mothers may consider the newborn unclean and prefer that a baby is washed before placing skin-to-skin. Campaigns to gain acceptance of skin-to-skin care in regions with low use but high rates of neonatal mortality remain a priority.

Additional low-cost, low-tech options are considered by the ILCOR, including use of plastic wraps or placement in clean food-grade bags up to the level of the neck. These interventions have been shown to reduce hypothermia and rates of early mortality.[45–48]

Resuscitation with Room Air

The 2015 ILCOR guidelines reaffirm that resuscitation of the term infant should start with room air and introduce the new recommendation that starting with 21% to 30% oxygen is reasonable for preterm infants as well, with titration of oxygen by pulse oximetry.[44] Although the administration of blended oxygen is difficult in many LMICs, the use of room air during resuscitation is both feasible and has been the practice long before it was considered standard of care in developed countries.

Structure of Educational Programs

The 2015 ILCOR guidelines emphasize a need for simulation and refresher training as a component of resuscitation education. Although frequency of training has not been demonstrated to affect patient outcomes, improved performance, knowledge, and confidence in cardiopulmonary resuscitation have been documented.[49–52] Use of refresher training courses, booster training, or low-dose and high-frequency skills practice have all shown improved retention of content of training programs.[53] The ILCOR recommendations for inclusion of simulation and refresher training highlight the need for well-coordinated efforts to implement structured and sustainable training programs.

IMPROVING THE QUALITY OF RESUSCITATIVE CARE

Despite the gains made in reducing rates of early neonatal mortality and stillbirth, performance gaps and bottlenecks still exist which training in neonatal resuscitation alone will not mitigate.[18,54] Focused quality improvement strategies have been suggested to overcome these quality gaps. Hill and colleagues[55] provide a framework for understanding the major categories of health system and quality gaps that serve as barriers to effective basic resuscitation services. Strategies to improve resuscitative care need to address gaps in provider competencies, essential commodities, quality improvement processes, and health information systems, as well as governance and national policies.

Provider Competencies: Current Status of Resuscitation Education

Several educational programs for teaching newborn resuscitation exist, including but not limited to the WHO's Essential Newborn Care, the American Academy of Pediatrics' (AAP) Neonatal Resuscitation Program, and the United Kingdom Resuscitation Council's Newborn Life Support Program. Because these programs assume access to intensive care and equipment, simplified versions have been designed and investigated in LRSs.[12,56,57] Most notable in these efforts has been widespread distribution of simplified resuscitation education through the *Helping Babies Breathe* (HBB) program.

HBB is a low-cost, portable, skills-based educational program intended for use in LRSs. The training materials are largely pictorial with simplified text, supporting inclusion of a wider community of providers (**Fig. 3**). The development of HBB was coordinated with the ILCOR 2010 guidelines with a commitment to bringing the latest in resuscitation science to all babies simultaneously. The algorithm for care focuses on assessment, stimulation, airway clearance, and assisted ventilation within the first minute after birth (The Golden Minute) but does not address use of oxygen, chest compressions, intubation, or medications. However, the algorithm segues directly into these interventions when required and available.

Since the launch of HBB in 2010, more than 300,000 providers have been trained in 77 countries globally with translation of materials into 26 languages (**Box 1**). To increase access, all teaching materials, including translations, are available online (http://www.helpingbabiesbreathe.org or http://internationalresources.aap.org). Preliminary studies on the efficacy, cost-effectiveness, and sustainability of HBB have identified the following:

- **Efficacy:** Implementation trials have demonstrated reduction in early newborn mortality rates as well as rates of stillbirth. Specifically, HBB programing in Tanzania resulted in a 47% reduction in neonatal mortality in the first 24 hours of life and a 24% reduction in fresh stillbirths.[13] Similar findings were noted in India where a 24% reduction in all stillbirths was demonstrated with a 46% reduction in those considered to be recent or fresh.[14] These data suggest that numerous infants previously assumed to be stillborn were misclassified since they responded to simple resuscitative measures provided with HBB.
- **Cost-effectiveness:** Analysis of HBB programing performed at a rural hospital in Tanzania implied that costs per life saved and life year gained were approximately US$233 and US$4.20, respectively. Once programing was established, costs of maintaining programs were brought down to approximately US$80 and US$1.40 per life saved and life year gained, respectively.[58] Additional evaluation in Indonesia and Brazil estimated costs of US$42 and US$88 per life saved.[59,60] Although application of cost analysis is limited by variable training strategies and equipment, the cost per life saved from these examples seems to be well below current acceptable benchmarks for cost-effectiveness of 1 to 3 times the gross domestic product per capita.[15]

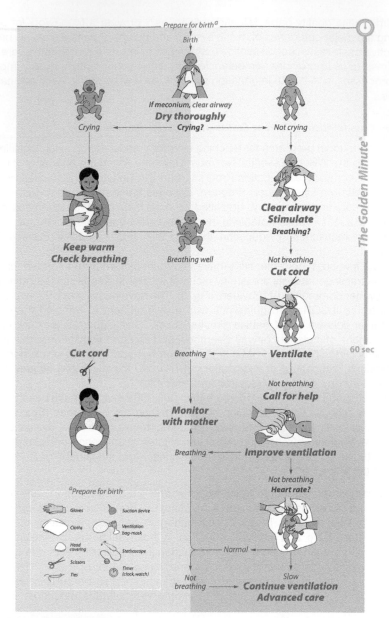

Fig. 3. Helping Babies Breathe Action Plan. (*Courtesy of* American Academy of Pediatrics (AAP), Elk Grove, IL, USA. Available at: http://internationalresources.aap.org/; with permission.)

- **Sustainability:** One-day HBB training courses in Tanzania were sufficient to improve performance in simulated scenarios several months after training. However, this did not translate into improved delivery room management.[53,61] Subsequent low-dose and high-frequency practice, refresher training, and review or debriefing of cases by clinical leadership resulted in change in provider performance and reduction in stillbirth and neonatal death. Currently, questions remain regarding the optimal approach to frequency of training and the role of refresher training.

Box 1		
Helping Babies Breathe translations		
Arabic	Kannada	Spanish
Bangla	*Karen*	Swahili
Burmese	Khmer	*Tajik*
Chinese	Laotian	Thai
Dari	Mongolian	*Tibetan*
French	Nepali	Vietnamese
Georgian	Pashto	*Urdu*
Haitian Creole	Portuguese	*Uzbek*
Indonesian	Sindhi	
Translations in italics are not yet posted online.		

Current status of HBB programming

HBB has recently been revised to update and align content with the 2015 ILCOR guidelines, with plans for release of a second edition in 2016. Notable changes to the content of HBB include the following:

- *Elimination of the conditional action step for meconium in amniotic fluid.* The action of suctioning before thorough drying when meconium is present will be removed from the action plan and teaching materials.
- *De-emphasis of suctioning.* Suctioning should be limited to use for airway obstruction or if there is meconium in the amniotic fluid and an infant is not responsive to stimulation. Discussion of the hazards of prolonged or vigorous suctioning will now be included.
- *Inclusion of ventilation with intact cord.* Although DCC was already recommended for crying infants, the possibility of resuscitation with an intact cord will now be included.
- *Inclusion of content emphasizing equipment reprocessing, implementation, ongoing practice, and quality improvement.*

Essential Commodities: Current Status of Resuscitation Equipment

Resuscitation programs require access to, investment in, and maintenance of equipment both for teaching and clinical care. These materials include newborn simulators for use as teaching aids, as well as equipment to clear the airway and provide ventilation. Although access to and upkeep of equipment remains a barrier, notable advances have been made in the development of low-cost equipment for use in LRSs.

Devices for clearing the airway

In 2011, the Program for Appropriate Technology in Health (PATH) evaluated a range of suction devices that were labeled for use in newborns.[62] A total of 20 devices were evaluated, ranging from $2 to $10 in price. Devices that can be opened offer a distinct advantage for reprocessing and reuse. One such suction device excelled in durability and options for cleaning at that time; however, additional low-cost devices that open have been developed since 2011.

Alternatives to bulb suction include the use of a mucus extractors or a cloth to clear the airway. Mucus extractors have a 1-way valve to reduce infectious risks; however, faulty equipment or improper use can result in exposure. Clearing the airway with a

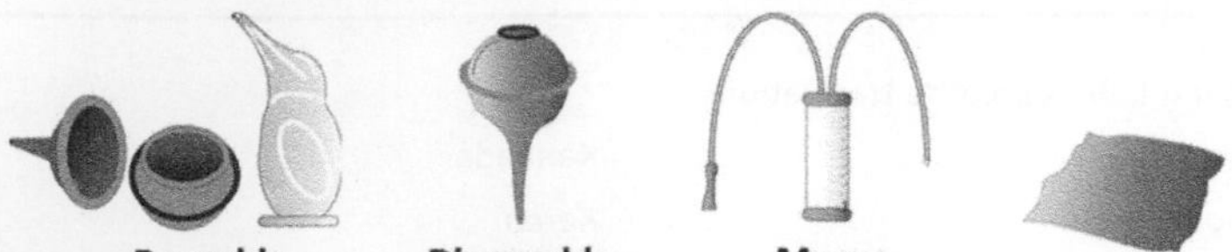

Fig. 4. Comparative characteristics of devices to clear the airway. Number of plus signs represents relative cost, efficacy, ease of cleaning, ease of use, portability, or infectious risks for a provider associated with use. All devices pose additional risk to infants if reused and improperly cleaned. Minus sign, negligible; NA, nonapplicable if disposed. (*Illustrations provided by* Satyan Lakshminrusimha, MD.)

cloth is also practiced because cloth has negligible cost and is widely available. However, this practice is of questionable efficacy and may induce mucosal injury (**Fig. 4**).

Devices for providing ventilation
Heightened awareness via the 1990 MDGs and widespread implementation of HBB has accelerated distribution of high-quality, affordable bag-mask ventilation (BMV) devices for use in newborn resuscitation. Comparative assessment of available equipment was published in 2010 (with an updated assessment pending) by PATH and the WHO.

Six distributors were producing BMV for less than US$20 at that time.[62] The lowest cost equipment was listed at US$12 to 15 and performed favorably with respect to function and usability. Notable advances since 2010 include development of an upright (vertical) resuscitator to improve ease of use, reduce costs, and simplify cleaning. Early simulation studies suggest improved delivery of adequate ventilation, although concerns remain for delivery of excessive volumes.[63,64] Additional lower cost devices have been developed since 2010; however, questions remain regarding their quality and function.

Alternatives to BMV, including mouth-to-mouth (or barrier), mouth-to-mask, and tube-and-mask, remain in use when ventilation equipment is not available.[15] Although early studies implied mouth-to-mask may be as effective as BMV,[65] simulation data questioned efficacy with unreliable delivery of pressure and volume.[66] Additional clinical studies raised concerns for increased mortality with mouth-to-mask and questioned ease of use.[29] Costs of these alternatives remain only slightly less than BMV devices (US $9–15) and manufacturing is severely limited.[62] As a result, use of BMV has been prioritized and recommended (**Fig. 5**).

Newborn simulators
ILCOR guidelines recommend use of simulation-based training with newborn resuscitation education. However, a systematic review found limited evidence to support this practice.[67] At present, there are no randomized controlled trials assessing clinical

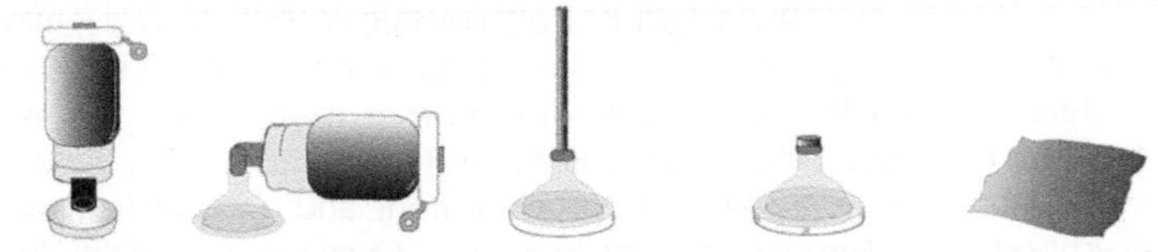

Mode of Ventilation	Upright BMV	Standard BMV	Tube-to-Mask	Mouth-to-Mask	Mouth-to-Cloth
Costs	+++	+++	++	++	-
Efficacy	+++	+++	++	++	-
Ease of cleaning	++	+	+++	+++	NA
Ease of use	+++	++	+	+	+++
Portability	+	+	++	++	+++
Infectious risk	-	-	++	++	+++

Fig. 5. Comparative characteristics of ventilation devices. Number of plus signs represents relative cost, efficacy, ease of cleaning, ease of use, portability, or infectious risk for a provider associated with use. All devices pose additional risk to infants if improperly cleaned. Minus sign, negligible; NA, nonapplicable if disposed. (*Illustrations provided by* Satyan Lakshminrusimha, MD.)

outcomes following simulation-based training in either a low-resourced or well-resourced setting. Educational evaluation specific to HBB noted improved knowledge and skills post-training but inadequate mastery of BMV after the workshop alone. These data suggest that integration of skills into clinical practice may not be achieved in the classroom setting without additional practice, continued learning, and active mentoring.[68]

A range of neonatal simulators exist, most of which are impractical for use in LRSs. A low-cost, water-filled simulator was purpose-designed to assist in teaching basic skills of newborn resuscitation, including stimulation, airway clearance, BMV, and assessment of respirations and pulse (**Fig. 6**). The NeoNatalie simulator manufactured by Laerdal (Stavenger, Norway) has been widely distributed for use with HBB and has been integrated into training provided by the WHO Basic Newborn Resuscitation Guide and the UK Resuscitation Council's Newborn Life Support.[24] NeoNatalie is currently sold at cost for US$60 if used in 1 of the 75 MDG countries.

Barriers to accessing resuscitation equipment
Access to critical resuscitation equipment remains a challenge in LRSs. Shipping costs may exceed those of the supplies themselves, arguing for distribution centers

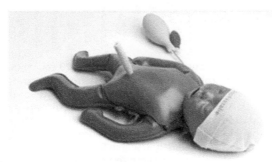

Fig. 6. NeoNatalie newborn simulator. (*Courtesy of* Laerdal Global Health, Stavanger, Norway; with permission.)

in areas of highest need. Imported equipment often requires national approval and inclusion on country essential devices lists. Although WHO Global Health Observatory data suggest that only 59% of countries have developed recommended lists of medical devices,[69] inclusion of BMV on those that exist would support national investment in equipment, facilitate procurement, and potentially avoid additional tariffs with importation. Beyond lack of inclusion on essential devices lists, complex procurement processes, and expectation of private exchange of funds may complicate access.

Unfortunately, resuscitation equipment may represent a lower priority resource in many less-resourced countries. A survey performed in 2012 identified that 18 of 20 countries depended on financial support from nongovernmental organizations and donors to purchase resuscitation equipment (**Fig. 7**). Future strategies to increase access should include improved distribution practices as well as increased demand to lower costs. Expansion of the highly successful model of public-private partnerships developed with HBB should be considered.[18]

Barriers to maintaining resuscitation equipment

Numerous challenges exist with respect to reprocessing of resuscitation equipment. Improper disinfection has been observed with subsequent damage to equipment.[70] Common challenges identified include insufficient disassembly, improper disinfection, and inadequate rinse after disinfection. To address these issues, PATH is developing neonatal resuscitation equipment reprocessing recommendations, which should be finalized in 2016. Online demonstrations have also been developed to assist in the proper upkeep and care.[70]

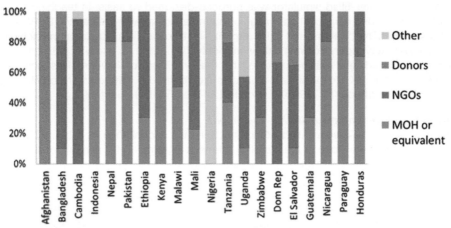

Fig. 7. Funding distribution for resuscitation equipment in 20 countries. Data from a 2012 survey demonstrate the large role of financial support from nongovernmental organizations (NGOs), Ministries of Health (MOH) and donors. Other: private for-profit and nonprofit organizations. Donors: USAID, World Bank, Swiss Aid, Australian Aid, United Nations Agencies, Laerdal Foundation. NGOs: Latter-Day Saint Charities, Management Sciences for Health, Plan, the Reproductive and Child Health Alliance, Save the Children, UNICEF, the United Nations Population Fund, University Research Co. LLC/Health Care Improvement Project, WHO. (*From* Coffey P, Kak L, et al. Newborn resuscitation devices, United Nations Commission on life-saving commodities for women and children. American Academy of Pediatrics (Elk Grove, IL, USA), 2012; with permission.)

Improvement Capacity: Current Status of Quality Improvement Processes

Dissemination of training and equipment for neonatal resuscitation does not equate to quality care at birth. Paramount to effective programming is quality assurance as well as improvement projects in response to ongoing monitoring and evaluation of data collected on newborn care and outcomes. Quality improvement initiatives are highly applicable to LRSs despite challenges of implementation. The past decade has heightened awareness and discussion of optimal approaches to assuring quality care. Processes such as mentoring, data acquisition and review, refresher training, and low-dose and high-frequency skills practice may all play an important role in strengthening both training and newborn care. A recent publication from a tertiary center in Nepal highlighted marked reduction in stillbirth and first-day mortality when HBB was paired with a quality improvement cycle.[71] This study described a multifaceted approach, including use of quality improvement teams, goals, objectives, and standards, as well as resuscitation training with weekly review, daily skills checks, self-evaluation checklists, and refresher training.

Health Information Services: Monitoring of Outcomes at Birth

Health information management systems and uniform data collection play a critical role in both documenting and ultimately improving care at birth. Standardization of key process and outcome indicators provides data to determine whether progress is being achieved, most notably the reduction of neonatal mortality.

Despite efforts to improve data collection in developing regions, the WHO MDGs 2015 report suggests slow progress.[72] Critical gaps remain in both quality and timeliness of data. Both policy changes and efforts to advance resuscitative care require accurate data on all deliveries. However, many lack presence of a skilled attendant to document care needed at delivery. Other births may be entirely undocumented in LRSs. Half of the world's newborns never receive a birth certificate and most neonatal deaths are not documented with death certificates.[19]

Recent advances in cellular and online technologies represent unprecedented opportunity for improved data collection and dissemination. Online data registries of midwifery care have been validated,[73] and mobile phones have been used to collect health information on pregnant women and newborns in Africa.[74,75] New applications for data collection using the internet or mobile telephones will accelerate access to and use of real-time data.

Governance: Resuscitation Policy in Low-Resource Settings

Improved care at birth requires consistent national policies with respect to both newborn resuscitation training and care. These guidelines may not exist in many LMICs or, if available, may be poorly implemented or accessed. The public health agenda remains complex in many countries, potentially leaving newborn resuscitation and newborn care at birth a lower priority.

Numerous lessons have been learned from dissemination of newborn resuscitation education using HBB.[18] Successful implementation efforts need to be locally owned and tailored to their specific context, looking beyond dissemination of training and equipment to systems components and sustainability. Although government leadership is key to affecting change, health professional associations may play an important role in providing influential and respected voices to advocate for and train others in resuscitation.

SUMMARY

Despite gradual reduction in global rates of newborn mortality, significant challenges remain in providing all infants optimal or appropriate resuscitative care at birth. Simplified resuscitation programs reduce rates of stillbirth and early neonatal mortality in LRSs; however, millions of babies are born in absence of a skilled provider or the equipment needed to provide care. Future progress in reducing the burden of birth asphyxia needs to address numerous barriers to care, including but not limited to the high rate of home deliveries, inadequate or ineffective training and equipment, and inadequate data collection for monitoring and evaluation. These data are critical to improving care, as well as in determining long-term outcomes after resuscitation. Although studies document improved survival in LRSs, the potential for increased risk of neurodevelopmental sequelae in resuscitated infants remains unknown.

Future efforts to improve access to neonatal resuscitation may include expanding coverage to frontline health providers, including health extension workers, skilled or traditional birth attendants, and midwives. Introducing skills-based education in resuscitation into preservice education may further exposure, complemented by mentoring and frequent skill practice to assure quality. Low-cost, simple task trainers, such as the augmented infant resuscitator (AIR) that provides feedback on resuscitation technique, are being developed to improve skills acquisition and delivery.

Timely and improved obstetrical responses in LRSs may also be facilitated by access to low-cost fetal heart rate monitors, potentially reducing the burden of stillbirth and asphyxia.[76] Ongoing development of equipment for airway management and monitoring during resuscitation has the potential to improve the safety and efficacy of interventions.[77] Numerous lower cost technologies for provision of respiratory and nutritional support exist and may be accessed through development of safe newborn transport systems. Ultimately, improved long-term outcomes may be influenced by improved access to regionalized specialty care.

Best practices

What is the current practice?

Simple resuscitative care, including stimulation, airway suctioning when needed, and bag-mask ventilation for nonbreathing infants, as well as avoidance of hypothermia, have been shown to reduce neonatal mortality in LRSs.

What changes in current practice are likely to improve outcomes?

Current practices need to assure the presence of a skilled provider and clean, functional equipment at all deliveries. Resuscitation education needs to address overuse of unneeded interventions (ie, suctioning) and inadequate use of those deemed beneficial (ie, DCC, skin-to-skin care). Resuscitation training needs to consistently address skills retention, monitoring, evaluation, and quality improvement.

Is there a clinical algorithm?

Clinical algorithms
  The ILCOR conducts evidence evaluation leading to a consensus on science and treatment recommendations. The WHO also reviews the quality of evidence for resuscitation interventions in LRSs and develops guidelines. The HBB Action Plan provides an algorithm for neonatal resuscitation in LRSs based on the ILCOR consensus on science.

Rating for the strength of the evidence
  Strong

Bibliographic sources

Perlman JM, Wyllie J, Kattwinkel J, et al. Part 7: Neonatal resuscitation: 2015 international consensus on cardiopulmonary resuscitation and emergency cardiovascular care science with treatment recommendations. Circulation 2015;132(16 Suppl 1):S204–241.

Msemo G, Massawe A, Mmbando D, et al. Newborn mortality and fresh stillbirth rates in Tanzania after helping babies breathe training. Pediatrics 2013;131(2):e353–360.

Goudar SS, Somannavar MS, Clark R, et al. Stillbirth and newborn mortality in India after helping babies breathe training. Pediatrics 2013;131(2):e344–352.

Summary statement

The past decade has seen significant progress in the widespread distribution of resuscitation education and equipment in LRSs. Further progress in achieving goals established by the ENAP calls for renewed national and global commitments to addressing gaps in quality of newborn resuscitative care.

REFERENCES

1. Oestergaard MZ, Inoue M, Yoshida S, et al. Neonatal mortality levels for 193 countries in 2009 with trends since 1990: a systematic analysis of progress, projections, and priorities. PLoS Med 2011;8(8):e1001080.

2. WHO global heath observatory Every Newborn Action Plan. Geneva, Switzerland: World Health Organization; 2014. Available at: http://www.everynewborn.org/Documents/Every_Newborn_Action_Plan- EXECUTIVE_SUMMARY-ENGLISH_updated_July2014.pdf. Accessed January 6, 2016.

3. Lawn JE, Wilczynska-Ketende K, Cousens SN. Estimating the causes of 4 million neonatal deaths in the year 2000. Int J Epidemiol 2006;35(3):706–18.

4. Liu L, Johnson HL, Cousens S, et al. Global, regional, and national causes of child mortality: an updated systematic analysis for 2010 with time trends since 2000. Lancet 2012;379(9832):2151–61.

5. Lee AC, Cousens S, Wall SN, et al. Neonatal resuscitation and immediate newborn assessment and stimulation for the prevention of neonatal deaths: a systematic review, meta-analysis and Delphi estimation of mortality effect. BMC Public Health 2011;11(Suppl 3):S12.

6. Kamath-Rayne BD, Griffin JB, Moran K, et al. Resuscitation and obstetrical care to reduce intrapartum-related neonatal deaths: a MANDATE Study. Matern Child Health J 2015;19(8):1853–63.

7. Lawn JE, Blencowe H, Waiswa P, et al. Stillbirths: rates, risk factors, and acceleration towards 2030. Lancet 2016;387(10018):587–603.

8. Barber CA, Wyckoff MH. Use and efficacy of endotracheal versus intravenous epinephrine during neonatal cardiopulmonary resuscitation in the delivery room. Pediatrics 2006;118(3):1028–34.

9. Palme-Kilander C. Methods of resuscitation in low-Apgar-score newborn infants–a national survey. Acta Paediatr 1992;81(10):739–44.

10. Perlman JM, Risser R. Cardiopulmonary resuscitation in the delivery room. Associated clinical events. Arch Pediatr Adolesc Med 1995;149(1):20–5.

11. Ersdal HL, Singhal N. Resuscitation in resource-limited settings. Semin Fetal Neonatal Med 2013;18(6):373–8.

12. Gill CJ, Phiri-Mazala G, Guerina NG, et al. Effect of training traditional birth attendants on neonatal mortality (Lufwanyama Neonatal Survival Project): randomised controlled study. BMJ 2011;342:d346.

13. Msemo G, Massawe A, Mmbando D, et al. Newborn mortality and fresh stillbirth rates in Tanzania after helping babies breathe training. Pediatrics 2013;131(2): e353–60.
14. Goudar SS, Somannavar MS, Clark R, et al. Stillbirth and newborn mortality in India after helping babies breathe training. Pediatrics 2013;131(2):e344–52.
15. Wall SN, Lee AC, Niermeyer S, et al. Neonatal resuscitation in low-resource settings: what, who, and how to overcome challenges to scale up? Int J Gynaecol Obstet 2009;107(Suppl 1):S47–62. S63–44.
16. Blencowe H, Cousens S, Chou D, et al. Born too soon: the global epidemiology of 15 million preterm births. Reprod Health 2013;10(Suppl 1):S2.
17. Enweronu-Laryea C, Dickson KE, Moxon SG, et al. Basic newborn care and neonatal resuscitation: a multi-country analysis of health system bottlenecks and potential solutions. BMC Pregnancy Childbirth 2015;15(Suppl 2):S4.
18. Kak LJ, McPherson R, Keenan W, et al. Helping babies breathe: lessons learned guiding the way forward. Global Developmental Alliance Report. 2015. Available at: http://www.helpingbabiesbreathe.org/docs/HBB-Report-2010-2015.pdf. Accessed January 20, 2016.
19. Lawn JE, Blencowe H, Oza S, et al. Every newborn: progress, priorities, and potential beyond survival. Lancet 2014;384(9938):189–205.
20. Meaney PA, Topjian AA, Chandler HK, et al. Resuscitation training in developing countries: a systematic review. Resuscitation 2010;81(11):1462–72.
21. Niermeyer S. From the neonatal resuscitation program to helping babies breathe: global impact of educational programs in neonatal resuscitation. Semin Fetal Neonatal Med 2015;20(5):300–8.
22. Wyckoff MH, Aziz K, Escobedo MB, et al. Part 13: neonatal resuscitation: 2015 American Heart Association guidelines update for cardiopulmonary resuscitation and emergency cardiovascular care. Circulation 2015;132(18 Suppl 2):S543–60.
23. Guidelines on basic newborn resuscitation. Geneva, Switzerland: World Health Organization; 2012. Available at: http://apps.who.int/iris/bitstream/10665/75157/1/9789241503693_eng.pdf?ua=1. Accessed January 5, 2016.
24. Coffey P, Kak L, et al. Newborn resuscitation devices, United Nations Commission on life-saving commodities for women and children. Elk Grove, IL: American Academy of Pediatrics; 2012.
25. Postnatal care for mothers and newborns: highlights from world health organization 2013 guidelines. Geneva, Switzerland: World Health Organization; 2013. Available at: http://www.who.int/maternal_child_adolescent/documents/postnatal-care- recommendations/en/. Accessed January 6, 2016.
26. Montagu D, Yamey G, Visconti A, et al. Where do poor women in developing countries give birth? A multi-country analysis of demographic and health survey data. PLoS One 2011;6(2):e17155.
27. Kumar A, Nestel D, Stoyles S, et al. Simulation based training in a publicly funded home birth programme in Australia: a qualitative study. Women Birth 2016;29(1): 47–53.
28. Titaley CR, Dibley MJ, Roberts CL. Utilization of village midwives and other trained delivery attendants for home deliveries in Indonesia: results of Indonesia Demographic and Health Survey 2002/2003 and 2007. Matern Child Health J 2011;15(8):1400–15.
29. Bang AT, Bang RA, Baitule SB, et al. Management of birth asphyxia in home deliveries in rural Gadchiroli: the effect of two types of birth attendants and of resuscitating with mouth-to-mouth, tube-mask or bag-mask. J Perinatol 2005;25(Suppl 1):S82–91.

30. Mehta R, Mavalankar DV, Ramani KV, et al. Infection control in delivery care units, Gujarat state, India: a needs assessment. BMC Pregnancy Childbirth 2011;11:37.
31. Dickson KE, Kinney MV, Moxon SG, et al. Scaling up quality care for mothers and newborns around the time of birth: an overview of methods and analyses of intervention-specific bottlenecks and solutions. BMC Pregnancy Childbirth 2015;15(Suppl 2):S1.
32. Wax JR, Lucas FL, Lamont M, et al. Maternal and newborn outcomes in planned home birth vs planned hospital births: a metaanalysis. Am J Obstet Gynecol 2010;203(3):243.e1–8.
33. Snowden JM, Tilden EL, Snyder J, et al. Planned out-of-hospital birth and birth outcomes. N Engl J Med 2015;373(27):2642–53.
34. Lindback C, Kc A, Wrammert J, et al. Poor adherence to neonatal resuscitation guidelines exposed; an observational study using camera surveillance at a tertiary hospital in Nepal. BMC Pediatr 2014;14:233.
35. Sobel HL, Silvestre MA, Mantaring JB 3rd, et al. Immediate newborn care practices delay thermoregulation and breastfeeding initiation. Acta Paediatr 2011; 100(8):1127–33.
36. Rabe H, Reynolds G, Diaz-Rossello J. Early versus delayed umbilical cord clamping in preterm infants. Cochrane Database Syst Rev 2004;(4):CD003248.
37. Garofalo M, Abenhaim HA. Early versus delayed cord clamping in term and preterm births: a review. J Obstet Gynaecol Can 2012;34(6):525–31.
38. Hosono S, Mugishima H, Fujita H, et al. Umbilical cord milking reduces the need for red cell transfusions and improves neonatal adaptation in infants born at less than 29 weeks' gestation: a randomised controlled trial. Arch Dis Child Fetal Neonatal Ed 2008;93(1):F14–9.
39. Katheria AC, Leone TA, Woelkers D, et al. The effects of umbilical cord milking on hemodynamics and neonatal outcomes in premature neonates. J Pediatr 2014; 164(5):1045–50.e1.
40. March MI, Hacker MR, Parson AW, et al. The effects of umbilical cord milking in extremely preterm infants: a randomized controlled trial. J Perinatol 2013;33(10): 763–7.
41. Bhatt S, Alison BJ, Wallace EM, et al. Delaying cord clamping until ventilation onset improves cardiovascular function at birth in preterm lambs. J Physiol 2013;591(Pt 8):2113–26.
42. Ersdal HL, Linde J, Mduma E, et al. Neonatal outcome following cord clamping after onset of spontaneous respiration. Pediatrics 2014;134(2):265–72.
43. Ersdal HL, Linde J, Auestad B, et al. Timing of cord clamping in relation to start of breathing or ventilation among depressed neonates-an observational study. BJOG 2015. [Epub ahead of print].
44. Perlman JM, Wyllie J, Kattwinkel J, et al. Part 7: Neonatal resuscitation: 2015 International Consensus on Cardiopulmonary Resuscitation and Emergency Cardiovascular Care Science with Treatment Recommendations. Circulation 2015; 132(16 Suppl 1):S204–41.
45. Leadford AE, Warren JB, Manasyan A, et al. Plastic bags for prevention of hypothermia in preterm and low birth weight infants. Pediatrics 2013;132(1):e128–34.
46. Belsches TC, Tilly AE, Miller TR, et al. Randomized trial of plastic bags to prevent term neonatal hypothermia in a resource-poor setting. Pediatrics 2013;132(3): e656–61.
47. Marin Gabriel MA, Llana Martin I, Lopez Escobar A, et al. Randomized controlled trial of early skin-to-skin contact: effects on the mother and the newborn. Acta Paediatr 2010;99(11):1630–4.

48. Nimbalkar SM, Patel VK, Patel DV, et al. Effect of early skin-to-skin contact following normal delivery on incidence of hypothermia in neonates more than 1800 g: randomized control trial. J Perinatol 2014;34(5):364–8.

49. Kaczorowski J, Levitt C, Hammond M, et al. Retention of neonatal resuscitation skills and knowledge: a randomized controlled trial. Fam Med 1998;30(10): 705–11.

50. Oermann MH, Kardong-Edgren SE, Odom-Maryon T. Effects of monthly practice on nursing students' CPR psychomotor skill performance. Resuscitation 2011; 82(4):447–53.

51. Su E, Schmidt TA, Mann NC, et al. A randomized controlled trial to assess decay in acquired knowledge among paramedics completing a pediatric resuscitation course. Acad Emerg Med 2000;7(7):779–86.

52. Sutton RM, Niles D, Meaney PA, et al. Low-dose, high-frequency CPR training improves skill retention of in-hospital pediatric providers. Pediatrics 2011;128(1): e145–51.

53. Mduma E, Ersdal H, Svensen E, et al. Frequent brief on-site simulation training and reduction in 24-h neonatal mortality–an educational intervention study. Resuscitation 2015;93:1–7.

54. Dickson KE, Simen-Kapeu A, Kinney MV, et al. Every Newborn: health-systems bottlenecks and strategies to accelerate scale-up in countries. Lancet 2014; 384(9941):438–54.

55. Hill K, Clark P, Narayanan I, et al. Improving quality of basic newborn resuscitation in low-resource settings: a framework for managers and skilled birth attendants. USAID ASSIST Project. Bethesda, MD: University Research Co, LLC (URC); 2014.

56. Bookman L, Engmann C, Srofenyoh E, et al. Educational impact of a hospital-based neonatal resuscitation program in Ghana. Resuscitation 2010;81(9): 1180–2.

57. Carlo WA, Goudar SS, Jehan I, et al. Newborn-care training and perinatal mortality in developing countries. N Engl J Med 2010;362(7):614–23.

58. Vossius C, Lotto E, Lyanga S, et al. Cost-effectiveness of the "helping babies breathe" program in a missionary hospital in rural Tanzania. PLoS One 2014; 9(7):e102080.

59. Vidal SA, Ronfani L, da Mota Silveira S, et al. Comparison of two training strategies for essential newborn care in Brazil. Bull World Health Organ 2001;79(11): 1024–31.

60. PATH. Reducing birth asphyxia through the Bidan di Desa Program: Final report submitted by Program for Appropriate Technology in Health (PATH) to Save the Childrens US at Jakarta, Indonesia, March 15 2006.

61. Ersdal HL, Vossius C, Bayo E, et al. A one-day "Helping Babies Breathe" course improves simulated performance but not clinical management of neonates. Resuscitation 2013;84(10):1422–7.

62. PATH. Practical selection of neonatal resuscitators: a field guide (version 3). 2010. Available at: http://www.path.org/publications/files/TS_nnr_field_guide_v3_print.pdf. Accessed January 5, 2016.

63. Coffey PS, Saxon EA, Narayanan I, et al. Performance and acceptability of two self-inflating bag-mask neonatal resuscitator designs. Respir Care 2015;60(9): 1227–37.

64. Thallinger M, Ersdal HL, Ombay C, et al. Randomised comparison of two neonatal resuscitation bags in manikin ventilation. Arch Dis Child Fetal Neonatal Ed 2015. [Epub ahead of print].

65. Massawe A, Kilewo C, Irani S, et al. Assessment of mouth-to-mask ventilation in resuscitation of asphyxic newborn babies. A pilot study. Trop Med Int Health 1996;1(6):865–73.
66. Terndrup TE, Warner DA. Infant ventilation and oxygenation by basic life support providers: comparison of methods. Prehosp Disaster Med 1992;7(1):35–40.
67. Rakshasbhuvankar AA, Patole SK. Benefits of simulation based training for neonatal resuscitation education: a systematic review. Resuscitation 2014; 85(10):1320–3.
68. Singhal N, Lockyer J, Fidler H, et al. Helping Babies Breathe: global neonatal resuscitation program development and formative educational evaluation. Resuscitation 2012;83(1):90–6.
69. Global health observatory data, Lists of medical devices. Geneva, Switzerland: World Health Organization; 2013. Available at: http://www.who.int/gho/health_technologies/medical_devices/en/. Accessed January 22, 2016.
70. Eslami P, Bucher S, Mungai R. Improper reprocessing of neonatal resuscitation equipment in rural Kenya compromises function: recommendations for more effective implementation of Helping Babies Breathe. Resuscitation 2015;91:e5–6.
71. KC A, Wrammert J, Clark R, et al. Reducing perinatal mortality in Nepal using Helping Babies Breathe. Pediatrics 2016;157(6):e1–10.
72. The millennium developmental goals report. New York: United Nations; 2015. Available at: http://www.un.org/millenniumgoals/2015_MDG_Report/pdf/MDG%202015%20rev%20(July%201).pdf. Accessed January 7, 2016.
73. Stapleton SR. Validation of an online data registry for midwifery practices: a pilot project. J Midwifery Womens Health 2011;56(5):452–60.
74. van Heerden A, Norris S, Tollman S, et al. Collecting maternal health information from HIV-positive pregnant women using mobile phone-assisted face-to-face interviews in Southern Africa. J Med Internet Res 2013;15(6):e116.
75. Gisore P, Shipala E, Otieno K, et al. Community based weighing of newborns and use of mobile phones by village elders in rural settings in Kenya: a decentralised approach to health care provision. BMC Pregnancy Childbirth 2012;12:15.
76. Safer births: research and development to save newborn lives. Moyo introduced in Tanzania. Available at: http://www.saferbirths.com/wp-content/uploads/2015/10/DSC_2646_HD1.jpg. Accessed February 2, 2016.
77. Elsevier.com. When seconds count - finding a new way to prevent newborn deaths. 2016. Available at: https://www.elsevier.com/connect/when-seconds-count-finding-a-new-way-to-prevent- newborn-deaths/_nocache#comment-2491829535. Accessed January 28, 2016.

Global Burden, Epidemiologic Trends, and Prevention of Intrapartum-Related Deaths in Low-Resource Settings

Shabina Ariff, MBBS, FCPS[a], ANNE CC LEE, MD, MPH[b],
Joy Lawn, FRCPCH, MPH, PhD[c], Zulfiqar A. Bhutta, FRCPCH, PhD[a,d,*]

KEYWORDS

- Intrapartum related neonatal deaths (IRND) • Neonatal encephalopathy (NE)
- Skilled birth attendant (SBA) • Helping Babies Breathe (HBB)
- The live saved tool (LiST) • Low and middle income countries (LMIC)
- Birth asphyxia (BA)

KEY POINTS

- The nonspecific term "birth asphyxia" needs to be replaced by more precise terminology "intrapartum-related neonatal death" so that more accurate estimates can be collected.
- Two-thirds of intrapartum-related deaths occur in South Asia and Africa where there is lack of competent skilled care providers and provision of basic and emergency obstetric care.
- Enhancement of facility delivery along with provision of a skilled birth attendant equipped with appropriate resources can reduce the burden of "birth asphyxia."
- Limited skilled care providers, lack of medical supplies and equipment, and lack of access to health services are specific bottlenecks hindering the effective implementation of interventions.
- Effective leadership, targeted resource allocation, enhanced human resources, and a well-organized health care system can save many lives.

All authors declare no competitive interests.
[a] Department of Paediatrics and Child Health, The Aga Khan University, Stadium Road, PO Box 3500, Karachi 74800, Pakistan; [b] Department of Pediatric Newborn Medicine, Brigham and Women's Hospital, 75 Francis Street, Thorn 229A, Boston, MA 02115, USA; [c] London School of Hygiene and Tropical Medicine, 103B Keppel Street, London WC 1E 7HT, UK; [d] Research Centre for Global Child Health, Toronto, Ontario, Canada
* Corresponding author. Department of Paediatrics and Child Health, The Aga Khan University, Stadium Road, PO Box 3500, Karachi 74800, Pakistan.
E-mail address: Zulfiqar.bhutta@sickkids.ca

Clin Perinatol 43 (2016) 593–608
http://dx.doi.org/10.1016/j.clp.2016.05.001
0095-5108/16/$ – see front matter © 2016 Elsevier Inc. All rights reserved.

perinatology.theclinics.com

INTRODUCTION

The term 'birth asphyxia' was introduced by the World Health Organization (WHO) in 1997 to describe the clinical condition of a newborn who either "fails to establish or sustain regular breathing at birth."[1] "Birth asphyxia" therefore implies a condition or a state of the newborn that requires immediate assistance to establish breathing. However, the term is imprecise and does not indicate a diagnosis or the causal pathology, which may vary from an intrapartum-related hypoxic event to a physiologic condition, such as prematurity, congenital structural abnormality of the brain, or maternal conditions. To add to the complexity, there is no gold standard test for the diagnosis. Over the decades, many clinical and biochemical markers such as cord pH, acidemia, Apgar scores, and fetal distress have been used to evaluate the intrapartum injury but the controversies and limitations remain.[2]

DEFINITIONS AND TERMINOLOGY

Over the past few years, the epidemiologic measurements of "birth asphyxia" have changed from nonspecific process and symptom-based diagnosis (obstructed labor, low Apgar scores, or fetal distress) to outcome-based proxy measures, such as early neonatal mortality, neonatal encephalopathy (NE), and seizure estimates.[3,4] These outcome measures have resulted in better correlations with the etiology and have improved the predictive value for long-term outcomes.

Three consensus statements were released in 1996 from leading academic institutes addressing the inappropriate use of the terminology and diagnosis of "birth asphyxia."[3] All reaffirm that birth asphyxia, fetal distress, perinatal asphyxia, and hypoxic-ischemic encephalopathy are nonspecific diagnoses and should not be used unless specific indicators of intrapartum insults are available. The terminology suggested in the consensus statement was "neonatal deaths associated with acute intrapartum events." Despite 2 decades, the uptake of the terminology has been slow and "birth asphyxia" continues to be the terminology in national and international estimation of disease burden.[5]

In this review article, "intrapartum stillbirth" is defined as late fetal death during labor, commonly assumed to be predominantly associated with intrapartum hypoxic-ischemic injury.[3] For neonatal deaths, previously called "birth asphyxia," we use the term "intrapartum-related neonatal death," which refers to live-born infants who die in the first 28 days of life from NE or who die before onset of NE and have evidence of intrapartum injury (**Box 1**).

GLOBAL BURDEN
How Many?

Intrapartum-related neonatal death (birth asphyxia) is a leading cause of neonatal mortality, particularly in low-income countries and also closely linked to a high burden of stillbirths.[6] According to Child Health Epidemiology Reference Group (CHERG) estimates in 2012, the number of global intrapartum deaths was 884,000 (uncertainty range [UR] 759–1,057,000) in 2000, which decreased to 717,000 (UR 610–876,000) in 2010, with an average annual rate reduction of 2.4%.[7] The latest CHERG (now MCEE [Maternal and Child Epidemiology Estimation group]) estimates report that in 2013, intrapartum-related neonatal deaths were the third leading cause of death in children younger than 5 years, accounting for 662,000 deaths (95% confidence interval [CI] 670,000–1.68 million), or 10.5% of deaths in children younger than 5 years and 24% of neonatal deaths.[8]

Box 1
Paradigm shift in the terminology of birth asphyxia.

Mortality outcomes

- *Early neonatal death:* Death in the first 7 days of life.
  - *Fetal death:* An infant born with no signs of life after 22 weeks of gestation (equivalent to 500 g). Late fetal death is an infant born dead after 28 weeks of gestation (equivalent to 1000 g)
  - *Stillbirth:* This will be taken as equivalent to late fetal death, which is an infant who is born with no signs of life after 28 weeks of gestation (equivalent to 1000 g)
  - *Intrapartum-related stillbirth:* A stillborn infant (shows no signs of life at delivery and weighs more than 500 g or is >22 weeks of gestation) with intact skin and no signs of disintegration in utero. The death is assumed to have occurred in the 12 hours before delivery and was most likely due to an intrapartum hypoxic event. Babies with severe congenital abnormalities are not included (based on the Wigglesworth classification)
- Intrapartum-related neonatal deaths (previously called "birth asphyxia" deaths):
  - Neonatal deaths of term infants with neonatal encephalopathy (NE) (see the next section) or who cannot be resuscitated (or for whom resuscitation is not available). Where possible, other causes should be excluded, such as lethal congenital malformations and preterm birth complications (less than 34 completed weeks of gestation or birth weight <2000 g).
  - Also includes a smaller group of infants who die from birth injury without hypoxic brain injury; for example, organ rupture

Morbidity outcomes

- NE:
  - "A disturbance of neurologic function in the earliest days of life in the term infant manifested by difficulty initiating and maintaining respiration, depression of tone and reflexes, abnormal level of consciousness and often by seizures" [[95], [96]], which may follow an intrapartum hypoxic insult or be due to another cause. NE is usually separated into 3 grades (mild, moderate, severe) by clinical findings during the first week of life. Virtually all infants with mild NE who are normal at the end of the first week of life will be free of long-term neurologic damage. Most infants with severe NE will die or manifest severe neurologic impairment.
- Hypoxic-ischemic encephalopathy (HIE):
  - A syndrome of abnormal neurologic behavior in the neonate, which is frequently associated with multisystem dysfunction and follows severe injury before or during delivery. There are several systems for categorizing HIE (most commonly into mild, moderate, severe). Most authorities now prefer the term "neonatal encephalopathy" and then specifying if the encephalopathy is associated with intrapartum injury.

Need for resuscitation

- *"Nonbreathing baby":* Infant with perinatal respiratory depression after birth that may be due to any of a multitude of causes, including but not restricted to intrapartum hypoxia, respiratory distress syndrome-preterm birth, infection, general anesthesia during labor, meconium, intracranial disease, and neuromuscular disease. Some clinicians use the term depressed baby or "perinatal depression."

From Lawn JE, Lee AC, Kinney M, et al. Two million intrapartum-related stillbirths and neonatal deaths: where, why, and what can be done? Int J Gynaecol Obstet 2009;107:S7; with permission.

Closely linked to intrapartum neonatal deaths are those intrapartum stillbirths that occur during childbirth.[9] In 2015, an estimated 1.3 million (UR 1.2–1.6 million) infants died during the intrapartum period (after the onset of labor) each year in Africa and South Asia.[10] Most of these stillbirths are preventable and approximately 98% occur in LMIC. Most, almost 75%, occur in the Sub-Saharan region and are due to obstetric complications or lack of skilled birth attendants (SBAs).[11] Global stillbirth rate reported in 2015 was 18.4 per 1000 live births compared with 24.7 in 2000.[12]

Intrapartum-Related Impairment and Neonatal Encephalopathy

One-tenth of all disability adjusted life years (DALY) arise from events during the first 28 days of life.[13] The major consequence of intrapartum-related hypoxic events is a stillbirth, neonatal death, or NE. NE is manifested by altered neurologic behavior, depression of tone and reflexes, and varying levels of consciousness, often accompanied by seizures.[14] The risk of NE increases in LMIC, where approximately 50 million births take place at homes without an SBA and where emergency obstetric care is inaccessible.[15]

The WHO world health report 2005 estimated that approximately 1 million neonates who had survived "birth asphyxia" may develop cerebral palsy and cognitive abnormalities, including difficulty in learning.[15,16] In 2010, there were an estimated 1.2 million infants (uncertainty interval 0.89–1.60 million) who developed NE associated with intrapartum events, 96% of those in LMICs. Of these 233, 000 (163,000–342,000) developed moderate to severe neurodevelopmental impairment and 181,000 (82,000–319,000) developed milder impairments. Intrapartum-related conditions accounted for 50.2 million DALY and 6.1 million years lived with disability in 2010.[15]

WHERE DO THE INTRAPARTUM-RELATED DEATHS OCCUR?

The highest intrapartum-related neonatal deaths and third-trimester stillbirth rates (SBRs) occur in countries with most births and the slowest progress in reducing the neonatal mortality rates. In a recent estimation of cause-specific mortality rate, the rates of intrapartum-related neonatal deaths were as low as 0.5 per 1000 live births in regions in which the neonatal mortality rate was less than 5, whereas in regions with neonatal mortality rates greater than 45 per 1000, the rates of intrapartum-related deaths were 24-fold higher, reflecting the need for interventions targeted during child birth and immediate postnatal period.[17]

Two-thirds of the world's intrapartum-related neonatal deaths occur in South Asia and Africa,[3,18] whereas 10 lower-income countries in the regions are responsible for 65% of all intrapartum-related neonatal deaths. They include countries with the largest number of births and deaths: India, China, Republic of Congo, Pakistan, Nigeria, Bangladesh, Ethiopia, Indonesia, Afghanistan, and Tanzania. High-income countries with improved access to skilled care have a low incidence of "asphyxia"-related deaths, at approximately 12%.[19]

INEQUITIES IN DISTRIBUTION OF INTRAPARTUM-RELATED DEATHS

There remains a noticeable disparity in the estimated number of intrapartum-related neonatal deaths within a country.[20] This is largely due to socioeconomic diversity (eg, poverty, large family size, cultural beliefs) that enables a smaller portion of the population to have access to basic obstetric and postnatal care.[21] The vast majority of deaths due to intrapartum-related hypoxic events occur in socioeconomically deprived environments, highly prevalent in LMIC where access to basic maternal and newborn skilled health care is almost nonexistent. Gender inequity and selected infanticide of female fetuses is also one of the sad practices deeply inhabited in certain societies and cultures in South Asia.[22]

CHALLENGES IN GLOBAL ESTIMATES OF INTRAPARTUM-RELATED NEONATAL DEATH

Complete lack of reliable vital registration in high mortality settings makes estimates of intrapartum-related neonatal deaths challenging.[23] Information regarding intrapartum and other causes of death for more than 97% of neonatal deaths is insufficient in countries that lack SBA coverage and reporting systems. More than 60% of births take place outside facilities and skilled care is absent in approximately two-thirds of the deliveries.[24] This is the major reason why there remains a noticeable lack of reliable data on neonatal deaths. Absence of basic postnatal care and skilled staff in a home setting leads to misclassification of a "live-born baby," who does not breathe at birth, as "stillbirth."[25] Therefore, a considerable amount of uncertainty surrounds the true estimated value of intrapartum-related deaths.[26]

The major source of mortality data is secondary and collected by reviewing intermittent large household surveys, demographic surveillance and clinical records. Stillbirths may be miscounted in retrospective surveys by a margin of 20%.[12] These surveys mostly rely on live birth histories and simple questions regarding stillbirths.[27] In developed countries, cause-specific data related to stillbirths are available through national perinatal surveillance systems. For example, in the United Kingdom, one such system works efficiently and is known as the United Kingdom Confidential Enquiry into Maternal and Child Health.[28] South Africa, a middle-income country, specifically stands out for having a National Confidential Enquiry for Maternal Deaths and also a voluntary perinatal audit system that contains the data of 40% of the births. The system provides data on direct causes of stillbirths and neonatal deaths.[29]

Verbal autopsies are commonly used to collect data regarding stillbirths or neonatal deaths in LMICs.[30] Only 2 developing countries, including Egypt and Pakistan, submitted national assessments of causes of stillbirths in a verbal autopsy follow-up to their Demographic Health Surveys.[31] Accurate estimation of the number of neonatal deaths and distinction from stillbirths is also hindered because many stillbirths remain "invisible" at the policy level.[32]

RISK FACTORS FOR INTRAPARTUM AND ANTEPARTUM-RELATED DEATHS

Newborn health is closely linked to maternal well-being.[20,33] The associations of pregnancy and intrapartum risk factors for intrapartum stillbirths and/or perinatal deaths are shown in **Tables 1** and **2**. Complications during the intrapartum period have the strongest associations with perinatal mortality.[25] The risks of complications during childbirth (malpresentation,[34] obstructed labor,[35] maternal fever[8,36]) are linked with up to 85-fold increased risk of intrapartum death. Other maternal causes, such as antepartum hemorrhage, pregnancy-induced hypertension eclampsia, and prolonged rupture of membranes are also significantly associated with increased risk of neonatal death.[37] Obstructed or prolonged labor is the most common preventable cause of fetal mortality affecting 3% to 6% of live births and accounting for approximately 43,000 maternal deaths annually.[35] The incidence is particularly high in settings with no skilled birth attendance and frequently results in hypoxic events that can eventually lead to developmental delays, cerebral palsy, and neonatal death.[38] A study in Nigeria documented a stillbirth rate of 23% in pregnancies complicated with obstructed labor.[39] Maternal fever, rapid heartbeat, and tender uterus following an intra-amniotic infection were found to be associated with preterm rupture of membranes and preterm labor, brain injury, and NE.[40] Maternal fever alone has proven to be an independent factor for intrapartum-related mortality with an adjusted odds ratio of 10-fold.[41] Umbilical cord complications, such as prolapse, nuchal cord, and cord

Table 1
Adjusted odds ratio for risk factors for all-cause neonatal/perinatal deaths reported from population-based studies

Time Period	Risk Factor	Adjusted Odds Ratio[a]	Approximate Range
Before pregnancy	*Maternal age*		Approximate range 1–5
	<18 y	1.1–2.0	
	>35 y	1.3–2.0 (NS in 2 studies)	
	Maternal size		
	Height <150 cm	1.3–5.0	
	Pre-pregnancy weight <47 kg	1.1–2.0	
	Parity		
	Primigravida	1.3–2.2	
	Parity >6	1.4–1.5	
	Poor obstetric history (previous perinatal death or instrumental delivery)	1.6–4.0	
During pregnancy (antenatal)	Multiple pregnancy	2.0–7.0	Approximate range 2–14
	Maternal anemia		
	(PCV <0.34)	NS in 4 studies	
	(PCV <0.21)	2–4	
	Maternal jaundice/cholestasis	2–8	
	Hypertensive disorders		
	Preeclampsia	2–4	
	Eclampsia	3–14	
	Diabetes	2–11	
	Syphilis (perinatal death)	1.7–6.0	
	Maternal malaria (blood test positive)	2–4	
	HIV	1.1–3.0	
	HIV and malaria	5	
	Postterm (>42 wk gestation)	1.5	
	Preterm birth (<37 wk gestation)	2–4	
During labor and childbirth (intrapartum)	Obstructed labor/dystocia	7–85	Approximate range 2–85
	Prolonged second stage	3–5	
	Meconium staining of liquor	12	
	Malpresentation		
	Breech	6–15	
	Other	8–34	
	Bleeding per vagina after 8th month	3–6	
	Maternal fever during labor (>38°C)	10–11	
	Rupture of membranes >24 h	1.8–7.0	

Figures rounded to the nearest whole number unless less than 2.

Abbreviations: HIV, human immunodeficiency virus; NS, not significant; PCV, packed cell volume.

[a] Odds ratios included are statistically significant and from population-based studies adjusting for major confounders (parity and socioeconomic status) and significantly associated with intrapartum stillbirth and/or neonatal death or perinatal death.

Adapted from Lawn JE, Cousens S, Zupan J. 4 million neonatal deaths: when? where? why? Lancet 2005;365(9462):896.

stricture, make a significant contribution to intrapartum fetal death. Intrapartum hemorrhage also increases the risk of fetal death.[7,12]

Antepartum conditions, such as hypertension, malnutrition, short stature, and anemia, are also linked with perinatal morbidity and mortality, with risks in the range

Table 2
Summary of Grading of Recommendations Assessment, Development and Evaluation (GRADE) recommendations for care in childbirth to reduce intrapartum-related adverse outcomes

Strongly Recommended	Conditionally Recommended	Weakly Recommended (Effectiveness, Feasibility or Risk-Benefit Concerns)	Possible Options: Not Currently Recommended; More Research Needed
Clinical intrapartum care interventions			
• Use of the partograph • Intermittent assessment of fetal heart rate • *In utero* resuscitation • Simplified umbilical artery Doppler • Symphysiotomy • Maneuvers to manage shoulder dystocia • Emergency laparotomy plus uterine repair or hysterectomy for uterine rupture • External cephalic version for breech presentation • Early delivery for severe preeclampsia or eclampsia • Early delivery for placental abruption • Antibiotics and early delivery for intra-amniotic infection	• Instrumental delivery • Planned cesarean for breech presentation • Anticonvulsant drugs for preeclampsia/eclampsia • Ultrasound confirmation of placenta previa with planned cesarean delivery	• Active management of labor • Use of Doptone • Fetal scalp blood sampling • Amnio-infusion for meconium-stained amniotic fluid and umbilical cord compression • Antihypertensive drugs for severe hypertension • Cervical cerclage for suspected placenta previa • Membrane sweeping for postterm pregnancy[a] • Routine induction for postterm pregnancy[a]	• Fundal pressure • Clinical fetal arousal tests • Amniotic fluid assessment • Induction for suspected macrosomia[a]
Intrapartum care provision strategies			
• Obstetric drills on labor wards with high-fidelity simulations (for shoulder dystocia, cesarean delivery) • Rapid response teams • Safety checklists (surgical safety, cesarean, general childbirth) • Continuous intrapartum support from a familiar individual	Task-shifting to nurse practitioners for cesarean delivery, anesthesia, and intrapartum monitoring	—	—

[a] Provided that early-gestation ultrasound dating is available.

From Hofmeyr GJ, Haws RA, Bergström S, et al. Obstetric care in low-resource settings: What, who, and how to overcome challenges to scale up? Int J Gynaecol Obstet 2009;107:S21–44; with permission.

of 2-fold to 14-fold. Intra-amniotic infection has been linked with neurologic damage and NE.[40] Hypertensive disease is one of the most common contributors to the perinatal mortality in LMIC.[42] Uncontrolled hypertension, preeclampsia, and eclampsia not only pose a great danger to the mother for cerebrovascular accidents but also to the fetal demise and NE.[43]

Antepartum hemorrhage is a significant contributor to maternal and fetal mortality and complicates 3.5% to 5.0% of all pregnancies, especially during the second and third trimester.[44] Most of the cases result from placenta previa or placental abruption.[43] Pregnant mothers with diabetes introduce a substantial risk of enlarged neonatal size in accordance to the gestational age, which results in increased risk of intrapartum injury and birth asphyxia/intrapartum-related neonatal death.[45]

WHAT CAN BE DONE? EVIDENCE-BASED INTERVENTIONS TO REDUCE INTRAPARTUM-RELATED DEATHS

The Lives Saved Tool (LiST) was designed to evaluate the impact of various interventions around the continuum of care and provide an estimate of number of mothers and newborns who could be saved. It is used to estimate the impact in lives saved and the cost of scaling up various interventions. The LiST includes all evidence-based interventions that have a direct impact on neonatal mortality. The interventions can be modified to see the impact on lives saved and cost incurred to save more mothers and newborns.[46]

A similar computer model developed by the Maternal and Neonatal Directed Assessment of Technology (MANDATE) initiative estimated the potential of current and new interventions to reduce intrapartum asphyxia in Sub-Saharan Africa and India. Introduction of basic neonatal care, increase in facility births, and scaling up of emergency obstetric care at all levels had an estimated reduction in intrapartum-related neonatal mortality rate by 2.5 per 1000 live births.[47]

IMPACT OF INTERVENTIONS AROUND LABOR AND DELIVERY MANAGEMENT
Basic and Comprehensive Emergency Obstetric Care

In the Lives Saved analysis,[48,49] full coverage of labor and delivery management during childbirth resulted in the largest reduction in intrapartum deaths, averting an estimated 70% of intrapartum deaths (**Fig. 1**). Presence of skilled maternity services at delivery is associated with lower neonatal mortality rates.[27] To ensure safe delivery and child birth, WHO recommends the availability of Basic and Comprehensive Emergency obstetric care (CEmOC) and skilled childbirth. Presently CEmOC coverage is extremely low in the regions with high burden of birth and deaths, especially in remote rural areas (5% in rural South Asia and 1% rural Sub-Saharan Africa).[50]

WHO defines basic emergency obstetric care as an essential care package that should be available at first-level health facilities to provide safe delivery and newborn assessment. It includes provision of parenteral antibiotics for infections, oxytocic drugs for preterm labor, anticonvulsants for preeclampsia or eclampsia, assisted vaginal delivery (including vacuum or forceps assistance for delivery, episiotomy, advanced skills for manual delivery of shoulder dystocia, skilled vaginal delivery of the breech infant), manual removal of the placenta, and removal of retained products. CEmOC also includes availability of a blood bank service, anesthesia, and cesarean delivery.

Historical reports from Malaysia and Finland show significant reduction in the neonatal mortality rate with provision of obstetric and neonatal care. In Malaysia, training of village midwives in basic obstetric care and gradual shifts to facility birth

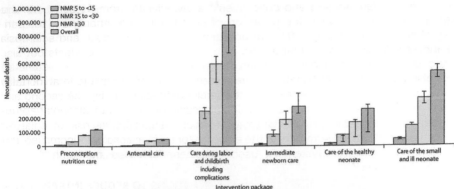

	Preconception nutrition care	Antenatal care	Care during labour and childbirth including complications	Immediate newborn care	Care of the healthy neonate	Care of the small and ill neonate
Estimated maternal lives saved by 2025	0	7500 (6700–9100)	150,000 (137,100–158,900)	NA	NA	NA
Estimated stillbirths prevented by 2025	23,000 (17,800–26,500)	240,000 (150,800–374,500)	550,000 (432,500–531,400)	NA	NA	NA
Estimated neonatal lives saved by 2025	110,000 (111,800–118,300)	43,000 (36,500–46,900)	790,000 (588,500–865,000)	190,000 (136,300–280,400)	230,000 (64,300–261,500)	580,000 (531,000–621,000)
Estimated additional child lives (post-neonatal) saved by 2025	7500	1200	0	0	1900	0
Costs by 2025 (in billion US$)	1·88	0·4	2·29	0·035	0·11	0·96
Costs (billion US$) per 100 000 maternal and newborn lives, and stillbirths saved	1·38	0·16	0·15	0·02	0·05	0·17
Costs (billion US$) per 100 000 newborn babies saved	1·65	0·92	0·29	0·02	0·05	0·17

Fig. 1. Estimated impact of interventions on the intrapartum-related neonatal deaths. NA, not applicable. (*From* Bhutta ZA, Das JK, Bahl R, et al. Can available interventions end preventable deaths in mothers, newborn babies, and stillbirths, and at what cost? Lancet 2014;384(9940):362; with permission.)

with provision of emergency obstetric care in 1985 to the 1990s resulted in a significant decline in the neonatal mortality rate from 75.5 in 1957 to 14.8 in 1991.[51] A more recent initiative in Burkina Faso brought a reduction in the perinatal mortality rate from 33 per 1000 live births to 27.5 per 1000 live births with the increase in availability and accessibility to CEmOC services.[52]

Skilled Birth Attendant

In addition to availability of obstetric services, WHO mandates the presence of SBAs to manage delivery and provide postnatal care.[51] An SBA is defined as an accredited health professional, such as a midwife, doctor, or nurse, who has been educated and trained to proficiency in the skills needed to manage uncomplicated pregnancies, childbirth, and newborn care and in the identification, management, and referral of complications.[53] It includes primary prevention via recognition and prompt referral for childbirth complications and secondary prevention via management of a nonbreathing infant with appropriate newborn care and neonatal resuscitation.

A review by Goldenberg and colleagues[54] analyzed data from 51 countries and established a link between the provision of skilled birth and intrapartum stillbirth. They observed a decrease of 0.27 intrapartum stillbirth per thousand births for each 1% increase in skilled birth attendance.

Access to CEmOC including cesarean delivery is estimated to prevent an estimated 85% of intrapartum-related deaths.[51] The presence of an SBA[55] and provision of basic emergency obstetric care can reduce intrapartum birth asphyxia by 40%.[56]

In a recent systematic review of individual/specific obstetric interventions to avert intrapartum deaths, the GRADE (Grading of Recommendations Assessment, Development and Evaluation) summary of the evidence for interventions in childbirth is summarized. The GRADE System is used to assess evidence quality and make recommendations.[50]

IMPACT OF INTERVENTIONS AROUND IMMEDIATE AND POSTNATAL CARE
Neonatal Resuscitation in Low-Resource Setting

Transition from fetal to neonatal period involves significant changes in the circulatory and respiratory physiology that is essential for normal transition. Some newborns are unable to adapt to these changes and require assistance in breathing and maintaining adequate circulation. The set of interventions or assistance provided to the newborn to establish breathing and circulation is called resuscitation.[57] Approximately 10% of all births require some form of resuscitation to establish regular breathing and circulation.[58] Basic resuscitation, such as stimulation and bag-and-mask ventilation, alone is sufficient to resuscitate as many as 6 million newborns each year.

Fewer than 1% require advanced resuscitation, such as chest compressions, endotracheal intubation, and medications.[59] The use of oxygen during resuscitation does not offer any added benefits for outcome.[60] Therefore, competency in basic resuscitation skills and extensive coverage should be the priority in LMICs with high burden of intrapartum-related deaths. Newborns that are resuscitated necessitate ongoing intensive care, which is mostly unavailable in LMICs.[58]

In a systematic review of the effectiveness of neonatal resuscitation,[58] 24 studies were identified that reported mortality outcomes (20 observational, 2 quasi-experimental, 2 cluster randomized controlled trials). A meta-analysis of 3 before-after facility-based studies of neonatal resuscitation training found a 30% reduction of intrapartum-related neonatal deaths (relative risk [RR] = 0.70, 95% CI 0.59–0.84) following resuscitation training. Data from community-based trials were identified in 8 studies; however, the data were not pooled due to heterogeneity of study design. An expert group estimated that community-based resuscitation may reduce intrapartum-related neonatal mortality by 20%.

The International Liaison Committee on Resuscitation defines the international consensus statements regarding resuscitation standards, intended for high-resource settings with skilled personnel. However, over the past decade, several resources have been developed for training specifically in low-resource settings. The WHO guide "Basic newborn resuscitation: a practical guide" targets first-referral level in low-resource settings.[61]

Helping Babies Breathe, an initiative of the American Academy of Pediatrics in collaboration with other public-private partners of a Global Development Alliance, is a simplified neonatal resuscitation training program aimed at training birth attendants in low-resource settings. The program includes basic neonatal care, initiation of breathing and resuscitation, including bag-and-mask ventilation, thermoregulation, and initiation of early breastfeeding.[62,63] In Tanzania, the extensive implementation of the HBB program led to a significant reduction in early neonatal deaths (RR with training 0.53; 95% CI 0.43–0.65; P = .0001) and rates of fresh stillbirth (RR with training 0.76; 95% CI 0.64–0.90; P = .001).[64]

Even though neonatal resuscitation has proven to be a high-impact intervention, its effective implementation in LMICs is hindered by a number of factors. In a recent analysis of health systems "bottlenecks" for *every newborn action plan"* conducted in 12 countries, identified several substantial barriers, including limited skilled care providers, lack of appropriate tools and medical products (bag-mask equipment), technologies and challenges regarding delivery service.[65] The local government and the leaders should work together and introduce strategies to overcome these barriers and improve information systems to monitor progress more closely and reduce intrapartum-related mortality.[49]

To achieve substantial gains in saving mothers and newborns, extensive antenatal care coverage, and standardized management around labor and delivery, are as good as neonatal interventions, especially in terms of returns of investment. **Fig. 2** projects lives saved with interventions across continuum of care.

Post Resuscitation Care

Most newborns following effective resuscitation require monitoring and evaluation for breathing,[66] metabolic problems, such as low glucose and calcium levels,[67] oxygenation, acidemia, temperature, and seizure control.[68] Effective post resuscitation care can improve the survival and neurodevelopment outcomes. However post resuscitation, reperfusion injuries are common and without adequate care vital organs such as lungs, kidneys, heart and liver are at risk of severe injuries. Post resuscitation care is possible only at the facility level where adequate equipment and expertise are available.

DISCUSSION

Intrapartum-related neonatal deaths continue to be one of the major causes of early neonatal deaths in the LMIC.[69,70] The confusion and clutter around the terminology

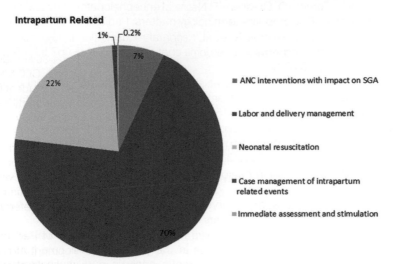

Fig. 2. Lives that could be saved by 2025 with universal coverage of care. (*From* Bhutta ZA, Das JK, Bahl R, et al. Can available interventions end preventable deaths in mothers, newborn babies, and stillbirths, and at what cost? Lancet 2014;384(9940):347–70; with permission.)

of "asphyxia" requires urgent clarity, consensus, and uptake by clinicians, researchers, and policymakers alike.[71] At present we have adequate knowledge and evidence on major interventions that can prevent intrapartum hypoxia-related morbidities and mortality.[72-74] Countries and global partners have recognized the need for greater attention to maternal, newborn, and child health. We also know the cost of implementation of the proposed interventions.[75,76] Immediate attention is required toward reducing specific bottlenecks in implementation so that interventions can have the maximum impact. Effective leadership-targeted funding, enhanced human resource performance and utilization, and well-organized health care facilities are required. With the announcement of Sustainable Development Goals and global Every Newborn Action Plan, there is a hope that interventions around continuum of care will save lives.[49,77,78]

ACKNOWLEDGMENTS

We are thankful to Batha Tariq for her contribution in literature search and editing the manuscript.

REFERENCES

1. Lincetto O. Birth asphyxia summary of the previous meeting and protocol overview. Geneve (Switzerland): World Health Organization; 2007.
2. American Academy of Pediatrics. The Apgar score. Adv Neonatal Care 2006; 6(4):220–3.
3. Lawn JE, Lee AC, Kinney M, et al. Two million intrapartum-related stillbirths and neonatal deaths: where, why, and what can be done? Int J Gynaecol Obstet 2009;107:S5–19.
4. Lawn J, Shibuya K, Stein C. No cry at birth: global estimates of intrapartum stillbirths and intrapartum-related neonatal deaths. Bull World Health Organ 2005; 83(6):409–17.
5. Dammann O, Ferriero D, Gressens P. Neonatal encephalopathy or hypoxic-ischemic encephalopathy? Appropriate terminology matters. Pediatr Res 2011;70(1):1–2.
6. Wall SN, Lee AC, Niermeyer S, et al. Neonatal resuscitation in low-resource settings: what, who, and how to overcome challenges to scale up? Int J Gynaecol Obstet 2009;107:S47–64.
7. Liu L, Johnson HL, Cousens S, et al. Global, regional, and national causes of child mortality: an updated systematic analysis for 2010 with time trends since 2000. Lancet 2012;379(9832):2151–61.
8. Liu L, Oza S, Hogan D, et al. Global, regional, and national causes of child mortality in 2000–13, with projections to inform post-2015 priorities: an updated systematic analysis. Lancet 2015;385(9966):430–40.
9. WHO U. Why are 4 million newborn babies dying each year? Lancet 2004;364: 399–401.
10. Lawn JE, Kerber K, Enweronu-Laryea C. 3.6 million neonatal deaths—what is progressing and what is not? Seminars in perinatology 2010;34:371–86.
11. Blencowe H, Cousens S, Oestergaard MZ, et al. National, regional, and worldwide estimates of preterm birth rates in the year 2010 with time trends since 1990 for selected countries: a systematic analysis and implications. Lancet 2012;379(9832):2162–72.
12. de Bernis L, Kinney MV, Stones W, et al. Stillbirths: ending preventable deaths by 2030. Lancet 2016;387(10019):703–16.

13. Murray CJ, Vos T, Lozano R, et al. Disability-adjusted life years (DALYs) for 291 diseases and injuries in 21 regions, 1990–2010: a systematic analysis for the Global Burden of Disease Study 2010. Lancet 2013;380(9859):2197–223.

14. Takenouchi T, Kasdorf E, Engel M, et al. Changing pattern of perinatal brain injury in term infants in recent years. Pediatr Neurol 2012;46(2):106–10.

15. Lee AC, Kozuki N, Blencowe H, et al. Intrapartum-related neonatal encephalopathy incidence and impairment at regional and global levels for 2010 with trends from 1990. Pediatr Res 2013;74(S1):50–72.

16. Blencowe H, Lee AC, Cousens S, et al. Preterm birth-associated neurodevelopmental impairment estimates at regional and global levels for 2010. Pediatr Res 2013;74(Suppl):17–34.

17. Lawn JE, Cousens S, Zupan J, et al. 4 million neonatal deaths: when? Where? Why? Lancet 2005;365(9462):891–900.

18. Stanton C, Lawn JE, Rahman H, et al. Stillbirth rates: delivering estimates in 190 countries. Lancet 2006;367(9521):1487–94.

19. Lawn JE, Wilczynska-Ketende K, Cousens SN. Estimating the causes of 4 million neonatal deaths in the year 2000. Int J Epidemiol 2006;35(3):706–18.

20. Althabe F, Bergel E, Cafferata ML, et al. Strategies for improving the quality of health care in maternal and child health in low-and middle-income countries: an overview of systematic reviews. Paediatr Perinat Epidemiol 2008;22(Suppl 1): 42–60.

21. Darmstadt GL, Lee AC, Cousens S, et al. 60 million non-facility births: who can deliver in community settings to reduce intrapartum-related deaths? Int J Gynaecol Obstet 2009;107:S89–112.

22. de Hilari C, Condori I, Dearden KA. When is deliberate killing of young children justified? Indigenous interpretations of infanticide in Bolivia. Soc Sci Med 2009; 68(2):352–61.

23. Ersdal HL, Mduma E, Svensen E, et al. Birth asphyxia: a major cause of early neonatal mortality in a Tanzanian rural hospital. Pediatrics 2012;129(5):e1238–43.

24. Lawn JE, Blencowe H, Oza S, et al. Every newborn: progress, priorities, and potential beyond survival. Lancet 2014;384(9938):189–205.

25. Frøen JF, Friberg IK, Lawn JE, et al. Stillbirths: progress and unfinished business. Lancet 2016;387(10018):574–86.

26. Lawn JE, Blencowe H, Waiswa P, et al. Stillbirths: rates, risk factors, and acceleration towards 2030. Lancet 2016;387(10018):587–603.

27. Yakoob MY, Lawn JE, Darmstadt GL. Stillbirths: epidemiology, evidence, and priorities for action. Seminars in perinatology 2010;34(6):387–94.

28. Mander R, Smith GD. Saving mothers' lives: reviewing maternal deaths to make motherhood safer–2003–2005. Midwifery 2008;24(1):8–12.

29. Moodley J, Pattinson RC, Fawcus S, et al. The confidential enquiry into maternal deaths in South Africa: a case study. BJOG 2014;121(Suppl 4):53–60.

30. Byass P, Herbst K, Fottrell E, et al. Comparing verbal autopsy cause of death findings as determined by physician coding and probabilistic modelling: a public health analysis of 54 000 deaths in Africa and Asia. J Glob Health 2015;5(1): 010402.

31. Jafarey SN, Rizvi T, Koblinsky M, et al. Verbal autopsy of maternal deaths in two districts of Pakistan—filling information gaps. J Health Popul Nutr 2009;27(2):170.

32. Horton R, Samarasekera U. Stillbirths: ending an epidemic of grief. Lancet 2016; 387(10018):515–6.

33. PLoS Medicine Editors. Maternal health: time to deliver. PLoS Med 2010;7(6): e1000300.

34. Hutton EK, Hofmeyr GJ. External cephalic version for breech presentation before term. Cochrane Database Syst Rev 2015;(7):CD000084.

35. Dolea C, AbouZahr C. Global burden of hypertensive disorders of pregnancy in the year 2000. GBD 2000 Working Paper. Geneva (Switzerland): World Health Organization; 2003. http://www.who.int/evidence/bod.

36. Rouse DJ, Landon M, Leveno KJ, et al. The maternal-fetal medicine units cesarean registry: chorioamnionitis at term and its duration—relationship to outcomes. Am J Obstet Gynecol 2004;191(1):211–6.

37. Lee AC, Mullany LC, Tielsch JM, et al. Risk factors for neonatal mortality due to birth asphyxia in southern Nepal: a prospective, community-based cohort study. Pediatrics 2008;121(5):e1381–90.

38. Harrison MS, Ali S, Pasha O, et al. A prospective population-based study of maternal, fetal, and neonatal outcomes in the setting of prolonged labor, obstructed labor and failure to progress in low-and middle-income countries. Reprod Health 2015;12(Suppl 2):S9.

39. Nwogu-Ikojo E, Nweze S, Ezegwui H. Obstructed labour in Enugu, Nigeria. J Obstet Gynaecol 2008;28(6):596–9.

40. Blume HK, Li CI, Loch CM, et al. Intrapartum fever and chorioamnionitis as risks for encephalopathy in term newborns: a case-control study. Dev Med Child Neurol 2008;50(1):19–24.

41. Cooke R. Chorioamnionitis, maternal fever, and neonatal encephalopathy. Dev Med Child Neurol 2008;50(1):9.

42. Allanson ER, Muller M, Pattinson RC. Causes of perinatal mortality and associated maternal complications in a South African province: challenges in predicting poor outcomes. BMC Pregnancy Childbirth 2015;15(1):37.

43. Ananth CV, Basso O. Impact of pregnancy-induced hypertension on stillbirth and neonatal mortality in first and higher order births: a population-based study. Epidemiology 2010;21(1):118.

44. Ngeh N, Bhide A. Antepartum haemorrhage. Curr Obstet Gynaecol 2006;16(2):79–83.

45. Bale JR, Stoll BJ, Lucas AO, editors. Improving birth outcomes: meeting the challenge in the developing world. Institute of Medicine (US), Committee on Improving Birth Outcomes. Washington, DC: National Academies Press (US); 2003.

46. Walker N, Tam Y, Friberg IK. Overview of the lives saved tool (LiST). BMC Public Health 2013;13(Suppl 3):S1.

47. Kamath-Rayne BD, Griffin JB, Moran K, et al. Resuscitation and obstetrical care to reduce intrapartum-related neonatal deaths: a MANDATE study. Matern Child Health J 2015;19(8):1853–63.

48. Bhutta ZA, Das JK, Bahl R, et al. Can available interventions end preventable deaths in mothers, newborn babies, and stillbirths, and at what cost? Lancet 2014;384(9940):347–70.

49. Dickson KE, Kinney MV, Moxon SG, et al. Scaling up quality care for mothers and newborns around the time of birth: an overview of methods and analyses of intervention-specific bottlenecks and solutions. BMC Pregnancy Childbirth 2015;15(Suppl 2):S1.

50. Hofmeyr GJ, Haws RA, Bergström S, et al. Obstetric care in low-resource settings: what, who, and how to overcome challenges to scale up? Int J Gynaecol Obstet 2009;107:S21–45.

51. Lee AC, Cousens S, Darmstadt GL, et al. Care during labor and birth for the prevention of intrapartum-related neonatal deaths: a systematic review and Delphi estimation of mortality effect. BMC Public Health 2011;11(3):S10.
52. Hounton SH, Byass P, Brahima B. Towards reduction of maternal and perinatal mortality in rural Burkina Faso: communities are not empty vessels. Glob Health Action 2009;2.
53. Inter-agency Working Group on Reproductive Health in Crises. Manual. IAWG, WHO; 2010.
54. Goldenberg RL, McClure EM. Maternal mortality. American Journal of Obstetrics and Gynecology 2011;205(4):293–5.
55. Hounton S, Menten J, Ouédraogo M, et al. Effects of a skilled care initiative on pregnancy-related mortality in rural Burkina Faso. Trop Med Int Health 2008; 13(Suppl 1):53–60.
56. Harvey SA, Ayabaca P, Bucagu M, et al. Skilled birth attendant competence: an initial assessment in four countries, and implications for the Safe Motherhood movement. Int J Gynaecol Obstet 2004;87(2):203–10.
57. Wang CL, Anderson C, Leone TA, et al. Resuscitation of preterm neonates by using room air or 100% oxygen. Pediatrics 2008;121(6):1083–9.
58. Lee AC, Cousens S, Wall SN, et al. Neonatal resuscitation and immediate newborn assessment and stimulation for the prevention of neonatal deaths: a systematic review, meta-analysis and Delphi estimation of mortality effect. BMC Public Health 2011;11(3):S12.
59. Perlman JM, Wyllie J, Kattwinkel J, et al. Neonatal resuscitation: 2010 international consensus on cardiopulmonary resuscitation and emergency cardiovascular care science with treatment recommendations. Pediatrics 2010;126(5): e1319–44.
60. Tan A, Schulze A, O'Donnell C, et al. Air versus oxygen for resuscitation of infants at birth. Cochrane Database Syst Rev 2005;(2):CD002273.
61. World Health Organization. Basic newborn resuscitation: a practical guide. Geneva: WHO; 1997. Available at: http://www.who.int/reproductivehealth/publications/maternal_perinatal_health/MSM_98_1/en/index.html. Accessed July 6, 2009.
62. Carlo WA, Goudar SS, Jehan I, et al. Newborn-care training and perinatal mortality in developing countries. N Engl J Med 2010;362(7):614–23.
63. Sibley L, Sipe TA. What can a meta-analysis tell us about traditional birth attendant training and pregnancy outcomes? Midwifery 2004;20(1):51–60.
64. Afnan-Holmes H, Magoma M, John T, et al. Tanzania's countdown to 2015: an analysis of two decades of progress and gaps for reproductive, maternal, newborn, and child health, to inform priorities for post-2015. Lancet Glob Health 2015;3(7):e396–409.
65. Dickson KE, Simen-Kapeu A, Kinney MV, et al. Every newborn: health-systems bottlenecks and strategies to accelerate scale-up in countries. Lancet 2014; 384(9941):438–54.
66. Ramji S, Saugstad OD, Jain A. Current concepts of oxygen therapy in neonates. Indian J Pediatr 2015;82(1):46–52.
67. Burns CM, Rutherford MA, Boardman JP, et al. Patterns of cerebral injury and neurodevelopmental outcomes after symptomatic neonatal hypoglycemia. Pediatrics 2008;122(1):65–74.
68. Evans D, Levene M, Tsakmakis M. Anticonvulsants for preventing mortality and morbidity in full term newborns with perinatal asphyxia [Review]. Cochrane Database Syst Rev 2007;(3):CD001240.

69. Black RE, Cousens S, Johnson HL, et al. Global, regional, and national causes of child mortality in 2008: a systematic analysis. Lancet 2010;375(9730):1969–87.
70. Darmstadt GL, Kinney MV, Chopra M, et al. Who has been caring for the baby? Lancet 2014;384(9938):174–88.
71. Hankins GD, Speer M. Defining the pathogenesis and pathophysiology of neonatal encephalopathy and cerebral palsy. Obstet Gynecol 2003;102(3): 628–36.
72. Bhutta ZA, Darmstadt GL, Haws RA, et al. Delivering interventions to reduce the global burden of stillbirths: improving service supply and community demand. BMC Pregnancy Childbirth 2009;9(1):1.
73. Darmstadt GL, Yakoob MY, Haws RA, et al. Reducing stillbirths: interventions during labour. BMC Pregnancy Childbirth 2009;9(1):S6.
74. Haws RA, Yakoob MY, Soomro T, et al. Reducing stillbirths: screening and monitoring during pregnancy and labour. BMC Pregnancy Childbirth 2009;9(1):S5.
75. Stenberg K, Axelson H, Sheehan P, et al. Advancing social and economic development by investing in women's and children's health: a new Global Investment Framework. Lancet 2014;383(9925):1333–54.
76. Bhutta ZA, Yakoob MY, Lawn JE, et al. Stillbirths: what difference can we make and at what cost? Lancet 2011;377(9776):1523–38.
77. Mason E, McDougall L, Lawn JE, et al. From evidence to action to deliver a healthy start for the next generation. Lancet 2014;384(9941):455–67.
78. Lozano R, Wang H, Foreman KJ, et al. Progress towards Millennium Development Goals 4 and 5 on maternal and child mortality: an updated systematic analysis. Lancet 2011;378(9797):1139–65.

Index

Note: Page numbers of article titles are in **boldface** type.

Moving?

Make sure your subscription moves with you!

To notify us of your new address, find your **Clinics Account Number** (located on your mailing label above your name), and contact customer service at:

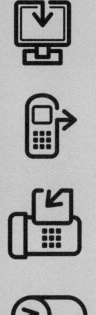

Email: journalscustomerservice-usa@elsevier.com

800-654-2452 (subscribers in the U.S. & Canada)
314-447-8871 (subscribers outside of the U.S. & Canada)

Fax number: 314-447-8029

Elsevier Health Sciences Division
Subscription Customer Service
3251 Riverport Lane
Maryland Heights, MO 63043

*To ensure uninterrupted delivery of your subscription, please notify us at least 4 weeks in advance of move.

Printed and bound by CPI Group (UK) Ltd, Croydon, CR0 4YY

07/10/2024

01040504-0005